Trauma-Informed Healthc

Megan R. Gerber
Editor

# Trauma-Informed Healthcare Approaches

A Guide for Primary Care

Springer

*Editor*
Megan R. Gerber, MD, MPH
Section of General Internal Medicine
Boston University School of Medicine
Veterans Affairs (VA) Boston Healthcare System
Boston, MA
USA

ISBN 978-3-030-04341-4     ISBN 978-3-030-04342-1  (eBook)
https://doi.org/10.1007/978-3-030-04342-1

Library of Congress Control Number: 2019934093

© Springer Nature Switzerland AG 2019, corrected publication 2019
This work is subject to copyright. All rights are reserved by the Publisher, whether the whole or part of the material is concerned, specifically the rights of translation, reprinting, reuse of illustrations, recitation, broadcasting, reproduction on microfilms or in any other physical way, and transmission or information storage and retrieval, electronic adaptation, computer software, or by similar or dissimilar methodology now known or hereafter developed.
The use of general descriptive names, registered names, trademarks, service marks, etc. in this publication does not imply, even in the absence of a specific statement, that such names are exempt from the relevant protective laws and regulations and therefore free for general use.
The publisher, the authors, and the editors are safe to assume that the advice and information in this book are believed to be true and accurate at the date of publication. Neither the publisher nor the authors or the editors give a warranty, express or implied, with respect to the material contained herein or for any errors or omissions that may have been made. The publisher remains neutral with regard to jurisdictional claims in published maps and institutional affiliations.

This Springer imprint is published by the registered company Springer Nature Switzerland AG
The registered company address is: Gewerbestrasse 11, 6330 Cham, Switzerland

*This book is dedicated to our patients who have taught us more about healing than any lecture or book and to our families who have been a bedrock for all of us as we have faced the difficult, tragic, unfathomable, and joyful aspects of caring for survivors of trauma. Thank you.*

# Preface

In recent years, trauma-informed care (TIC) has gained traction as an important set of principles that should guide optimal healthcare delivery. Our understanding of the profound impact traumatic exposure has on health is not new, but the recent #METOO movement has resulted in expanding interest in optimizing the healthcare response to interpersonal trauma. The literature contains many offerings on TIC in mental health, substance abuse, and pediatric care settings, but there has been comparably less published on TIC principles in general adult medical settings. There is a continuum from being trauma-aware to trauma-informed. Organizations may be *trauma-aware* and have outstanding *trauma-focused* care, but being trauma-informed is a process of infusing an entire organization or system with a guiding set of principles that reorders the environment to promote safety, empowerment, and healing for both patients and staff. A truly trauma-informed health system understands its community and collaborates with stakeholders, service providers, and relevant social services.

This book is geared toward general medical practitioners, healthcare administrators and leaders. While trauma has a profound impact on global health, this volume restricts its focus to the United States and similar countries. It begins with a broad overview of trauma and the suspected mechanisms by which it creates poor health. A discussion of practical applications of TIC principles is followed by an introduction to the concept of TIC as an important promoter of health equity through acknowledging and addressing trauma in individuals and communities. The World Health Organization (WHO) Commission on Social Determinants of Health (SDoH) (http://www.who.int/social_determinants/thecommission/finalreport/en/) described health systems as intermediary determinants of SDoH. Trauma is inextricably linked to many SDoH, so conceptualizing healthcare as having a role in mitigating SDoH is another way of understanding its role in achieving health equity and reducing disparities that often result from trauma.

The concept of cultural humility and its critical role in TIC is followed by a series of chapters (Part II) on selected special populations including men of color, gender nonconforming persons, and US military Veterans. While not all groups who are susceptible to trauma are covered, these chapters provide useful paradigms to apply/customize TIC principles to vulnerable populations.

Part III of the book is geared toward both clinicians and healthcare administrators. It covers practical clinical strategies for primary care (adult, adolescent and pediatric) and maternity care settings. Chapter 9 discusses adolescent and pediatric trauma-informed care through the lens of developing and extending trauma-informed systems. This chapter is relevant to all healthcare settings. Finally, a chapter on trauma-informed holistic nursing provides an overview on transforming nursing care across the health system. The book concludes with a chapter on fostering resilience and self-care for staff; an organization cannot transform into a truly trauma-informed system without understanding the needs of staff who treat survivors.

Boston, MA, USA											Megan R. Gerber, MD, MPH

# Acknowledgments

We are grateful to the Society of General Internal Medicine (SGIM) for providing a professional home to many of us and a platform over the years for discussing and advancing the needs of trauma survivors in general medical settings. We wish to especially acknowledge our colleagues in the Physicians Against Violence Interest Group for supporting us and shaping our collective "voice." William R. Bachman, MD; Christine J. Kolehmainen, MD, MS; and Aasia S. Romano, MD, provided invaluable assistance in content review and preparation of this book.

**Disclaimer** The views expressed in this book are those of the authors and do not necessarily reflect the position or policy of the Department of Veterans Affairs or the United States government.

# How to Use This Book

> Trying to implement trauma-specific clinical practices without first implementing trauma-informed organizational culture change is like throwing seeds on dry land.
>
> Sandra Bloom, MD
> Creator of the Sanctuary Model

The reader can access topics of interest and concern as the chapters can be read independently of one another. For administrators, we recommend using guidance from the *Substance Abuse and Mental Health Services Agency (SAMHSA)* (https://www.samhsa.gov/nctic/trauma-interventions) or the *Center for Healthcare Strategies (CHCS)* (http://www.chcs.org/media/ATC_whitepaper_040616.pdf) to determine where an organization is on the continuum of trauma informed care (TIC) implementation. Being "trauma aware" is a critical first step. There is no *"one size fits all"* approach to implementing TIC, and most experts do not offer one standard implementation checklist for this reason. Because it provides practical setting-based examples, this book can be a useful adjunct to implementing TIC using the guiding principles laid out by SAMHSA.

# Contents

**Part I   Introduction and Scope**

1   **An Introduction to Trauma and Health** .......................... 3
    Megan R. Gerber and Emily B. Gerber

2   **Trauma and Trauma-Informed Care** ............................ 25
    Leigh Kimberg and Margaret Wheeler

**Part II   Special Populations**

3   **Cultural Humility in Trauma-Informed Care** ................... 59
    Joseph Vinson, Ariel Majidi, and Maura George

4   **Trauma-Informed Care: A Focus on African American Men** ..... 69
    Marshall Fleurant

5   **Trauma-Informed Care of Sexual
    and Gender Minority Patients** ................................. 85
    Tyler R. McKinnish, Claire Burgess, and Colleen A. Sloan

6   **Trauma-Informed Care of Veterans** ........................... 107
    Megan R. Gerber

**Part III   Clinical Strategies**

7   **Trauma-Informed Adult Primary Care** ......................... 125
    Megan R. Gerber

8   **Trauma-Informed Maternity Care** ............................. 145
    Megan R. Gerber

## 9 Trauma-Informed Pediatrics: Organizational and Clinical Practices for Change, Healing, and Resilience ................................... 157
Emily B. Gerber, Briana Loomis, Cherie Falvey, Petra H. Steinbuchel, Jennifer Leland, and Kenneth Epstein

## 10 Trauma-Informed Nursing Care .......................... 181
Jay Ellen Barrett

## Part IV  Helping Providers

## 11 Trauma-Informed Care: Helping the Healthcare Team Thrive ....................... 197
Jessica Barnhill, Joslyn W. Fisher, Karen Kimel-Scott, and Amy Weil

**Correction to: Trauma-informed Care of Sexual and Gender Minority Patients**................................... C1

**Conclusion** ................................................. 215

**Index** ..................................................... 217

# About the Contributors

**Jessica Barnhill, MD**  Dr. Barnhill's research interests draw on her clinical experience as a family physician and her life experiences as a human being. Department of Physical Medicine and Rehabilitation, UNC-Chapel Hill, Chapel Hill, NC, USA.

**Jay Ellen Barrett, RN, BSN, MBA**  Ms. Barrett has been a leader in disseminating the concepts of whole health and holistic nursing care. She is the 2017 recipient of the Deborah Sampson Award which is presented to a Massachusetts resident whose military and community service is extraordinary. US Army Nurse Corps, Lieutenant Colonel (Retired), Nurse Manager Women's Health, Veterans Affairs (VA) Boston Healthcare System, Boston, MA, USA.

**Claire Burgess, PhD**  Dr. Burgess has expertise in assisting organizations with training considerations for transgender and gender nonconforming patients. Clinical psychologist, Harvard Medical School, Veterans Affairs (VA) Boston Healthcare System, Boston, MA, USA.

**Kenneth Epstein, PhD, LCSW**  Dr. Epstein has spent his career working to build and develop family-centered programs and services within the public system of care. Department of Psychiatry, University of California San Francisco, San Francisco, CA, USA.

**Cherie Falvey, MPH**  Ms. Falvey's research and public health career has focused on identifying tools and strategies that allow individuals, teams, and organizations to draw upon their inner resiliencies and strengths to collectively create places and spaces of reflection, growth, and healing. Trauma Transformed, East Bay Agency for Children, Oakland, CA, USA.

**Joslyn W. Fisher, MD, MPH, FACP**  Dr. Fisher has served as a primary care clinician and educator in a local county hospital for two decades. Her academic focus has been on fostering community engagement as well as helping survivors of intimate partner violence. Baylor College of Medicine, Houston, TX, USA.

**Marshall Fleurant, MD, MPH** Dr. Fleurant is a general internist with an interest in health disparities and health policy and studies how these interact to affect vulnerable populations. Emory University School of Medicine, Atlanta, GA, USA.

**Maura George, MD, FACP** Dr. George has always felt a calling to work for the underserved and has harmony between this goal and her love for teaching at the large, safety-net hospital where she works. Division of General Medicine, Emory University, Atlanta, GA, USA.

**Emily B. Gerber, PhD** Dr. Gerber has a career-long interest in transforming behavioral health, juvenile justice, child welfare, and education systems to promote health, equity, and well-being for all of our children, youth, and families. Mental Health, Kaiser Permanente, San Rafael, CA, USA.

**Megan R. Gerber, MD, MPH** Dr. Gerber is a general internist with an interest in improving the health of trauma-exposed women and healthcare-based interventions that enhance outcomes and healing. Section of General Internal Medicine, Boston University School of Medicine, Harvard Medical School, VA Boston Healthcare System, Boston, MA, USA.

**Leigh Kimberg, MD** Dr. Kimberg has been a primary care physician in the San Francisco safety net for more than two decades. She leads trauma-informed care and violence prevention programs in the San Francisco Health Network; she is committed to promoting social justice and health equity through medical education and healthcare-community partnerships. University of California, San Francisco, Program in Medical Education for the Urban Underserved (PRIME-US), San Francisco, CA, USA.

**Karen Kimel-Scott, MD** Dr. Kimel-Scott, a general internist, became interested in provider wellness specifically that of resident physicians while serving as a chief resident. University of North Carolina at Chapel Hill, Chapel Hill, NC, USA.

**Jennifer Leland, LMFT** Informed by her clinical and lived experience as a system-impacted adolescent, Ms. Leland transforms systems and prioritizes healing-centered approaches for staff, children, youth, and families to sustain practices that respond to trauma and offer radical healing in our work and in our communities. Trauma Transformed, East Bay Agency for Children, Oakland, CA, USA.

**Briana Loomis, PhD** Dr. Loomis has dedicated her career to understanding trauma psychology, with a special focus on children, youth, and families. Her recent work has focused on better serving vulnerable communities through trauma-informed systems and evaluating their outcomes and impacts. San Francisco Department of Public Health, San Francisco, CA, USA.

**Ariel Majidi, MD** Having served and worked with various immigrant and refugee communities, Dr. Majidi has a lifelong passion for providing culturally humble, patient-centered care to diverse populations and addressing the social determinants of health in medicine. Cambridge Health Alliance, Harvard Medical School, Cambridge, MA, USA.

**Tyler R. McKinnish, MD** Dr. McKinnish is an Obstetrics and Gynecology resident in St. Louis with interests in sexual and gender minority health, medical education, and healthcare quality improvement. Department of Obstetrics and Gynecology, Washington University/Barnes-Jewish Hospital, St. Louis, MO, USA.

**Colleen A. Sloan, PhD** Dr. Sloan provides direct clinical care, supervision, and education/training on sexual and gender minority health. She has published on topics of gender roles and sexual and gender minority health disparities, and she has developed significant interest regarding the utilization of evidence-based therapies for gender and sexual minority clients. Clinical Psychologist, Department of Psychiatry, Boston University School of Medicine, Veterans Affairs (VA) Boston Healthcare System, Boston, MA, USA.

**Petra H. Steinbuchel, MD** Dr. Steinbuchel has had a long-standing interest in trauma, and the interplay between physical and mental illness, as well as caregiver well-being. UCSF Department of Psychiatry, University of California, San Francisco, San Francisco, CA, USA.

**Joseph Vinson, MD** Dr. Vinson's current focus is on attempting to provide sound and compassionate psychiatric care, but he also has evolving interests in cultural issues, religion/spirituality, and psychotherapy. Department of Psychiatry and Behavioral Sciences, Emory University School of Medicine, Atlanta, GA, USA.

**Amy Weil, MD** Dr. Weil is a practicing general internist who has worked for two decades to improve education about the pervasiveness of trauma and its significant health effects. Her academic work also includes efforts to improve provider wellness, integrate behavioral health into primary care and improve the care, of vulnerable populations using innovative care models. UNC Chapel Hill School of Medicine, Beacon Child and Family Program, Chapel Hill, NC, USA.

**Margaret Wheeler, MD** Dr. Wheeler has been a primary care physician at San Francisco General Hospital for more than two decades. She is a leader in medical education and an expert in the care of the underserved. Dr. Wheeler is an editor of the textbook, 'Medical Management of the Vulnerable and Underserved Patient.' University of California, San Francisco Site Director, Medicine Clerkships, San Francisco General Hospital (SFGH) Co-Director, MODEL SFGH, San Francisco, CA, USA.

# Part I
# Introduction and Scope

# Chapter 1
# An Introduction to Trauma and Health

**Megan R. Gerber and Emily B. Gerber**

## Introduction: The Case for Trauma-Informed Care

Exposure to traumatic events is ubiquitous worldwide and has a well-established deleterious impact on health. Trauma can take many forms, and its impact varies based on the unique life circumstances, environment and resilience of the impacted individual. This volume is designed to enable clinicians – notably primary care providers (PCPs), nurses, and their extended care teams – to understand the potential impact of trauma on their patient population and the elements of a trauma-informed care (TIC) response. We believe that TIC is akin to "universal precautions" – front-line clinicians and health systems do not always know who has experienced, or currently is experiencing, trauma but can respond in an effective, patient-centered manner. The goal of this book is to inform implementation and sustainment of TIC across the individual patient encounter to health systems and communities at large. To lay the groundwork for understanding and implementing TIC, this chapter will provide a broad overview of common forms of interpersonal trauma experienced by patients and the ways in which traumatic experiences impact population health in the US.

---

M. R. Gerber (✉)
Section of General Internal Medicine, Boston University School of Medicine,
Veterans Affairs (VA) Boston Healthcare System, Boston, MA, USA
e-mail: meggerber@post.harvard.edu

E. B. Gerber
Kaiser Permanente, San Rafael, CA, USA

© Springer Nature Switzerland AG 2019
M. R. Gerber (ed.), *Trauma-Informed Healthcare Approaches*,
https://doi.org/10.1007/978-3-030-04342-1_1

## Trauma Defined

Broadly defined, the medical definition of trauma refers to "an injury (such as a wound) to living tissue caused by an extrinsic agent, a disordered psychic or behavioral state resulting from severe mental or emotional stress or physical injury, an emotional upset" [1]. The word "trauma" is derived from the Greek word for "wound," and accounts of interpersonal trauma date back to antiquity [2]. Judith Herman in her seminal work, "Trauma and Recovery," provides historical context leading up to the publication of the 5th Edition of the Diagnostic and Statistical Manual of Mental Disorders (DSM V) [3, 4]. In the late nineteenth century, Pierre Janet and Sigmund Freund provided the first accounts characterizing traumatic events and their clinical implications. Freud's work on the etiology of hysteria [3] in the twentieth century – notably experiences of psychological and sexual trauma – was met with such a degree of contention and censuring at that time, that contemporary trauma theories and definitions were largely derived from studies of male soldiers' experiences of war [2, 3]. After World War I, studies of traumatic stress and interventions emerged and then waned to some degree until the advent of the Vietnam war [2]. A shift occurred when society's attention was drawn to consequences of sexual and domestic violence as a result of the women's movement of the 1970s [3]. It was then recognized that the most common posttraumatic disorders are not those of war but "of women in civilian life;" Herman describes the history of psychological trauma as "one of episodic amnesia" [3]. This examination of violence and trauma on both the war-related and domestic/interpersonal fronts led to the groundbreaking inclusion of posttraumatic stress disorder (PTSD) in the DSM III in 1980 [5]. Prior to that, the DSM had characterized reactions to stressful experiences as "transient situational disturbances" that would wane over time.

Subsequently, DSM IV and DSM IV-TR ushered in a more inclusive definition of trauma (including varied events such as car accidents, natural disasters, or learning about the death of a loved one) that resulted in a marked expansion in trauma-related diagnoses [2, 6]. Contemporary theory conceptualizes trauma and responses to it as occurring along a continuum [2, 6]. It is clear that not all persons exposed to even highly traumatic events will go on to develop PTSD [7]; nonetheless, the experience of that trauma can still have a lasting impact on that individual.

## The Adverse Childhood Experiences (ACEs) Study

It was the landmark work of Felitti and Anda in the Adverse Childhood Experiences (ACEs) Study of the 1990s that ushered in a more mainstream understanding of the impact of childhood trauma on lifelong health [8]. Dr. Vincent Felitti, an internist and Director of Preventive Medicine at Kaiser Permanente, a health maintenance organization (HMO) in California, first made the connection between childhood abuse and adult health during an obesity research study he ran in the 1980s [9]. During a routine checkup, one of his patients mentioned that the year after she was raped, she gained 105 pounds. Felitti recalled what happened next: "She looked down at the carpet and muttered to herself, 'Overweight is overlooked. And, that's the way I needed to be'" [10]. In the obesity clinic at Kaiser, 50% of patients dropped out of treatment. Felitti interviewed these patients and found that a history of child sexual abuse was common [9]. The ACEs Study formally began in 1995 with an initial questionnaire sent to patients who presented for standardized wellness exams at the Kaiser Health Appraisal Clinic.

The initial study published in 1998 presented findings for 9,508 participants (eventually over 17,000 were enrolled) – all were insured patients at Kaiser Permanente – and provided groundbreaking evidence linking ACEs to morbidity and mortality in adulthood [8]. The initial study [8] found that patients reporting greater numbers of ACEs had increased risk for smoking, severe obesity, physical inactivity, depressed mood, and suicide attempts. Similar findings occurred for substance use and sexually transmitted infections. The greatest odds, or risk, of disease occurred in those who reported four or more ACEs. The researchers also found a dose–response relationship between the number of ACEs and ischemic heart disease, cancer, chronic bronchitis/emphysema, liver disease, skeletal fractures, and poor overall self-rated health. The initial study population, all insured, was mostly White and middle class. The authors posited that the resulting development of adverse health behaviors, like smoking, led to disease and called for increased communication and coordination across healthcare specialties and enhanced training of providers [8]; this was truly an early call for what we now know as trauma-informed care delivery.

## Trauma as a Process

A traumatic event or series of events results in physiologic changes, complex adaptations, and pathways that are linked to adverse health impacts. For example, the hypothalamic-pituitary-adrenal (HPA) axis serves as an important mediator after a stressor or under conditions of chronic stress [11]. The HPA axis is responsible for the release of stress hormones, notably glucocorticoids and cortisol. Under normal circumstances, the HPA axis is well-regulated and serves to enable a rapid response to stressful events with prompt return to a normal state. Chronic activation of this system is thought to damage the feedback loops that return stress hormones to their basal, or resting, levels [12, 13]. HPA axis function is determined by a number of factors including genetics, early-life environment [14], and current life stress [15]. The immune system is also involved, and chronic stress can lead to sustained levels of inflammation [13, 16]. An individual's genetic make-up and environment further modify and contribute to either enhancing or inhibiting these processes. Thus, two people may experience and react entirely differently to the same event objectively characterized as traumatic.

We now know that trauma should be conceptualized as a *process* that is dynamic and involves interaction between an event, or series of events, and the individual (and community's) level of vulnerability and resilience/protective factors [17]. Understanding resilience and protective factors is important in efforts to aid in prevention and recovery. Thus, trauma is less of an event, episode, or exposure and more of an interaction that may offer points of intervention, particularly in the healthcare setting. A brief review of the current understanding of factors that mediate the "process" of trauma follows.

## Allostatic Load

"Allostasis" refers to the highly integrated balance of the central nervous system (CNS), endocrine/metabolic, and immune systems which mediate the response to stress [11, 13, 18]. As discussed above, prolonged activation of these systems through chronic or repeated exposure to psychosocial stress and traumatic events has damaging consequences or "wear and tear on the body" [13]. The cumulative physiologic consequences of these result in "allostatic load" [11, 18]. Allostatic load is a contributor to cardiovascular disease [11], metabolic disorders [11], and accelerated cognitive decline [19] and has been consistently linked to lower socioeconomic status (SES) [11, 12]. Allostatic load is measured in different ways [11]; some studies use biomarkers such as urinary or salivary cortisol and epinephrine, while others use clinical measurements like laboratory data, for example, lipid measurements and hemoglobin A1c. Some studies combine these with measurements of blood pressure, heart rate, body mass index (BMI), or skinfold measurements [11].

Chronic toxic stressors, or traumatic experiences, that occur during childhood, and beyond, can have an enduring influence on allostatic load because they coincide with developmental windows [13], notably those of the brain [20]. ACEs appear to impact allostasis [13], resulting in the observed higher prevalence of disease and premature mortality observed in adulthood [8]. Allostatic load causes ill-health through both the primary biologic impact of stress and damaging behaviors like tobacco and alcohol consumption which are often used as methods of coping with stress [11]. Allostatic load increases with age [11], resulting in longitudinal, worsening health impact.

Racial disparities in allostatic load were demonstrated in data from National Health and Nutrition Examination Survey (NHANES); after controlling for SES [11], Black patients were more likely than Whites to have greater allostatic load at all ages [21]. Black women across all age groups had the highest allostatic load and accrued higher allostatic load at younger ages than all other women [11]. Allostatic load is a useful construct for conceptualizing mechanisms that underlie many health disparities [11].

## Environment and Epigenetics

Early life stress results in poor physical and mental health states. As discussed above, HPA axis and immune system changes play a major role in linking adversity early in life to poor health later on [13, 14]. Research has also focused on cellular-level changes, notably chromosomal changes. Telomeres are regions of nucleotide repeats – or repetitive deoxyribonucleic acid (DNA) – at the ends of chromosomes that protect them from damage during replication [22]. Telomeres progressively shorten with every replication cycle and are thus often used as a marker for biological aging [23]. A number of studies have consistently demonstrated a relationship between childhood maltreatment and telomere length [24, 25]. There appears to be a dose-dependent association between early-life stressors and telomere shortening [22]. It also appears that protective factors, such as parental responsiveness, are linked to longer telomeres [22].

## Socioeconomic Status and Cortisol: Biology and Injustice

Decreased SES has been consistently linked to poor health in the US [26] and worldwide [27]. The mechanisms that underlie this are multiple and complex. Persons of lower SES are exposed to more stressors and have a higher overall risk of lifetime trauma exposure and less access to mitigating or protective resources to buffer stressful events [11, 28]. As previously discussed, the HPA axis plays a key role in regulating the response to stressors. Cortisol is one of the most well-studied hormones produced by the HPA axis, in part because it exerts widespread effects on the CNS, metabolic, and immune systems [29], each of which contributes to allostasis [13]. Overexposure to cortisol has been hypothesized as one critical mechanism linking traumatic events to poor health outcomes. A review of these studies suggests that this association is inconsistent in part due to variability in measurement [12]. The body of research investigating the biologic mechanisms of trauma continues to grow and may soon provide opportunities to intervene at the molecular level to mitigate some of the health effects of these exposures.

## Posttraumatic Stress Disorder (PTSD) and Metabolic Syndrome

While not all who experience trauma develop PTSD, the addition of PTSD to the DSM III in 1980 [5] ushered in a new era in terms of traumatic studies. In 2013, the DSM V redefined PTSD and included it as part of a category designated as "Trauma and Stressor-Related Disorders" [4]. A detailed discussion of PTSD is beyond the scope of this chapter, but briefly defined, PTSD may develop after exposure to a serious traumatic event known as a "Criterion A" event (the person was exposed to: death, threatened death, actual or threatened serious injury, or actual or threatened sexual violence, through either direct exposure or witnessing the trauma) [4]. It consists of the following symptoms: re-experiencing the traumatic event, avoidance, arousal/reactivity, and changes in cognition and mood for at least 1 month after the event. Many effective, evidence-based PTSD treatments have been developed since 1980 when PTSD was first included in the DSM III [30].

PTSD has received attention as a critical mediator between trauma exposure and health [31] and is known to be linked to allostatic load [32]. While poor health is observed among trauma-exposed persons who *do not* develop PTSD, studies have consistently shown poorer health after a traumatic event for persons with PTSD compared to those without it [31]. As research has consistently shown linkages between trauma and chronic disease outcomes [8, 31, 32], attention has been focused on PTSD as a mediator between exposure to traumatic stress and poor health [31].

One of the most well-studied health outcomes associated with PTSD is metabolic syndrome, a group of medical risk factors that signal abnormal underlying pathophysiological processes that increase risk for morbidity (notably hypertension, type II diabetes, and cardiovascular disease) and, eventually, mortality [32]. Some of the markers of metabolic syndrome are also used to estimate allostatic load [11], and PTSD has been consistently linked to increased risk of metabolic syndrome [32]. PTSD manifests variably among individuals, in keeping with the concept of trauma as a "process." One proposed causal mechanism is through alterations in neuropeptide Y (NPY), a stress-activated cardiovascular and metabolic regulating hormone that is variably expressed based on genetic makeup [32]. This is another pathway for which ongoing research may yield important points of potential therapeutic intervention after traumatic exposure.

In summary, traumatic events set off a myriad of biological responses that vary among individuals and are still being elucidated. The pathways between traumatic experiences and adverse health effects are complex but indisputable and hold promise for future treatment and care for survivors.

## Prevalence of Common Traumatic Exposures

While it is beyond the scope of this volume to provide a detailed review of every form of interpersonal trauma, we will now provide an overview of the epidemiology of some of the traumatic exposures experienced by patients who seek US medical care. This summary will better equip both clinicians, administrators and systems of care with critical background knowledge to tailor patient care and develop/enhance trauma-informed practices. Most prevalance and background data on traumatic exposure come from either (1) population-based surveys, frequently conducted through random digit dialing in a limited number of languages (commonly English and Spanish at a minimum), (2) studies conducted in medical populations (which typically demonstrate higher rates of traumatic exposures than in general population-based surveys), and (3) surveillance data collected by government agencies and reporting systems such as law enforcement/justice department and child protective services referrals. Each of these forms of data has its own limitations. For example, often government agencies are mandated to collect certain data which depend, in part, on reporting. In cases involving child maltreatment; if a report is not made, the potential trauma to the child is not captured in that data source.

Many forms of traumatic exposures overlap in their definitions, and multiple exposures during the course of an individual's lifetime are unfortunately too common. Often patients will not self-identify as survivors of trauma, so familiarity with different

1  An Introduction to Trauma and Health

forms of trauma is key to TIC and to delivery of high-quality medical care (and related, critical social services). Trauma exposure in subgroups of patients who may need adaptations in their care to meet unique sets of needs is covered in Part III of this book. In addition, many of those who commit abusive, violent acts against others have themselves experienced abuse and trauma (as "victims") and also need understanding and care [33]. Table 1.1 summarizes key aspects of and, selected data sources for, each form of trauma reviewed below, it is intended to provide sample estimates and is not an exhaustive summary of all available data for each form of trauma.

**Table 1.1** Interpersonal trauma: Definitions and Data Examples

| Trauma type | Definition | Estimated prevalence | Selected data sources |
|---|---|---|---|
| Child neglect & physical abuse | When a parent or caregiver acts, or fails to act, in a way that results in physical injury to a child or adolescent even if unintentional [45] | Any maltreatment 30.1 per 1000 children (22% of maltreated children are referred to foster care) | Government Reporting Data: NCANDS, Child Maltreatment 2016 [94] https://www.acf.hhs.gov/cb/research-data-technology/reporting-systems/ncands |
| | | Any maltreatment: 25.6% | Population-based data: National Survey of Children's Exposure to Violence (NatSCEV/NatSCEV II) [35] |
| Child sexual abuse | An interaction between a child and an adult or child in which the child is used by the perpetrator for sexual stimulation (Includes touching and non-touching behavior) [34] | 8.5% sexual abuse | NCANDS [94] |
| | | Sexual assault 4.2% (2.5% for males and 5.9% for females) | NatSCEVII [35] |
| Intimate partner violence | Physical violence, sexual violence, stalking, and psychological aggression (including coercive tactics) by a current or former intimate partner (i.e., spouse, boyfriend/girlfriend, dating partner, or ongoing sexual partner) [95] | 1 in 3 women (35.6%) 1 in 4 men (28.5%) Sexual IPV: 16.9% of women 8.0% of men | National Intimate Partner and Sexual Violence Survey (NISVS) [96] |
| Sexual assault | Sexual violence refers to any sexual activity in which consent is not obtained or freely given [95] | Rape: 19.3% of women 1.7% of men All forms of sexual violence: 43.9% of women 23.4% of men | NISVS [96] |

(continued)

**Table 1.1** (continued)

| Trauma type | Definition | Estimated prevalence | Selected data sources |
|---|---|---|---|
| Community violence | Exposure to intentional acts of interpersonal violence committed in public areas. Common types include individual and group conflicts (e.g., bullying, fights among gangs and other groups, shootings in schools and communities) [48] | Varies by neighborhood/state<br><br>Violent crime: 21.1 victimizations per 1000 persons (1.3%)<br><br>8.8% of households experienced at least one property victimization.<br><br>Ages 12–34 had higher rates of violent victimization than persons age 35 or older (BJS) [97]<br><br>Victimization rates vary by income bracket (highest for persons in households earning less than $10,000 each year) (BJS) [97] | National Survey of Children's Exposure to Violence [35]<br><br>National Crime Victimization Survey https://www.icpsr.umich.edu/icpsrweb/NACJD/NCVS/<br><br>Youth Risk Behavior Surveillance System (YRBSS) [60]<br><br>National Neighborhood Crime Study (NNCS) [58]<br><br>Survey of Exposure to Community Violence (SECV) [56] |
| Human trafficking | The action or practice of illegally transporting people from one country or area to another, typically for the purposes of forced labor or commercial sexual exploitation [61] | 40.3 million worldwide as reported by the Polaris Project<br>Statistics are limited; research is scarce and challenging to conduct | Trafficking in Persons Report;<br>US Department of State [67]<br>Counter-Trafficking Data Collaborative (CTDC), The Polaris Project [98, 99] |
| Historical trauma | Cumulative emotional and psychological injury, as a result of group traumatic experiences transmitted across generations within a community [80] | Population-based prevalence rates are unavailable at this time | National Child Traumatic Stress Network [100] |

## Child Abuse and Maltreatment

Systems of care are not only treating acutely injured and abused children, but adult survivors of childhood maltreatment and the medical sequelae that develop as a result of these adverse experiences. Much of what we know about the prevalence of child abuse and maltreatment in the USA comes from reports made to social service and law enforcement. It is likely that these data are underestimates of the true prevalence of abuse in childhood. Widening the definition of childhood maltreatment to include household dysfunction, as Felitti did [8], yielded estimates similar to those published at the same time in the first national prevalence study of child sexual abuse [34].

In 1999, the Office of Juvenile Justice and Delinquency Prevention (OJJDP) created the Safe Start Initiative to prevent and reduce the impact of children's exposure to violence. As a part of this initiative, and with a growing need to document the full extent of children's exposure to violence, OJJDP launched the National Survey of Children's Exposure to Violence (NatSCEV) with the Centers for Disease Control and Prevention (CDC) [35]. The NatSCEV is a population-based survey that captures a wide range of violent exposures that range from peer and sibling victimization (emotional bullying or relational aggression), Internet/cell phone victimization, witnessing violence ("indirect victimization"), to sexual victimization and child maltreatment [35]. For the NatSCEV II, conducted in 2011 [35], telephone interviews were conducted with a nation-wide sample of 4503 children and youth ages 1 month to 17 years (or their caregivers for children younger than age 10). Estimates from that survey indicate a lifetime rate of any child mistreatment of 25.6% and sexual assault in childhood of 4.2% (2.5% for males and 5.9% for females).

Government reporting data is collected through the National Child Abuse and Neglect Data System (NCANDS). NCANDS was established in 1988 as a national data collection and analysis program to make available state child abuse and neglect information. Data has been collected every year since 1991, and NCANDS now annually collects maltreatment data from child protective services agencies in the 50 states, the District of Columbia, and Puerto Rico [36]. In 2015, there were an estimated four million referrals alleging maltreatment to child protective services (CPS). Over half of those "screened in," i.e., became reports. 3.4 million children received an investigation or response and of those 676,000 (30.1 per 1000 children) were found to have been victimized. 1670 children died. Nearly 75% experienced neglect (18.2% physical abuse and 8.5% sexual abuse). Twenty-two percent of children found to have experienced maltreatment wound up in foster care services. Children often witness violence between their caregivers, guardians, and parents as well. In 2018, the forced separation of children from parents seeking asylum in the US prompted a global outcry and also raised concerns for longterm health effects from this form of child maltreatment [37].

## Intimate Partner Violence and Sexual Assault

The CDC has defined intimate partner violence (IPV) (also known as domestic violence) as including physical violence, sexual violence, stalking, and psychological aggression (including coercive tactics) by a current or former intimate partner (i.e., spouse, boyfriend/girlfriend, dating partner, or ongoing sexual partner) [38]. IPV is common in the US population, and over the last 20 years, programs to detect and respond to IPV in healthcare settings have proliferated. As with all forms of interpersonal trauma, IPV can have lasting health consequences.

The CDC conducts a national population-based telephone survey, the National Intimate Partner and Sexual Violence Survey (NISVS) [39]. Data from the NISVS show that more than one in three women (35.6%) and one in four men (28.5%) in the US have experienced rape, physical violence, and/or stalking by an intimate partner in their lifetime [39]. Nearly half of all women and men have experienced psychological aggression by an intimate partner in their lifetime (48.4% and 48.8%, respectively).

IPV risk is highest at younger ages; most female and male victims of rape, physical violence, and/or stalking by an intimate partner (69% of female victims; 53% of male victims) experienced some form of IPV for the first time before the age of 25 [39]. Nearly one in ten women in the US (9.4%) has been raped by an intimate partner in her lifetime, and an estimated 16.9% of women and 8.0% of men have experienced sexual violence other than rape by an intimate partner at some point in their lifetime. Some groups are at heightened risk of violence, for example approximately 4 out of every 10 women of non-Hispanic Black or American Indian or Alaska Native race/ethnicity (43.7% and 46.0%, respectively), and 1 in 2 multiracial non-Hispanic women (53.8%) have experienced rape, physical violence, and/or stalking by an intimate partner in their lifetime [39]. This further underscores that trauma impacts health disparities and equity. IPV and sexual violence commonly co-occur as sexual violence can be a form of IPV when committed by an intimate partner. Rates of IPV are elevated among sexual and gender minority individuals, almost one-third of sexual minority males and one-half of sexual minority women in the US report experiencing physical or psychological abuse in an intimate relationship [40]. The US Preventive Services Task Force (USPSTF) [41] and many major medical organizations recommend routine screening for IPV in medical settings [42–44].

## Sexual Assault

Sexual violence refers to any sexual activity in which consent is not obtained or freely given [45]. While the majority of those who experience sexual violence are female, anyone can experience or perpetrate sexual violence [39]. In the US, an estimated 19.3% of women and 1.7% of men have been raped during their lifetimes; 43.9% of women and 23.4% of men experienced other forms of sexual violence during their lifetimes [46]. Among female victims of completed rape, an estimated 78.7% experienced their first assault before age 25 (40.4% before age 18). Among male victims who were made to penetrate a perpetrator, an estimated 71.0% were assaulted before 25 (21.3% before age 18) [46]. Some racial and ethnic groups experience higher rates of sexual assault; in the NISVS, rates of lifetime reported rape were 32.3% for multiracial women and 27.5% for American Indian/Alaskan Native women [46]. The American College of Obstetricians and Gynecologists (ACOG) recommends that healthcare providers routinely screen all women for a history of sexual assault, paying particular attention to those who report pelvic pain, dysmenorrhea (painful menses), or sexual dysfunction [47].

## Community Violence

Violence outside the home or confines of a familial or intimate relationship is often referred to as community violence, which has been broadly defined as "exposure to intentional, interpersonal violent acts experienced directly (through victimization) or indirectly (witnessing others be victimized) in a public setting" [48]. Community-level risk factors for violence include unemployment, poverty, decreased levels of economic opportunity and community participation, lack of access to services, poor housing, and gang activity [49].

Accurately estimating the full scope of community violence exposure is challenging, and there is no single data source that accurately captures its full impact in the US. Among the many challenges of describing the scope and impact of community violence is the fact that studies have been hampered by limited consensus concerning its definition [50], use of unvalidated measures [50, 51], and lack of comparator populations [51]. Adult exposure to community violence is commonly measured using tools developed for children and adolescents [50]. These issues aside, it is clear that exposure to community violence adversely impacts health similarly to other forms of trauma; it is associated with adverse mental [52] and physical health in both children [51] and adults [50]. It is also associated with violence perpetration, substance use, and sexual risk-taking behavior among emerging adults [53].

A number of data sources report community violence. As reviewed above, the NatSCEV [35] provides important data on violence exposure in children and youth and some of the types of violence reported in it fall under the definition of community violence. Crime and justice system data are limited by the need for law enforcement to be involved, and even when they are, the community impact from the violence cannot be fully captured in the resulting estimates. The population-based National Crime Victimization Survey (NCVS) provides crime statistics annually; data are obtained from a nationally-representative sample of about 135,000 households (nearly 225,000 persons), on the frequency, characteristics, and consequences of criminal victimization in the US including whether the crime was reported to authorities [54]. According to the NCVS, fewer than half (42%) of all violent victimizations committed in 2016 were reported to the police, but this varied by type of crime: rape or sexual assault (23%) and simple assault (38%) were less likely to be reported to the police than robbery (54%) and aggravated assault (58%) [55]. The Survey of Exposure to Community Violence (SECV) is another commonly referenced survey measure of community violence exposure [51, 56] that demonstrates highest exposures in poor urban communities [57].

Community violence commonly occurs in lower SES neighborhoods, but the empirical basis for this is not well-understood. Peterson and Krivo conducted the landmark National Neighborhood Crime Study (NNCS) to overcome the common bias of single-city research [58]. The NNCS compiled crime and other data for 9,593 neighborhoods in 91 large cities and found that violence is five times as high for the average African American neighborhood as for the typical White urban community. Furthermore, only about one-fifth of African American areas have violence levels that are as low as those for 90% of White areas. The authors emphasize that racial composition of neighborhoods is not a causal factor in accounting for crime patterns. Instead, it is appears to be a correlate of the concentration of unequal resources in separate contexts that also produces varied responses from outside agencies and actors [58]. Healthcare systems function as actors and provide such resources to communities, underscoring the need for responsive systems of care that are trauma-informed and seek to understand and respond to community needs and culture. More work is needed to identify the correlates of community violence exposure, as well as the mitigating (protective) factors that foster resilience and healing such as family, community, and religious organizations.

Community violence disproportionately impacts younger persons (homicide is the leading cause of death for Black boys and men ages 15–34 and the second leading cause for ages 10–14) [59]. This is especially concerning because trauma impacts the developing brain. For this reason, the CDC funds Youth Violence Prevention Centers (YVPCs) to design, implement, and evaluate community-based youth violence prevention programs and to monitor surveillance data from many sources including the Youth Risk Behavior Surveillance System (YRBSS), a biennial survey the agency conducts [60]. Clinicians and healthcare systems that serve areas with high rates of community violence should remain aware of these programs and data sources; trauma-informed care for youth is discussed in detail in Chapter 9 of this book.

Healthcare is provided not only to individuals but to social networks, neighborhoods, and communities. It is critical that frontline clinical teams, and health system administrators understand their locality and the burden of community violence experienced by patients and families in order to provide outstanding, culturally appropriate, responsive TIC which includes listening to patients, advocates, community voices and stakeholders.

## Human Trafficking

Human trafficking (HT) is an under-recognized form of interpersonal trauma, and there is great potential for healthcare professionals to make a significant impact through screening and intervention. It is defined as "the recruitment, transportation, transfer, harboring, or receipt of persons," by means of threat, force, coercion, abduction, fraud, deception, the abuse of power, or payments, "for the purpose of exploitation" [61]. Victims are most commonly trafficked for sexual exploitation [62] and for domestic servitude and forced labor [63]. Labor exploitation (also known as "labor trafficking") occurs in agricultural and fishing industry work, repetitive labor, domestic servitude, debt bondage, and other forms of slavery [64]. HT has been described as "modern slavery" [65]; its prevalence is vastly underestimated and its victims are hard to recognize [66]. Approximately 40 million people are trafficked worldwide [62] and the US Department of State reports a steady increase in cases investigated and prosecuted in the US and worldwide [67]. Victims, including men, women, children, refugees, migrants, and members of the lesbian/gay/bisexual/transgender (LGBT) community, may be trafficked locally or moved across borders [64]. Rates of trafficking appear to be higher within communities of color, further driving health disparities [68]. HT encompasses and employs many of the forms of violence reviewed above, notably child maltreatment and sexual assault.

The overall prevalence of HT victims in the general US population is likely very low, but survivors commonly describe medical encounters that, in retrospect, should have aroused suspicion among the treating clinicians [69]. The majority of those trafficked in the US are women and girls [62], close to half are minors. The Polaris Project, a non-profit organization that runs a hotline and services for trafficked persons, estimates a 13% increase in US cases between 2016 and 2017 and has received over 40,000 calls in the last decade [62]. Unlike other forms of interpersonal trauma, HT is commonly committed by women against other women; in some European countries women comprise the majority of offenders [70].

Trafficked individuals may commonly present in medical settings [66]; one study found that 50% of female trafficking survivors interviewed reported visiting a physician while trafficked [69]; these visits present a window of opportunity to aid these patients. A number of authors have described characteristics of patients that should raise concern for HT [66, 69], and an increasing body of evidence describes best practices for working with survivors [71–73]. Presentations and signs that should raise suspicion for trafficking when patients access healthcare or social services are listed in Table 1.2 [69, 74].

As trafficked patients are typically not allowed access to routine, ongoing preventive care, emergency departments are a common point of entry into healthcare, and tools for identification have been created for these settings [75]. As for survivors of other forms of trauma, engagement in healthcare services is often a challenge [76], further underscoring the importance of a TIC environment for these patients. When trafficked persons do access healthcare, they present with an increased risk of human immunodeficiency virus (HIV), sexually transmitted infections, as well as somatic symptoms such as headaches, back pain, and abdominal pain, resembling those seen among survivors of other forms of interpersonal trauma [63].

Research on HT is scarce, challenging, and potentially dangerous to undertake [63, 66]. Research with survivors has demonstrated that HT utilizes psychological methods to coerce victims into bondage, including isolation, monopolization of perception, induced debility, occasional indulgences, threats, and degradation [77]. Participants are typically people recruited from post-trafficking support services whose experiences may not generalize to those in captivity [63]. Ravi et al. interviewed a cohort of previously trafficked incarcerated women with substance use histories to determine their preferences for healthcare [78], most (71%) identified as a member of a racial/ethnic minority and more than half had not completed high school. The trafficking survivors' suggestions for ideal care included having rapport with the front desk and support staff. They also suggested that providers be aware of their reactions to a disclosure and expression of empathy. In essence, these survivors of HT described a preference for TIC.

Clinicians and care systems can develop routine processes that are trauma-informed and can aid in detecting trafficked persons [69] including:

- Training of healthcare personnel and staff (including physicians, nurses, dentists, medical assistants, technicians, and receptionists) to increase awareness of trafficking and coercion.
- Provision of professional interpreters.

**Table 1.2** Potential signs of HT [69, 74]

| |
|---|
| **In the medical setting** |
| *Poor mental health or abnormal behavior* |
|    Is fearful, anxious, depressed, submissive, tense, or nervous/paranoid |
|    Exhibits unusually fearful or anxious behavior after topic of law enforcement is brought up |
|    Avoids eye contact |
| *Poor physical health* |
|    Lacks healthcare |
|    Appears malnourished |
|    Shows signs of physical and/or sexual abuse, physical restraint, confinement, or torture |
| *Lack of control* |
|    The person accompanying the patient will not leave them alone |
|    Is not in control of his/her own identification documents (ID or passport) |
|    Is not allowed or able to speak for themselves (a third party may insist on being present and/or translating) |
|    Has few or no personal possessions |
|    Is not in control of his/her own money, no financial records, or bank account |
| *Other* |
|    Claims of just visiting and inability to clarify where he/she is staying/address |
|    Lack of knowledge of whereabouts and/or do not know what city they are in is in |
|    Loss of sense of time |
|    Has numerous inconsistencies in story |
| **Other social histories** |
| *Common work and living conditions: The individual(s) in question* |
|    Is not free to leave or come and go as s/he, they wish |
|    Is under 18 and is providing commercial sex acts |
|    Is in the commercial sex industry and has a pimp/manager |
|    Is unpaid, paid very little, or paid only through tips |
|    Works excessively long and/or unusual hours |
|    Is not allowed breaks or suffers under unusual restrictions at work |
|    Owes a large debt and is unable to pay it off |
|    Was recruited through false promises concerning the nature and conditions of work |
|    High security measures exist in the work and/or living locations (e.g. opaque windows, boarded-up windows, bars on windows, barbed wire, security cameras, etc.) |
|    Owes employer money |

- Interviewing/ examining all patients privately at some point during their medical visit (away from whomever may have accompanied them).
- Incorporating social, work, home history, and intimate partner violence screening questions into routine intake.
- Carefully observing body language and the communication style of patients and those who accompany them.

In summary, the practice of HT is widespread and challenging to detect. HT deploys forms of violence reviewed previously but has its own unique power and control dynamics that can render victims invisible and impossible to locate. Healthcare settings, as frequent points of contact, offer hope; training does improve provider knowledge and report of recognition of victims of trafficking [66, 79]. Any trauma-informed system of care must remain aware of and respond to trafficked persons.

## Historical Trauma

Like HT, historical trauma has been less commonly appreciated in medical settings. The term refers to a complex and collective trauma that is experienced over time and across generations by a group of people who share an identity, affiliation or circumstance [80]. Informed by theories of social epidemiology, historical trauma is linked to health through psychosocial stressors that create susceptibility to disease as well as act as direct pathogenic mechanisms. Political, economic, and structural determinants of health and disease such as unjust power dynamics and social inequality [81] play a critical role in creating, and perpetuating, poor health for populations.

Initially, historical trauma was conceptualized in reference to the children of Holocaust survivors [82] and this cohort remains the most studied to date. Mohatt et al. note that over the last 2 decades, the range of groups to whom the term has been applied include indigenous peoples [83], African Americans [84], Armenian and other refugees [85], Japanese American survivors of internment camps [86], Mexican Americans [87], and many other cultural groups that share a history of massive group trauma exposure and oppression [80]. As discussed earlier in this chapter, trauma is a psychological *process* that is distinct from the traumatic event itself. As such, a number of authors refer to trauma as a "representation" of a traumatic event [80, 88]. Scholarly work around both validated measurement and intervention is emerging on the topic of historical trauma [83].

Historical trauma has been linked to health effects, and an emerging literature reflects this. The mechanisms for this are complex, and a variety of pathways have been proposed. Sotero [81] describes four distinct assumptions that link historical trauma and adverse health: (1) mass trauma is deliberately and systematically inflicted upon a population by a dominant group, (2) trauma is not limited to a single catastrophic event but continues over an extended period of time, (3) traumatic events resonate for the entire population creating a universal experience of trauma, and (4) the enormity of the trauma experience deranges the population's natural, projected historical course, resulting in physical, psychological, social, and economic disparities that span generations. Some examples of this follow below.

Estrada [87] set forth a conceptual model for the Mexican American population that is likely applicable to other minority groups in the US; he suggests that historical and social events have created institutions and perceptions that are racist and discriminatory toward Mexicans and Mexican Americans. This, in turn, negatively influenced their eligibility for health insurance coverage and access and availability to healthcare through cultural or institutional barriers that prevent them from obtaining care when needed. Over time, with limited or no access to healthcare, generations of Mexicans and Mexican Americans have begun to show increased rates of substance abuse, hypertension, metabolic syndrome, anti-social personality disorders, and type 2 diabetes mellitus. In turn, these diseases are influenced by the psychosocial stressors (e.g., anti-Mexican sentiment, discrimination, and racism) that generations of Mexicans and Mexican Americans have experienced from the dominant culture [87].

Other examples suggest that historical trauma impacts health and well-being by disrupting or jeopardizing culture-based resilience and protective factors, like social support and parenting knowledge, resulting in mass unresolved grief [80, 89]. To illustrate this concept, research among indigenous peoples in North America ("Native Americans") has shown that historical trauma, in part mediated by the mid-nineteenth-century practice of forcing children into boarding schools, may be in part responsible for substance use and health disparities [89, 90].

Some have found evidence to support epigenetic changes [80, 91] similar to the findings discussed above that linked early life stress to telomere shortening [22, 25]. For example, children of Holocaust survivors have been shown to be more vulnerable to PTSD [82] and to have overall lower basal cortisol levels [92]. Thus, understanding the potential for historical trauma in populations is essential not only for clinicians but for systems of care which must tailor services that are mindful of the collective experiences of the community members they serve. Systems of care will be discussed in detail in the next part of this book.

# Conclusion

In sum, while trauma is a part of the human experience, we can see from the breadth and depth of data presented above that we are in the midst of a public health crisis. Healthcare clinicians, administrators and leaders have a critical role to play in responding through identification and prevention of poor health outcomes for their patients. As with any other highly contagious disease, we recommend that foundational knowledge and understanding of trauma be part of healthcare education at all levels and disciplines. This must be coupled with universal trauma precautions [93] to prevent retraumatization in medical settings and to mitigate transmission and spread between individuals, within families, among communities, and in the healthcare workforce.

To do this requires a commitment on the part of our healthcare institutions and systems of care to regular training on trauma including, its current definitions and concepts, prevalence, the mechanisms through which it manifests in the body and drives disparities. This knowledge must be continuously reinforced and applied to enhance and sustain trauma-informed practices.

# References

1. "Trauma". Miriam-Webster, [Internet]. 2018. Accessed 17 April 2018. Available from: https://www.merriam-webster.com/dictionary/trauma.
2. Jones LK, Cureton JL. Trauma redefined in the DSM-5: rationale and implications for counseling practice. Prof Couns. 2014;4(3):257–71.
3. Herman J. Trauma and recovery. New York: Basic Books; 2015.
4. American Psychiatric Association. Trauma- and stressor-related disorders. diagnostic and statistical manual of mental disorders. 5th ed. Washington, DC: American Psychiatric Association; 2013.
5. American Psychiatric Association. Diagnostic and statistical manual of mental disorders. 3rd ed. Washington, DC: American Psychiatric Association; 1980.
6. Breslau N, Kessler RC. The stressor criterion in DSM-IV posttraumatic stress disorder: an empirical investigation. Biol Psychiatry. 2001;50(9):699–704.
7. Yehuda R, McFarlane AC, Shalev AY. Predicting the development of posttraumatic stress disorder from the acute response to a traumatic event. Biol Psychiatry. 1998;44(12):1305–13.
8. Felitti VJ, Anda RF, Nordenberg D, Williamson DF, Spitz AM, Edwards V, et al. Relationship of childhood abuse and household dysfunction to many of the leading causes of death in adults. The Adverse Childhood Experiences (ACE) Study. Am J Prev Med. 1998;14(4):245–58.
9. Felitti VJ. Childhood sexual abuse, depression, and family dysfunction in adult obese patients: a case control study. South Med J. 1993;86(7):732–6.
10. Lester C. How childhood trauma affects health, July 13, 2017. Accessed 28 April 2018. Available from: http://blogs.wgbh.org/innovation-hub/2017/7/13/felitti-ace/.
11. Beckie TM. A systematic review of allostatic load, health, and health disparities. Biol Res Nurs. 2012;14(4):311–46.
12. Dowd JB, Simanek AM, Aiello AE. Socio-economic status, cortisol and allostatic load: a review of the literature. Int J Epidemiol. 2009;38(5):1297–309.
13. Danese A, McEwen BS. Adverse childhood experiences, allostasis, allostatic load, and age-related disease. Physiol Behav. 2012;106(1):29–39.
14. Gillespie, CF, Phifer, J, Bradley, B, Ressler, KJ. Risk and resilience: Genetic and environmental influences on development of the stress response. Depression and Anxiety. 2009; 26 (11):984-992
15. Stephens MA, Wand G. Stress and the HPA axis: role of glucocorticoids in alcohol dependence. Alcohol Res. 2012;34(4):468–83.
16. Dougall AL, Baum A. Psychoneuroimmunology and trauma. In: Schnurr PP, Green BL, editors. Trauma and health: physical consequences of exposure to extreme stress. Washington, DC: American Psychological Association (APA); 1999. p. 129–55.
17. Kimberg L. Trauma and trauma-informed care. In: King TE, Wheeler MB, editors. Medical management of vulnerable and underserved patients: principles, practice and populations. 2nd ed. New York: McGraw-Hill Education; 2016.
18. McEwen, BS. Stress, Adaptation, and Disease: Allostasis and Allostatic Load. Annals of the New York Academy of Sciences. 1999; 840 (1):33-44
19. Juster RP, McEwen BS, Lupien SJ. Allostatic load biomarkers of chronic stress and impact on health and cognition. Neurosci Biobehav Rev. 2010;35(1):2–16.
20. McEwen BS. Allostasis and the epigenetics of brain and body health over the life course: the brain on stress. JAMA Psychiat. 2017;74(6):551–2.
21. Geronimus AT, Hicken M, Keene D, Bound J. "Weathering" and age patterns of allostatic load scores among blacks and whites in the United States. Am J Public Health. 2006;96(5):826–33.
22. Asok A, Bernard K, Roth TL, Rosen JB, Dozier M. Parental responsiveness moderates the association between early-life stress and reduced telomere length. Dev Psychopathol. 2013;25(3):577–85.

23. Rizvi S, Raza ST, Mahdi F. Telomere length variations in aging and age-related diseases. Curr Aging Sci. 2014;7(3):161–7.
24. Tyrka AR, Price LH, Kao HT, Porton B, Marsella SA, Carpenter LL. Childhood maltreatment and telomere shortening: preliminary support for an effect of early stress on cellular aging. Biol Psychiatry. 2010;67(6):531-4.
25. Li Z, He Y, Wang D, Tang J, Chen X. Association between childhood trauma and accelerated telomere erosion in adulthood: a meta-analytic study. J Psychiatr Res. 2017;93:64–71.
26. Nandi A, Glymour MM, Subramanian SV. Association among socioeconomic status, health behaviors, and all-cause mortality in the United States. Epidemiology. 2014;25(2):170–7.
27. Lago S, Cantarero D, Rivera B, Pascual M, Blazquez-Fernandez C, Casal B, et al. Socioeconomic status, health inequalities and non-communicable diseases: a systematic review. Z Gesundh Wiss. 2018;26(1):1–14.
28. Baum A, Garofalo JP, Yali AM. Socioeconomic status and chronic stress. Does stress account for SES effects on health? Ann N Y Acad Sci. 1999;896:131–44.
29. Miller GE, Chen E, Zhou ES. If it goes up, must it come down? Chronic stress and the hypothalamic-pituitary-adrenocortical axis in humans. Psychol Bull. 2007;133(1):25–45.
30. National Center for PTSD. PTSD Treatment White River Junction, VT. 2017, August 18. Accessed 15 May 2018. Available from: https://www.ptsd.va.gov/public/treatment/therapy-med/treatment-ptsd.asp.
31. Green BL, Kimerling R. Trauma, posttraumatic stress disorder, and health status. In: Schnurr PP, Green BL, editors. Trauma and health: physical consequences of exposure to extreme stress. Washington, DC: American Psychological Association; 2004. p. 13–42.
32. Rasmusson AM, Schnurr PP, Zukowska Z, Scioli E, Forman DE. Adaptation to extreme stress: post-traumatic stress disorder, neuropeptide Y and metabolic syndrome. Exp Biol Med (Maywood). 2010;235(10):1150–62.
33. Latta RE, Blanco S. Contextual intimate partner violence therapy: holistic, strengths-based treatment for veterans who use violence. Bedford, MA: Veterans Integrated Service Network 1, VA New England, Veterans Health Administration; 2012.
34. Finkelhor D, Hotaling G, Lewis IA, Smith C. Sexual abuse in a national survey of adult men and women: prevalence, characteristics, and risk factors. Child Abuse Negl. 1990;14(1):19–28.
35. Finkelhor D, Turner HA, Shattuck A, Hamby SL. Violence, crime, and abuse exposure in a national sample of children and youth: an update. JAMA Pediatr. 2013;167(7):614–21.
36. U.S. Department of Health & Human Services, Administration for Children and Families, Administrationon Children, Youth and Families, Children's Bureau. (2017). Child Maltreatment 2015. Accessed 28 April 2018. Available from: http://www.acf.hhs.gov/programs/cb/research-data-technology/statistics-research/child-maltreatment.
37. Teicher, MH. Childhood trauma and the enduring consequences of forcibly separating children from parents at the United States border. BMC Medicine. 2018; 16 (1).
38. Breiding MJ, Basile KC, Smith SG, Black MC, Mahendra RR. Intimate Partner Violence Surveillance: Uniform Definitions and Recommended Data Elements, Version 2.0. Atlanta, GA: National Center for Injury Prevention and Control, Centers for Disease Control and Prevention; 2015. Accessed 29 April 2018. Available at https://www.cdc.gov/violenceprevention/pdf/ipv/intimatepartnerviolence.pdf.
39. Black MC, Basile KC, Breiding MJ, Smith SG, Walters ML, Merrick MT, Chen J, & Stevens MR. (2011). The National Intimate Partner and Sexual Violence Survey (NISVS): 2010 Summary Report. Atlanta, GA: National Center for Injury Prevention and Control, Centers for Disease Control and Prevention. Accessed 29 April 2018. Available at http://www.cdc.gov/ViolencePrevention/pdf/NISVS_Report2010-a.pdf.
40. Walters ML, Chen J, & Breiding MJ. The National Intimate Partner and Sexual Violence Survey (NISVS): 2010 Findings on Victimization by Sexual Orientation. Atlanta, GA: National Center for Injury Prevention and Control,Centers for Disease Control and Prevention. 2013. Accessed 16 December 2018. Available from: https://www.cdc.gov/ViolencePrevention/pdf/NISVS_SOfindings.pdf.

41. Curry SJ, Krist AH, Owens DK, Barry MJ, Caughey AB, Davidson KW, et al. Screening for Intimate Partner Violence, Elder Abuse, and Abuse of Vulnerable Adults: US Preventive Services Task Force Final Recommendation Statement. JAMA. 2018;320(16):1678-87.
42. American Academy of Family Practice. Intimate partner violence. Leawood, KS; 2002, 2014 (COD). Accessed 22 June 2018. Available at https://www.aafp.org/about/policies/all/intimate-partner-violence.html.
43. Council on Ethical and Judicial Affairs (CEJA)/American Medical Association. Amendment to opinion E-2.02, "Physicians' obligations in preventing, identifying, and treating violence and abuse". Chicago, IL; 2007.
44. The American College of Obstetricians and Gynecologists (ACOG). Committee Opinion No. 518: Intimate partner violence. Obstet Gynecol. 2012;119(2 Pt 1):412-7.
45. Basile KC, Smith SG, Breiding MJ, Black MC, Mahendra RR. Sexual violence surveillance: uniform definitions and recommended data elements, Version 2 Atlanta, GA; 2014. Accessed 29 April 2018. Available from: https://www.cdc.gov/violenceprevention/pdf/sv_surveillance_definitionsl-2009-a.pdf.
46. Breiding MJ, Smith SG, Basile KC, Walters ML, Chen J, Merrick MT. Prevalence and characteristics of sexual violence, stalking, and intimate partner violence victimization–national intimate partner and sexual violence survey, United States, 2011. MMWR Surveill Summ. 2014;63(8):1–18.
47. American College of Obstetricians and Gynecologists (ACOG). Sexual assault. Committee opinion no. 592. Obstet Gynecol. 2014;123:905–9.
48. Kliewer W. Community violence. In: Bornstein M, editor. The SAGE encyclopedia of lifespan human development. New York: Sage; 2016.
49. American Psychological Association (APA). Violence and socioeconomic status 2018. Accessed 12 May 2018. Available from: http://www.apa.org/pi/ses/resources/publications/violence.aspx.
50. DeCou CR, Lynch SM. Assessing adult exposure to community violence: a review of definitions and measures. Trauma Violence Abuse. 2017;18(1):51–61.
51. Wright AW, Austin M, Booth C, Kliewer W. Systematic review: exposure to community violence and physical health outcomes in youth. J Pediatr Psychol. 2017;42(4):364–78.
52. Fowler PJ, Tompsett CJ, Braciszewski JM, Jacques-Tiura AJ, Baltes BB. Community violence: a meta-analysis on the effect of exposure and mental health outcomes of children and adolescents. Dev Psychopathol. 2009;21(1):227–59.
53. Motley R, Sewell W, Chen YC. Community violence exposure and risk taking behaviors among black emerging adults: a systematic review. J Community Health. 2017;42(5):1069–78.
54. Bureau of Justice Statistics. National Crime Victimization Survey (NCVS)/ Criminal Victimization, 2016. 2017, December. Accessed 30 July 2018. Available from: https://www.bjs.gov/content/pub/pdf/cv16_sum.pdf.
55. Ahn R, Alpert EJ, Purcell G, Konstantopoulos WM, McGahan A, Cafferty E, et al. Human trafficking: review of educational resources for health professionals. Am J Prev Med. 2013;44(3):283–9.
56. Richters JE, Saltzman W. Survey of exposure to community violence: self-report version. Rockville, MD: National Institute of Mental Health. (NIMH) 1990
57. Richters JE, Martinez P. The NIMH community violence project: I. Children as victims of and witnesses to violence. Psychiatry. 1993;56(1):7–21.
58. Peterson R, Krivo L, Hagan J. Divergent social worlds: neighborhood crime and the racial-spatial divide. New York: Russell Sage Foundation; 2010.
59. Heron M. Deaths: leading causes for 2015. Hyattsville, MD: National Center for Health Statistics; 2017.
60. Masho SW, Schoeny ME, Webster D, Sigel E. Outcomes, data, and indicators of violence at the community level. J Prim Prev. 2016;37(2):121–39.

61. United Nations Office on Drugs and Crime. Human trafficking 2018. Accessed 16 May 2018. Available from: https://www.unodc.org/unodc/en/human-trafficking/what-is-human-trafficking.html.
62. Polaris Project. 2017 Statistics from the National Human Trafficking Hotline and BeFree Textline Washington, DC; 2018. Accessed 12 December 2018. Available from: https://polarisproject.org/2017statistics.
63. Ottisova L, Hemmings S, Howard LM, Zimmerman C, Oram S. Prevalence and risk of violence and the mental, physical and sexual health problems associated with human trafficking: an updated systematic review. Epidemiol Psychiatr Sci. 2016;25(4):317–41.
64. Gordon M, Fang S, Coverdale J, Nguyen P. Failure to identify a human trafficking victim. Am J Psychiatry. 2018;175(5):408–9.
65. Logan TK, Walker R, Hunt G. Understanding human trafficking in the United States. Trauma Violence Abuse. 2009;10(1):3–30.
66. Dovydaitis T. Human trafficking: the role of the health care provider. J Midwifery Womens Health. 2010;55(5):462–7.
67. United States Department of State. Trafficking in persons report 2018. Washington, DC; 2017. Accessed 30 June 2018. Available from: https://www.state.gov/j/tip/rls/tiprpt/2018/index.htm.
68. Rollins R, Gribble A, Barrett SE, Powell C. Who is in your waiting room? Health care professionals as culturally responsive and trauma-informed first responders to human trafficking. AMA J Ethics. 2017;19(1):63–71.
69. Baldwin SB, Eisenman DP, Sayles JN, Ryan G, Chuang KS. Identification of human trafficking victims in health care settings. Health Hum Rights. 2011;13(1):E36–49.
70. United Nations Office on Drugs and Crime (UNODC), Global report on trafficking in persons. New York, NY; 2016. Accessed 12 December 2018. Available from: https://www.unodc.org/documents/data-and-analysis/glotip/2016_Global_Report_on_Trafficking_in_Persons.pdf.
71. Hemmings S, Jakobowitz S, Abas M, Bick D, Howard LM, Stanley N, et al. Responding to the health needs of survivors of human trafficking: a systematic review. BMC Health Serv Res. 2016;16:320.
72. Dell NA, Maynard BR, Born KR, Wagner E, Atkins B, House W. Helping survivors of human trafficking: a systematic review of exit and postexit interventions. Trauma Violence Abuse. 2017; 1524838017692553.
73. Muraya DN, Fry D. Aftercare services for child victims of sex trafficking: a systematic review of policy and practice. Trauma Violence Abuse. 2016;17(2):204–20.
74. Polaris Project. Recognize the signs. Washington, DC; 2018. Accessed 25 June 2018. Available from: https://polarisproject.org/human-trafficking/recognize-signs.
75. Shandro J, Chisolm-Straker M, Duber HC, Findlay SL, Munoz J, Schmitz G, et al. Human trafficking: a guide to identification and approach for the emergency physician. Ann Emerg Med. 2016;68(4):501–8.e1.
76. Judge AM, Murphy JA, Hidalgo J, Macias-Konstantopoulos W. Engaging survivors of human trafficking: complex health care needs and scarce resources. Ann Intern Med. 2018;168(9):658–63.
77. Baldwin SB, Fehrenbacher AE, Eisenman DP. Psychological coercion in human trafficking: an application of Biderman's framework. Qual Health Res. 2015;25(9):1171–81.
78. Ravi A, Pfeiffer MR, Rosner Z, Shea JA. Trafficking and trauma: insight and advice for the healthcare system from sex-trafficked women incarcerated on Rikers Island. Med Care. 2017;55(12):1017–22.
79. Grace AM, Lippert S, Collins K, Pineda N, Tolani A, Walker R, et al. Educating health care professionals on human trafficking. Pediatr Emerg Care. 2014;30(12):856–61.
80. Mohatt NV, Thompson AB, Thai ND, Tebes JK. Historical trauma as public narrative: a conceptual review of how history impacts present-day health. Soc Sci Med. 2014;106:128–36.
81. Sotero M. A conceptual model of historical trauma: implications for public health practice and research. J Health Disparities Res Pract. 2006;1(1): 93-107.

82. Kellermann NP. Transmission of Holocaust trauma--an integrative view. Psychiatry. 2001;64(3):256–67.
83. Brave Heart MY, Chase J, Elkins J, Altschul DB. Historical trauma among indigenous peoples of the Americas: concepts, research, and clinical considerations. J Psychoactive Drugs. 2011;43(4):282–90.
84. Gump JP. Reality matters: the shadow of trauma on African American subjectivity. Psychoanal Psychol. 2010;27(1):42–54.
85. Karenian H, Livaditis M, Karenian S, Zafiriadis K, Bochtsou V, Xenitidis K. Collective trauma transmission and traumatic reactions among descendants of Armenian refugees. Int J Soc Psychiatry. 2011;57(4):327–37.
86. Nagata DK, Cheng WJ. Intergenerational communication of race-related trauma by Japanese American former internees. Am J Orthopsychiatry. 2003;73(3):266–78.
87. Estrada AL. Mexican Americans and historical trauma theory: a theoretical perspective. J Ethn Subst Abus. 2009;8(3):330–40.
88. Mestrović SG. A sociological conceptualization of trauma. Soc Sci Med. 1985;21(8):835–48.
89. Brave Heart MY, DeBruyn LM. The American Indian Holocaust: healing historical unresolved grief. Am Indian Alsk Native Ment Health Res. 1998;8(2):56–78.
90. Nutton J, Fast E. Historical trauma, substance use, and indigenous peoples: seven generations of harm from a "big event". Subst Use Misuse. 2015;50(7):839–47.
91. Kellermann NP. Epigenetic transmission of Holocaust trauma: can nightmares be inherited? Isr J Psychiatry Relat Sci. 2013;50(1):33–9.
92. Yehuda R, Teicher MH, Seckl JR, Grossman RA, Morris A, Bierer LM. Parental posttraumatic stress disorder as a vulnerability factor for low cortisol trait in offspring of holocaust survivors. Arch Gen Psychiatry. 2007;64(9):1040–8.
93. Raja S, Hasnain M, Hoersch M, Gove-Yin S, Rajagopalan C. Trauma Informed Care in Medicine. Family & Community Health. 2015;38(3):216–26.
94. Administration on Children/Youth and Families/Children's Bureau. Child maltreatment 2016. Washington, DC: US Department of Health & Human Services; 2018. Accessed 12 December 2018. Available from: https://www.acf.hhs.gov/cb/resource/child-maltreatment-2016.
95. Breiding MJ, Basile KC, Smith SG, Black MC, Mahendra RR. Intimate partner violence surveillance: uniform definitions and recommended data elements, Version 2.0 Atlanta, GA; 2015. Accessed 28 April 2018. Available from: https://www.cdc.gov/violenceprevention/pdf/ipv/intimatepartnerviolence.pdf.
96. Smith SG, Zhang, X. Basile, KC, Merrick, MT, Wang J, Kresnow M, Chen J. The national intimate partner and sexual violence survey (NISVS): 2015 data brief. Atlanta, GA: National Center for Injury Prevention and Control, Centers for Disease Control and Prevention; 2018.
97. Bureau of Justice Statistics. National Crime Victimization Survey (NCVS)/Criminal Victimization, 2016. 2018, October. Accessed 30 July 2018. Available from: https://www.bjs.gov/content/pub/pdf/cv16re.pdf.
98. Polaris Project. The Facts Washington, DC; 2016. Accessed 1 July 2018. Available from: https://polarisproject.org/human-trafficking/facts.
99. International organization for migration (IOM). UN Migration Agency, Polaris to Launch Global Data Repository on Human Trafficking. 9 September 2017. Accessed 16 December 2018. Available from: https://www.iom.int/news/un-migration-agency-polaris-launch-global-data-repository-human-trafficking.
100. The National Child Traumatic Stress Network (NCTSN). Conversations about historical trauma: part three Rockville, MD; 2014. Accessed 30 June 2018. Available from: https://www.nctsn.org/resources/conversations-about-historical-trauma-part-three.

# Chapter 2
# Trauma and Trauma-Informed Care

**Leigh Kimberg and Margaret Wheeler**

## Objectives

- Define trauma and resilience.
- Review the prevalence of trauma and the effects of trauma and resilience on health.
- Define trauma-informed care.
- Describe principles and components of trauma-informed care.
- Describe a practical approach to implementing trauma-informed care (4 Cs).
- Review qualities of trauma-informed healthcare systems.

*Eric Johnson is a 45-year-old man who is a landscape architect. He has poorly controlled hypertension and diabetes, untreated hepatitis C, undiagnosed chronic post-traumatic stress disorder, and drinks alcohol daily. During his childhood, an older cousin who used to take care of him while his parents were at work sexually abused Mr. Johnson. During a pediatric visit for his tetanus immunization at age 11, he felt like his mind left his body and he lost all control of his actions. Two healthcare staff held him down to give him his shot as he struggled and screamed. He has been terribly afraid of doctors' visits since then. He has never told anyone about the sexual abuse. He still gets frequent nightmares about this abuse; the nightmares have been getting worse since his cousin contacted him recently. Today, Mr. Johnson*

---

L. Kimberg (✉) · M. Wheeler
Division of General Internal Medicine, San Francisco General Hospital (SFGH), University of California, San Francisco (UCSF), San Francisco, CA, USA
e-mail: Leigh.Kimberg@ucsf.edu

© Springer Nature Switzerland AG 2019
M. R. Gerber (ed.), *Trauma-Informed Healthcare Approaches*,
https://doi.org/10.1007/978-3-030-04342-1_2

*has his first appointment with Dr. Melissa Jones in the Redwood Health System Adult Medical Clinic.*

## Introduction

Traumatic events are common and can have lasting effects on a person's life and health and a community's well-being. The effects of trauma go far beyond its immediate psychological and physical effects. Experiencing trauma can alter individual biology and behavior over the life course; these changes have an impact on interpersonal and intergenerational relationships. Ultimately, traumatic events alter the well-being of not only individuals but also our communities and society. How a person responds to trauma is complex and dependent on many factors, including the resources of the individual and their supporting community. Trauma's effects can be mitigated by protective factors and resiliencies or compounded by other risk factors and vulnerabilities. Trauma experienced in childhood is particularly damaging. Childhood exposure to trauma can alter development and have particularly profound and lasting effects on health and well-being, including resulting in the development of chronic illness in adulthood. Exposure to one traumatic event increases the vulnerability of individuals and communities to future trauma. Communities subjected to historical and structural violence are disproportionally afflicted by trauma and its effects. Understanding the devastating and multiplicative effects of trauma on health and well-being and addressing the consequences of trauma are crucially important for healthcare providers and the systems in which they work. Preventing trauma and mitigating its adverse effects promote health equity.

Because trauma is both ubiquitous [1] and associated with many chronic illnesses and high-risk behaviors, all healthcare providers will care for patients with histories of trauma. Survivors of trauma may be "triggered", consciously or unconsciously, by situations they encounter in the healthcare setting [2, 3]. The use of physical restraints and the need to undress, undergo invasive procedures, wait in a room with a closed door, or see blood are all concrete ways that patients may be re-traumatized while obtaining medical care. Traumatic memories, provoked by healthcare encounters, may make medical care intolerable to a patient and contribute to worsened health outcomes [4]. Most importantly, the power imbalance between patient and provider can trigger a traumatic response. Effective and compassionate treatment for trauma survivors depends upon the healthcare setting becoming "trauma-informed." In this chapter, we present a practical model of care, "trauma-informed care," to respond to the multifaceted needs of people and communities exposed to trauma. Because trauma affects all of us directly and indirectly, "trauma-informed care" benefits us all.

## Definition of Trauma and Types of Traumatic Events

It can be difficult to pin down a definition of trauma. The word trauma is often used to refer to both injurious events themselves and to their outcomes. Certainly, the outcomes of traumatic experiences vary greatly from person to person based on a wide spectrum of circumstances including genetic, epigenetic, biological, psychological, environmental, family, community, societal, historical, and other factors. How a person responds to a harmful event, or series of events, is now thought of as a process resulting from the interaction between the events themselves and the person, ameliorated or further undermined by their individual, familial, and community resilience or vulnerability and resources or lack thereof. When the harmful event causes lasting suffering, the event is considered traumatic. Trauma ruptures relationships, with oneself and others.

The Substance Abuse and Mental Health Services Administration (SAMHSA) defines individual trauma: "Individual trauma results from an event, series of events, or set of circumstances that is experienced by an individual as physically or emotionally harmful or threatening and that has lasting adverse effects on the individual's functioning and physical, social, emotional, or spiritual well-being." [5] *"Complex trauma" or "complex psychological trauma" is defined as "resulting from exposure to severe stressors that (1) are repetitive or prolonged, (2) involve harm or abandonment by caregivers or other ostensibly responsible adults, and (3) occur at developmentally vulnerable times in the victims' life, such as early childhood:..."* [6] *but can also occur later in life* [6]. The concept of historical trauma refers to complex traumatic experiences that affect an entire community or cultural group over multiple generations [7, 8].

Individuals as well as entire communities or cultural groups can be traumatized. Catastrophic events and forces that traumatize both individuals and communities may be environmental disasters, famine, war, genocide, torture, human trafficking, terrorism, forced migration, mass incarceration, police violence [9], poverty, and "structural violence" involving systematic oppression or discrimination (e.g., racism, sexism, homophobia, transphobia, mistreatment and persecution of immigrants, etc.). Trauma can be conceptualized as being "contagious"; it may be passed on through individuals, families, communities, and society, often inter-generationally. Trauma's mode of transmission is most often through adverse power dynamics. When one searches for the origins, means of perpetuation, and factors that worsen trauma, ultimately one uncovers various forms of structural violence involving systematic oppression or discrimination. Interpersonal violence including family violence, abuse and neglect, and life events that reduce trust or a sense of safety and security, like the death of loved ones, divorce of one's parents, major illness, or other life upheavals are detrimental to individuals. Broader cultural, political, and societal factors that contextualize the trauma also need to be recognized and understood to promote healing and prevent future trauma.

## Resilience and Protective Factors

Resilience is "the ability of an individual, family, or community to cope with adversity and trauma, and adapt to challenges or change [10]." Resilience has been described as acting to maintain health and equilibrium despite adversity by allowing people or communities to withstand, adapt to, and, then, recover from adversity [11]. Individual resilience is often conceptualized as being related to fixed intrinsic factors (genetics, temperament), but we now understand that even those factors are affected by our experiences and those of our forbearers through epigenetic, biological, and relational factors. Thus, resilience, like trauma, is best conceived of as a process that is constructed relationally and inter-generationally. Protective factors contributing to resilience occur at every level of the socioecological model, including the individual, family, community, or societal level [12]. Individual and family factors that protect against childhood maltreatment and violence, for example, include a child's IQ, a nurturing parent, grandparent or other supportive adults, parental employment, housing stability, and access to health and social services [13–15].

The Harvard Center for the Developing Child has created a visual model to help us understand that resilience occurs when the balance between adverse experiences or factors and positive experiences or factors "tips" in favor of positive outcomes. Positive experiences that support resilience include "facilitating supportive adult-child relationships, building a sense of self-efficacy and perceived control, providing opportunities to strengthen adaptive skills and self-regulatory capacities, and mobilizing sources of faith, hope, and cultural traditions [16]." The single most significant protective factor in preventing both childhood trauma and its adverse outcomes is the presence of a safe, stable, nurturing adult caregiver consistently present in a child's life [17]. The presence of a safe, stable, nurturing adult provides the attunement, support, and protection that buffer children from the adverse effects of traumatic experiences. Safe, stable, and nurturing relationships can effectively break the intergenerational transmission of abuse [18]. These resiliency-promoting, caregiving relationships flourish most fully in supportive communities; communities that focus on preventing abuse and supporting parents and caregivers also protect children from maltreatment [19]. In turn, communities thrive when they are supported by equitable and just societal policies. Across the US, communities are becoming "trauma-informed" in order to develop policies and programs that promote resilience and healing [20].

## Early Trauma

One of the largest, most comprehensive studies of the effects of childhood trauma on adulthood disease, the "Adverse Childhood Experiences" (or "ACE Study"), highlighted the high prevalence of several types of trauma occurring during childhood (ACES) [21] including childhood emotional, sexual, and physical abuse, neglect, and family dysfunction (i.e., witnessing of parental domestic violence, parental separation or divorce, parental mental illness, parental substance use, or parental incarceration). Even in the predominantly white, middle class study population, 63.9% of the participants had experienced at least one ACE category and 12.5% had experienced four or more ACE categories.

Communities where poverty and lack of access to optimal educational opportunities, employment, healthy food, and sufficient housing are prevalent have higher rates of adverse childhood events [22, 23]. ACEs differ not only by place (state) but also by race and ethnicity, with the prevalence of ACEs lowest among Asian non-Hispanic children in all regions and highest among black non-Hispanic children in most regions [24]. The original ACE study did not measure multiple forms of adversity and trauma experienced by children [25]. For example, the US General Accounting Office (GAO) has found that black students, boys, and children with disabilities experience disproportionate rates of discipline in US schools [26]. These disproportionate rates of discipline, inhumane forms of discipline, and educational quality disparities later increase the risk of poor social outcomes, like poverty or incarceration, and poor health outcomes [27, 28]. The burden of overall trauma in urban and rural underserved communities is thought to approach that of conflict-ridden developing countries [29]. The Institute for Safe Families in Philadelphia has developed an "Urban ACE score" that includes measures of witnessed community violence, adverse neighborhood experiences, bullying, and discrimination [30]. The World Health Organization has developed and is validating an "ACE International Questionnaire" that includes additional questions related to forced marriage, peer violence, exposure to community violence and war, and collective violence [31].

Because our experiences and relationships, in constant interplay with our genetic makeup, build our biology including our brains [32], adversity and trauma have profound health effects. Childhood trauma and adversity are at the root of many adulthood high-risk behaviors and diseases that often occur decades after the trauma (Fig. 2.1). Additionally, adverse experiences may have an effect on poor health out-

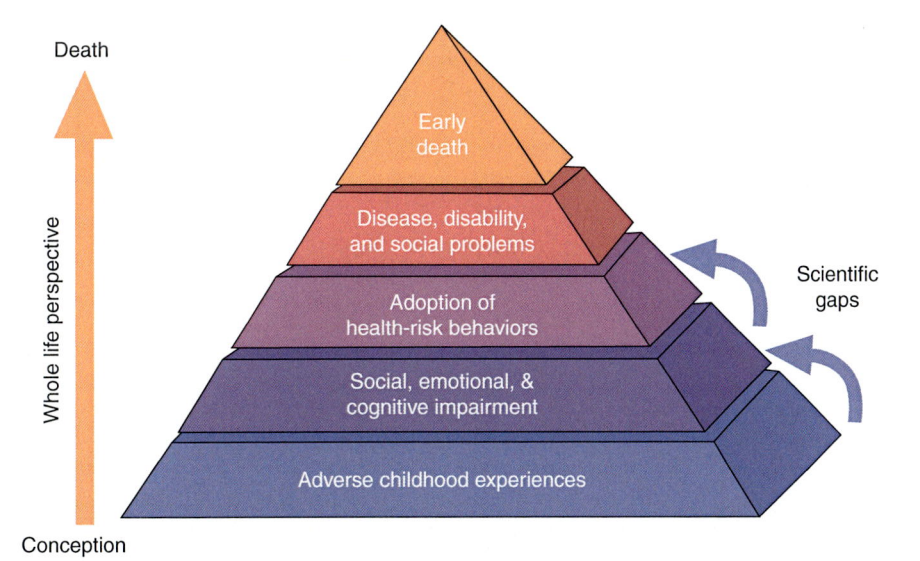

**Fig. 2.1** Adverse childhood experience and lifetime health. From http://www.cdc.gov/violenceprevention/acestudy/pyramid.html

comes that is independent of adverse coping behaviors [33]. Retrospective and prospective studies have demonstrated that childhood trauma and adversity are associated with a risk of premature mortality [34, 35]. When considering the devastating health effects and adverse social outcomes associated with ACEs like lower educational attainment, graduation rates, teen pregnancy, and even higher incarceration rates, it is hard to fathom the longevity and pervasive effects of trauma [36].

## Protective Factors and Resilience

Fortunately, protective factors like supportive relationships and resilience factors can mitigate the behavioral and health outcomes of ACEs [11, 13, 37]. In a recent study of both individual ACEs and social adversity, researchers found that having support from an adult that the child trusts can mitigate the impacts of childhood adversity. In this retrospective study, the presence of an "always available adult" (AAA), trusted during childhood, was associated with a lower prevalence of unhealthy behaviors (poor diet, smoking, and alcohol use) and poor mental health in adulthood. Having an AAA in one's life also mitigated the effects of ACEs on unhealthy behaviors and on poor mental health status [13].

In another retrospective study, childhood community resilience assets—including knowing where to get help, having opportunities to apply one's skills, being treated fairly, enjoying community culture, having supportive friends, having people to look up to, and having a trusted adult available—were found to be associated with better childhood health and high school attendance. These community resilience assets were also associated with mitigation of the negative effects of ACEs on the prevalence of childhood illnesses. Interestingly, different resilience factors were associated with mitigation of the prevalence of different childhood illnesses [37]. Thus, promoting community resilience promises to not only prevent ACEs but also to mitigate the harmful effects of ACEs once they have occurred. Promoting resilience through healthcare, as well as through multi-sector partnerships involving healthcare, is essential to achieving healthcare and health equity [11]. Table 2.1 provides an overview of these risk and protective factors for trauma and the conditions associated with trauma.

## Trauma-Informed Care

Trauma-informed care has been defined as "a strengths-based service delivery approach that is grounded in an understanding of and responsiveness to the impact of trauma, that emphasizes physical, psychological, and emotional safety for both providers and survivors, and that creates opportunities for survivors to rebuild a sense of control and empowerment [38]." There is emerging evidence that adopting trauma-informed care may improve patient and workplace outcomes [2, 39, 40]. *How can we build systems of trauma-informed care that promote resilience and healing?*

**Table 2.1** Trauma-related conditions, risk and protective factors

| Risk Factors | Conditions related to trauma | Protective Factors |
|---|---|---|
| Lack of safe, stable, nurturing relationships | Psychiatric illnesses (anxiety, depression, PTSD, cPTSD, suicidality) | Supportive family relationships |
| Young age | Chronic illnesses (heart, lung, liver and other diseases) | Well-resourced, safe communities |
| Female gender for intimate partner violence/sexual violence | | Financial security |
| | Sexually transmitted infections including HIV | Employment |
| Male gender for community violence | Sleep disorders | Stable housing |
| | Unwanted pregnancy and pregnancy at early age | Higher educational status |
| Minority status (Race, ethnicity, religion, sexual orientation, gender identity, other) | | Higher brain executive function |
| | Childhood learning and behavior problems | Community engagement |
| Psychiatric illness | Childhood learning and behavior problems | Good health |
| Substance use | Poor educational attainment | |
| Disability (physical and mental) | Substance use | |
| Family history of violence | Homelessness | |
| Homelessness | Premature death (due to poor health, homicide, suicide) | |
| Poverty | Future victimization or perpetration of violence | |

**Table 2.2** San Francisco Department of Public Health Trauma-informed Principles and Competencies[a]

| |
|---|
| Trauma understanding |
| Cultural humility and responsiveness |
| Safety and stability |
| Compassion and dependability |
| Collaboration and empowerment |
| Resilience and recovery |

[a]http://www.leapsf.org/pdf/Trauma-Informed-Systems-Initative-2014.pdf

## Trauma-Informed Care Mission and Principles

Ideally, a trauma-informed system is an "ecosystem" that supports and promotes health and well-being for all people who interact within that system. Defining and adopting a shared mission and core foundational principles lays the groundwork for trauma-informed care and guides healthcare transformation. SAMHSA has developed and disseminated trauma-informed principles that have influenced health system transformation nationally and internationally [41]. The San Francisco Department of Public Health has adopted foundational principles, based upon the SAMHSA principles and others (Table 2.2).

These foundational principles can guide the process of trauma-informed systems and care transformation. These principles are based upon a deep understanding of how trauma affects human beings and their relationships. They describe how healing from trauma may occur through relationships and experiences that are safe, stable, compassionate, dependable, collaborative, empowering, and focused on the building of resilience.

Cultural humility [42], one of the principles adopted by the San Francisco Department of Public Health, is a particularly helpful concept in addressing the healthy and equitable relationship-building between physicians and patients or others that is a pre-requisite for preventing and mitigating traumatic experiences. Cultural humility [42], which stands in contrast to cultural competence, calls for each of us to commit to life-long learning about our own identities so that we can better understand our own complex cultural identities and aspects of power and privilege (or lack thereof) in society. The practice of cultural humility, then, asks us to use our self-awareness and respect for others' self-determined, always evolving cultural identities to interact in ways that recognize, minimize, and mitigate power differentials. Finally, cultural humility asks us to mitigate power differentials on an organizational level by holding our powerful institutions, like hospitals, accountable to the community. Directly addressing self-determination of identity and power differentials in relationships is a promising perspective to lead individuals and organizations toward becoming more trauma-informed and resiliency–promoting.

Becoming trauma-informed is a journey, rather than a fixed set of interventions, that is guided by one's trauma-informed mission and foundational principles. Healthcare providers, staff, and systems become more trauma-informed as they delve deeply into how each of these trauma-informed principles influence their relationships, experiences, and work. Multiple conceptual and practical models of trauma-informed care have been developed [2, 43–45]. Most organizations that have embarked on a path of trauma-informed systems transformation understand that it is a process of culture change. The Sanctuary Model ® [45], for example, describes itself as, "a theory-based, trauma-informed, trauma-responsive, evidence-supported, whole culture approach that has a clear and structured methodology for creating or changing an organizational culture." Culture change is never complete; it is always evolving. Ultimately, striving for social justice and health equity is fundamentally necessary to create the conditions through which all people can heal from past traumatic experiences, remain unexposed to re-traumatization, and participate in preventing the transmission of trauma to others.

## Trauma-Informed Care Is for Everyone

Trauma-informed care, built upon the foundational principles discussed above, creates an optimally healing environment for the patient, the patient's family, and the healthcare providers and staff [46, 47]. When all providers and staff in a clinic or hospital have been trained to understand that trauma and its sequelae can affect everyone (including each of their co-workers) and that many forms of trauma are hidden, it can deepen respect for the resilience of both patients and colleagues. Developing a shared understanding that maladaptive behaviors or ways of relating often have their roots in traumatic experiences promotes a climate of compassion and respect. The devastating traumatic impacts of various forms of structural violence like racism can be highlighted and directly addressed. The legacy of historical trauma and its ongoing manifestations in affected communities can be integrated into the response to trauma [48]. Once healthcare providers and organizations understand that highly hierarchical and non-collaborative decision-making processes and policies or management practices perpetuate the dynamics of trauma and run counter to the principles of trauma-informed care, they can build more healing systems of care.

Creating an environment that exudes calm, safety, and compassion is a goal of trauma-informed systems. In trauma-informed systems, respectful approaches that earn patients' and communities' trust and cultivate resilience, positive coping strategies, and a sense of control are emphasized. Educational materials about trauma and resilience are made easily accessible. Programs to help mitigate the difficulties that traumatized patients may have in accessing care such as peer advocacy, patient navigation [49, 50], case management, and community outreach, improve the quality of care and extend treatment beyond the walls of the clinic or hospital [43, 50, 51]. Models of care using proactive outreach to patients and practical assistance to increase access and adherence to treatment result in increased care for patients [29], reduced violence recidivism, and improved cost-effectiveness [52]. The healthcare organization attends to their relationship with and impact in the community to examine institutional accountability for the perpetuation of inequities and commits to equitable partnerships that support community resilience and social justice.

Trauma-informed systems also build and support the resilience of providers and staff. Provider and staff well-being are required to maintain safety and compassion for patients. In particular, attending to the personal traumatic experiences of providers and staff and the phenomenon of "vicarious traumatization" (VT), defined as "the negative transformation in the helper that results from empathic engagement with trauma survivors and their trauma material, combined with a commitment or responsibility to help them," [53] is regarded as critically important to allowing providers and staff to respond with empathy to patient stories of interpersonal and structural acts of cruelty and betrayal.

## Practical Application of Trauma-Informed Principles to Clinical Care: The 4 Cs

Maintaining a calm, supportive, non-judgmental, and resiliency-promoting demeanor that is stabilizing and reassuring to patients with a history of trauma can be challenging even for experienced clinicians; it requires a commitment to ongoing self-reflection, practice, and both individual and systems transformation. To help providers understand how to enact practices that support trauma-informed care transformation, one of the authors (LK) developed a simple 4 Cs paradigm in a concrete and memorable rubric. These 4 Cs are: *Calm, Contain, Care, and Cope*

**Table 2.3** The Four Cs of Trauma-informed Care

| |
|---|
| *Calm* |
| *Pay attention to how you are feeling when you are caring for the patient. Breathe deeply and calm yourself to model and promote calmness for the patient, yourself, and your co-workers* |
| Practice calming exercises (deep breathing, grounding) with patients |
| Cultivate understanding of trauma and its effects to promote a calm, patient attitude toward others (patients and co-workers) |
| Re-design healthcare environments, policies, and practices to reduce chaos and promote calmness |
| Cultivate understanding of how resilience, justice, and equity build peaceful, calm communities and environments |
| *Contain* |
| *Limit trauma history detail to maintain emotional and physical safety. Provide education, resources, and referrals to trauma-specific care without requiring disclosure of trauma* |
| Model healthy relationship boundaries and earn trust by behaving reliably |
| Monitor patients' emotional and physical responses to education and inquiry about trauma |
| Practice calming techniques to help patient (or parent/caregiver and child dyad) regain composure |
| Normalize fear of returning to the healthcare setting if the triggering of a trauma response occurs; invite the patient to share what changes would make visits more tolerable and healing |
| Enact healthcare policies and practices that minimize re-traumatization of patients and staff |
| Form multi-disciplinary and multi-sector partnerships that reduce re-traumatization for patients and staff |
| *Care* |
| *Practice self-care and self-compassion while caring for others* |
| Share messages of support when patients disclose trauma or trauma symptoms |
| Normalize and de-stigmatize trauma symptoms and harmful coping behaviors (as common sequelae of trauma) |
| Practice cultural humility [42] |
| Adopt behaviors, practices, and policies that minimize and mitigate power differentials to reduce trauma and structural violence |
| Enact healthcare policies that promote self-care, compassion, and equity |
| Form equitable partnerships to extend CARE into the community |
| *Cope* |
| *Emphasize coping skills, positive relationships, and interventions that build resilience* |
| Inquire about practices that help the patient feel better and more hopeful |
| Document a "Coping Strategies" list instead of only "Problem Lists" and include patient's own words of wisdom and good self-advice in the "after-visit" summary |
| Improve identification and treatment of the mental health, substance use, and other sequelae of trauma |
| Connect patients and families with community organizations to increase social support and access to necessary resources |
| Promote equity within healthcare organizations, communities, and society |

(Table 2.3). These 4Cs emphasize key concepts in trauma-informed care and can serve as touchstones to guide immediate and sustained behavior change. In this chapter, the 4Cs paradigm is expanded to apply to not only individuals [54, 55] but also healthcare organizations and multi-sector partnerships.

## *Calm*

**Calm** Pay attention to how you are feeling when you are caring for the patient. Breathe deeply and calm yourself to model and promote calmness for the patient, yourself, and your co-workers. Practice calming exercises (deep breathing, grounding) with patients. Cultivate understanding of trauma and its effects to promote a calm, patient attitude toward others (patients and co-workers.)

*Dr. Jorge García, a beloved provider in a busy family practice clinic in the Redwood Health System, made it a regular practice to pause for just a second before entering each patient's room. He paused to breathe deeply and allow himself to feel a deep sense of gratitude that his next patient, despite many stressful life circumstances, had come to this appointment. As he washed his hands at the beginning and end of each visit, he noticed the soothing sensations of water on his hands and silently offered his wishes for the well-being of his patient and himself.*

Because human beings biologically "co-regulate" with one another [56, 57], healthcare providers and staff can use the relaxation of their own bodies and breath to create a calm, healing environment not only for patients but also for one another. Imagine how peaceful and healing a healthcare environment would feel if each person working within that environment practiced mindfulness, a practice of maintaining awareness of the current moment and gently acknowledging one's thoughts, emotions, and bodily sensations and breath. People can practice mindfulness in a myriad of different ways that are congruent with their cultural preferences. People who have experienced severe or chronic trauma may have difficulty regulating their emotional affect or staying present (and not dissociating) during stressful moments. Healthcare providers and staff who breathe peacefully with relaxed, expansive exhalations and speak calmly even when they encounter stressful situations model and spread a sense of calmness. Especially when paired with active compassion and self-awareness about power and privilege, this calmness can subtly assist a patient or co-worker who is responding to past or current trauma co-regulate into a less stressful physical and emotional state.

Whenever healthcare providers and staff are interacting with patients, it is important that they observe patients and their caregivers for signs of emotional dysregulation that could be indications of the triggering of traumatic memories or a trauma response. Observing when patients become anxious, talk more quickly or loudly or, conversely, stop talking or appear to be dissociating from the present moment can help healthcare providers and staff attend to adjusting their approach to make the healthcare visit more tolerable. When a healthcare provider observes that a patient seems dysregulated or overwhelmed, the healthcare team can elicit the patient's preferred calming practices and teach additional skills that activate the calming parasympathetic system [58]. Patients may utilize prayer, meditation, breathing techniques, visualization, repetition of a special word, muscle relaxation, music, self-care and meditation digital apps, and other skills to re-orient to the present moment and gain more calmness. It is critically important to normalize the fear of returning to an environment that the patient has found triggering and inquire as to how best to accommodate the patient to allow for continued engagement in healthcare.

In pediatric practice, observing the emotional regulation of the caregiver, the child, and the dyadic interactions of the caregiver and child can also provide clues to the healthcare provider about the effects of traumatic experiences on both the caregiver and child. Healthcare providers can coach caregivers in teaching their children calming practices and breathing exercises through playful shared activities like gently blowing soap bubbles, reading books together, or soothing touch to make the healthcare environment less triggering for both the caregiver and child [59]. By coaching a caregiver, rather than stepping in to calm a child, the healthcare provider can enhance a mutually healing relationship between caregivers and children to contribute to breaking the intergenerational cycle of trauma transmission [11, 18, 59–61].

Practicing mindfulness to promote a calm environment does not mean that healthcare providers and staff should avoid conflict. Human beings, our interactions, and relationships are complex and bound to result in conflict. Through practicing mindfulness, we can learn to move toward conflict more calmly rather than recoiling or reacting in ways that exacerbate stressful situations. Practicing mindfulness and remaining in touch with our thoughts, emotions, bodily sensations, and breath can render stress and trauma less contagious and damaging [62].

*Despite experiencing a high burden of trauma, the patients cared for by Dr. Jorge García have better diabetic control than the average for his health system. Dr. García understands that there are many evidence-based factors that contribute to these improved outcomes including his compassion, stellar clinical skills, attention to detail, Spanish language and cultural concordance with many of his Latino patients, the well-functioning team-based care in his clinic, and the excellent continuous quality improvement program. Yet, Dr. García also feels that his deep understanding of trauma-informed care and how to promote a calm, healing environment strongly contributes to the good outcomes for his patients and team.*

There are specific trauma-informed attitudes that help healthcare providers and staff maintain a calm perspective and demeanor. When one understands the near universal prevalence of trauma, one can recognize the importance of adopting trauma-informed care practices with everyone in the environment including one's co-workers and patients. When one deeply understands how trauma affects neurodevelopment and behavior, one does not expect behavior change to happen quickly (for oneself, one's patients, or co-workers). An understanding of the effects of trauma can support healthcare providers and staff in adopting evidence-based approaches like harm reduction and motivational interviewing with a more wholehearted sense of patience. When one understands neuroplasticity and the power of respectful, safe, stable, and nurturing relationships to promote healing from trauma, one can focus on patient-centered and colleague-centered resilience-building and relationship-building practices [58].

*The Redwood Health System decided to embark upon organizational culture transformation to become trauma-informed. Learning from other health systems, they realized that this transformation would require years of sustained focus. At the same time, they wanted to make some rapid changes that would promote a more healing environment. They held a series of meetings with key stakeholders to adopt foundational trauma-informed principles. They embarked on initiatives to teach and support mindfulness practices and prevent vicarious traumatization for their staff, including the behavioral health staff. They asked staff to begin each meeting with different evidence-based practices to promote well-being, like taking turns leading a brief gratitude exercise or 1 min guided meditation. The health system also decided to remodel their environment's physical spaces and staffing patterns to be more soothing and peaceful for patients and staff.*

Organizations that are in the process of becoming trauma-informed have recognized the importance of promoting a calm, peaceful environment through hiring practices, workforce development and support, management training, improved workflows, and alteration of the physical environment. Whenever possible the healthcare environment should be altered to minimize noise, harsh lighting, cramped and uncomfortable spaces, and chaos. Involving all of the stakeholders who will utilize a space in designing the physical and human environment is critically important. Aspects of the environment that promote a sense of peacefulness and security for one person may feel uncomfortable and, even threatening, to another person; for example, some staff and patients may be comforted by physical barriers between people or abundant security staff, and others may find these disturbing. Workflows that are clear and efficient can promote a calm environment as well. Addressing vicarious traumatization requires a multi-pronged approach that ideally includes offering all staff training in mindfulness-based stress reduction techniques.

*The Redwood Health System realized from the start of this process that if they really wanted to become trauma-informed and resiliency-promoting, they would need to focus on transforming their relationship with the community. They knew that they had a lot to learn from community members and the community-based organizations in their region. They immediately changed their policies to provide childcare and stipends to patient advisory board members to foster community stakeholder leadership. They began attending community meetings as listeners. They began a process of learning how they could support existing trauma-informed systems' work in their community. They quickly learned that the community was not satisfied with their hiring processes, pointing out that the Redwood Health System did not hire diverse staff from the community.*

Promoting peacefulness and healing in the community requires an explicit commitment to promoting equity. Inequitable power differentials are root causes of trauma and the mode of transmission of trauma [63]. Societal structures and policies that create and perpetuate these inequitable power differentials drive health and healthcare disparities. Large healthcare organizations wield a great deal of power in a community and, thus, have the opportunity and responsibility to behave as responsible, accountable anchor institutions. They can adopt best principles and practices of healthcare institution-community partnerships that can support and facilitate multi-sector trauma-informed systems initiatives [64]. When healthcare institutions fully embrace trauma-informed care, they can learn how to function as structural facilitators in building community resilience and equity.

## *Contain*

**Contain** Asking the level of detail of trauma history that will allow the patient to maintain emotional and physical safety, respects the timeframe of the healthcare interaction, and allows you to offer the patient important treatment options. Providing education, resources, and referrals to trauma-specific care without requiring disclosure of trauma details facilitates an interaction that does not emotionally overwhelm the provider or the patient.

*The medical assistants (MAs) in the Redwood Health System's women's clinic implemented a "universal education" protocol about interpersonal violence (IPV) and reproductive coercion that was based upon a program implemented and studied at Planned Parenthood [65]. Alicia Greene, an MA, invited a woman who came to the clinic to discuss birth control options into the exam room alone. Ms. Greene shared a wallet-sized educational card about IPV and reproductive coercion and said, "Our relationships affect our health. If we have stress in our relationships or someone is hurting us that can cause or worsen many health problems. We always share information about how partners can try to control whether you get pregnant by doing things like poking holes in condoms or throwing out birth control pills. At our clinic, we always offer hidden birth control methods like an IUD with the string cut short so your partner cannot feel it or a Depo-Provera shot that your partner won't know you had. Feel free to ask the provider for a hidden method of birth control. Also, if you or any of your family members or friends are being hurt by someone, this card explains how to get help. Would you like to take one or more of these cards to share with friends?"*

There is a paucity of evidence about patients' experiences with various models of trauma-informed care. One of the more robust areas of research has been the study of addressing intimate partner violence (IPV) with adult patients, especially women. Directly addressing adulthood IPV compassionately and non-judgmentally has been found to be safe, effective, and acceptable [70]. Once a patient discloses IPV, the patient receives brief counseling and referral to resources. Yet, in most healthcare settings, IPV screening rates are low and IPV disclosure rates after screening are far lower than the expected IPV prevalence [66]. Providers have reported many barriers to implementing IPV screening including a fear of opening "Pandora's Box" [67]. Patients may have many reasons for not disclosing IPV to providers including shame, lack of trust, fear of the person who has threatened and hurt them, fear about lack of confidentiality, fear about adverse consequences like imposed separation from children, and more [68]. Thus, with a "screening" model of care, only the small fraction of people who are experiencing IPV, and are screened and disclose IPV, ever receive education about life-saving resources.

In response to these barriers, a new approach called "Universal Education" (UE) has been developed and tested in reproductive healthcare; it was found to be effective in addressing reproductive coercion regardless of disclosure [65]. The UE approach has three main components. A healthcare provider relates an educational message about how trauma might relate to the patient's presenting complaint or concern, explicitly describes the trauma they are referring to (like IPV or reproductive coercion), and, then, offers resources without requiring disclosure. Because UE has been found to be successful in reproductive healthcare, all family planning visits should include UE about both reproductive coercion and IPV at least. More recently, leaders in promoting and studying a UE approach have discovered that many patients appreciate a fourth component of UE: offering a patient UE materials to "take for a family member, friend, or people in your community" engages the patient as an active stakeholder in preventing the transmission of violence and other forms of trauma. Altruism is powerfully healing; this participation of the patient in helping others can become a vital component in healing from traumatic experiences [69]. Because screening for IPV has been found to be safe and effective, one can also follow UE with direct inquiry about IPV [70]. To prevent misunderstandings and unexpected consequences of discussions about trauma, healthcare providers and systems should always explain the limits of confidentiality governing an interaction.

*Dr. Melissa Jones, a provider in the Redwood Health System Adult Medical Clinic, has a new patient, Mr. Eric Johnson, who looks nervous and smells of alcohol when she greets him. Dr. Jones, who has reviewed his chart, sees that his blood pressure and diabetes are poorly controlled and that he has untreated hepatitis C. Having been trained in providing trauma-informed care, she assumes that so many poorly controlled medical problems and alcohol use may have their roots in childhood trauma. She calms herself before entering his room. After she listens without interruption to his concerns and elicits that he began drinking alcohol at age 10, she gently reflects, "In my experience, when a patient tells me that he began drinking at age 10, it is often because he was experiencing very difficult things during childhood. We are just meeting each other for the first time today, so we don't need to go into those details right now. I do want you to know that I am open to discussing those things in the future or referring you to a counselor who specializes in helping people who have had difficult or painful circumstances in childhood if you think that would be helpful."*

Addressing childhood trauma or ACEs with adults is an area of current, active exploration [71]. For many patients, it can be so powerfully healing to reveal the weighty trauma burden that one has been carrying for decades to a trusted, reliable, and compassionate healthcare provider. Many patients may not consciously realize the connection between their distressing symptoms and prior or ongoing traumatic experiences; making this connection may provide new insights and motivation to seek healthier coping techniques and support. Yet, many patients may either not be ready to disclose detailed trauma histories (to themselves or others), or may be ambivalent about this, or even unsure of how they feel about disclosure. For people who have difficulties negotiating relationship boundaries due to childhood abuse, judging whether it feels safe or not to disclose a detailed trauma history may be challenging at best and re-traumatizing at worst.

In a recent study in a safety-net clinic with integrated behavioral health services, a majority of the patients surveyed believed that they would be comfortable completing an ACE questionnaire and a PTSD screening tool (the PC-PTSD) and having these results shared with a treating clinician. They also felt that their clinician would be able to provide helpful information [71]. This study and others do not yet elucidate the full experience of adult patients or healthcare providers after the administration of a trauma questionnaire. There remains controversy in adult medicine and pediatrics over whether to administer the ACE or other trauma questionnaires [72, 73] such as resilience or coping measures, screening tools to diagnose mental health or other sequelae of trauma [74, 75], or some combination of these to patients [76]. Although the UE approach described above has not been widely tested for all forms of trauma, the rationale and method are trauma-informed; patients can receive important educational messages about the impact of trauma on health, support, and resiliency-promoting referrals without having to disclose details about traumatic experiences.

*Dr. Melissa Jones notices that after she reflects about the possibility that Mr. Johnson could have experienced "very difficult things in childhood", he gets tears in his eyes, starts breathing much more quickly and sweating, and stares blankly at the wall. Dr. Jones has noticed that her remarks have triggered an emotional reaction. She also does not want to be forceful about asking Mr. Johnson to trust her upon their first meeting when he may have been hurt (and, thus, his trust betrayed) by a caregiver when he was a child; she wants to model earning his trust over time. She pauses and inquires, "Mr. Johnson, I wonder if we could both take a deep breath and allow ourselves to feel the weight of our bodies sinking into the healing energy of the earth. Let's feel our feet connecting firmly and solidly to the floor." After she and Mr. Johnson take a few deep breaths together, she explains, "I want this clinic to feel like a safe and healing place for you, so that you always feel like you can return for further appointments. Coming to a clinic can feel frightening for many people. Please let me know if there are things that I could do to help you feel as safe as possible here. And, please let me know if I could introduce you to one of our behavioral health clinicians who can support people in coping with stress, painful experiences, and feeling safer."*

Providers who are experienced in trauma-informed care pay close attention to the response of patients to education and questions about traumatic experiences. One way to obtain clues to the time of onset of traumatic events without explicitly inquiring about these events is to ask the age of onset of poor mental health and substance use. When a patient reveals that they began using alcohol or other drugs at a very young age, this is virtually pathognomonic for trauma and adversity. Sadly, many depressed patients who have experienced childhood trauma are unable to remember a time in their lives that they were not depressed. Even when patients feel relieved that they have revealed a traumatic event to a healthcare provider, they may still feel ambivalent about returning for another visit; they may feel that the intensity of the visit was difficult to tolerate, that the provider is judging them, or that they feel overexposed and vulnerable. Providers can reassure patients that it is normal to have all sorts of complicated feelings after disclosing a trauma history; providers can explicitly state that they are greatly looking forward to seeing the patient again and offer any possible accommodations.

Modelling reliable and trustworthy behavior is critically important. By definition, people who were cared for by unreliable or abusive caregivers likely experienced many broken promises and betrayals of trust. While it is natural for healthcare providers and staff to want to generously extend themselves to provide care to someone who has suffered immensely, a good rule of reliability is to not make any promises that one is not assured of being able to keep; under-promising and over-delivering are preferable.

*As part of their trauma-informed care transformation initiative, The Redwood Health System's Trauma-informed Advisory Board, consisting of inter-professional staff and patients who had experienced a high burden of trauma, examined all of their workflows and practices and asked themselves questions like, "How many times does a patient have to re-tell their trauma story to get the help they need in our system?", "How much information about sensitive trauma history details should be documented in the electronic health record and who should have access to this information?", "How can we provide information and access to trauma-specific services without requiring our patients to disclose trauma history details?", "How can we partner with the many other professionals serving our patients (lawyers, case managers, school administrators, advocates, police, etc.) in ways that don't re-traumatize our patients or staff?", and "How can our staff share experiences and information with one another in ways that don't traumatize one another?"*

## Care

**Care** Practice self-care and compassion for yourself, the patient, and your co-workers. Adopt a compassionate attitude toward oneself and others, sharing messages of support, de-stigmatizing adverse coping behaviors, and adhering to the practice of cultural humility to promote healing.

*Ms. Sullivan is a 32-year-old mother of two boys who recently completed her GED and started community college classes. When she first met Dr. Garcia, she suffered from severe bouts of pancreatitis due to alcohol use, was using heroin, and had lost custody of her sons during a recent incarceration. When he learned Ms. Sullivan had started drinking alcohol at age 11, Dr. Garcia assumed it was likely that she had a history of childhood trauma. He built rapport with her, referred her to behavioral health, a methadone program and a post-incarceration transitions program. After she transitioned to suboxone and enrolled in college classes, he referred her to a legal aid organization to re-gain custody of her sons. Over time, Dr. Garcia and the behavioral health clinicians learned about Ms. Sullivan's very severe childhood trauma. Dr. Garcia repeatedly reminded Ms. Sullivan, "Of course you started drinking at age 11. You were trying to cope with an impossibly painful situation." Ms. Sullivan attributes her recent accomplishments to her faith in God and the help she has obtained from the Redwood Health System Clinic. "They believed in me. For years, I have felt like a failure, like my life didn't matter. They helped me see that I was drinking and using dope to cope with the abuse and pain. They treated me with dignity…like I matter as a person and a mother. I still have nightmares and struggle a lot, but I have hope and dreams too."*

Understanding of the contribution of trauma to the development of illness, adverse coping behaviors, emotional regulation, and ways of relating is important to provide effective and trauma-informed care. Harmful coping behaviors are common in people with adverse experiences and range from smoking, over-eating, inactivity, alcohol and other drug use to reacting to stress with violence, avoidance to hyper-passivity [77, 78]. Traumatic experiences, which are existentially threatening by definition, often shatter a person's sense of safety, control, and self-worth. Following trauma, guilt, shame, anger, and difficulty regulating emotions [41] are not uncommon and can make seeking and receiving healthcare challenging, triggering, and destabilizing. Self-protective, but ultimately harmful, behavioral responses to trauma or the sequelae of trauma such as self-harm, or substance use may lead to estrangement from oneself or those who seek to be helpful. The immense burden of guilt and shame about both the experience of victimization and harmful coping behaviors can be compounded when the trauma itself or a person's responses are stigmatized. When the trauma involves painful experiences that breach trust in relationships, as happens in interpersonal violence, structural violence, and historical violence, the person or community who has experienced trauma may be particularly attuned to whether healthcare providers and staff are behaving in a trustworthy and compassionate manner. Because most forms of trauma are rooted in abuses of power and oppression and the medical profession has participated in many abuses of power throughout history, trust must be earned; any behaviors, procedures, or policies that create differentials in power may feel threatening and re-traumatizing.

So, how can we behave in ways that support resilience and healing? SAMHSA has suggested a fundamental paradigm shift in the approach to patients; they suggest that all healthcare providers, including those providing substance use services, should stop asking patients "What's wrong with you?" and, instead, help patients understand that their adverse emotional, behavioral, relational, and health outcomes stem from "What happened to you?" Reframing the approach to patients in this way reduces shame, guilt, and blame. This approach reaffirms the value and humanity of every patient (and staff member) and inspires compassion for oneself and others.

Emotional, behavioral, and psychological responses to the trauma such as substance abuse, over-eating, depression, and anxiety can be destigmatized by acknowledging them as attempts to deal with stress and suffering. Understanding that self-harm is a common post-traumatic coping strategy can be healing for patients. Indeed, this approach has been studied in mental health and substance use settings and has been shown to be more beneficial to patients than usual care [39]. Attending to the root causes of traumatic experiences (e.g., colonization, racism, misogyny, etc.) as conceptualized by a patient or community de-stigmatizes the adverse outcomes of trauma and honors resilience in the face of overwhelming structural and interpersonal violence [7, 8].

Responses to disclosures of current or past trauma can be simple, non-judgmental, and compassionate. When patients share past trauma, providers can state, "Thank you for sharing this with me. I am sorry that happened. We are here to help. Can you tell me how you feel this experience is still affecting you?" It is important to remember that patients may have extremely complicated feelings toward people who hurt them, especially if those people were caregivers or partners, and to refrain from any immediate criticism of the person who hurt the patient. There are excellent sources of information on responding to current interpersonal violence and assessing safety [79].

Adhering to the practice of cultural humility [42] is essential to providing trauma-informed care. Practicing cultural humility helps providers and other staff celebrate self-defined, complex cultural identities and understand how culture may affect trauma exposure, trauma responses, and available and appropriate resources. Practitioners of cultural humility, aware of how power and privilege affect our cultural experiences and identities, continually attempt to minimize power differentials in relationships. Because power imbalances and being or feeling powerless or dehumanized are central to the causes and experiences of trauma, the practice of cultural humility is foundational in building healing, resiliency-promoting relationships.

*After 2 years of the Redwood Health System's organizational culture transformation to become trauma-informed, staff and leadership are gratified that they have made some significant changes including teaching mindfulness skills to all staff and many patients, remodeling physical spaces to be more soothing and peaceful, and improving their integration of behavioral health into primary care. At the same time, this process of culture change raises many difficult issues for the Redwood Health System; they realize that it is not only the patients who feel traumatized in the health system but that many staff, especially those with less decision-making power, feel a heavy burden of stress at work. Many staff report that they do not feel fully respected. They describe a "culture of blame" in the workplace and unfair treatment of many staff and patients, especially those from racial/ethnic minority communities. The Redwood Health System re-addresses the composition of their Trauma-informed Advisory Board to include more patients and frontline staff from minority and marginalized communities in this leadership group. The newly formed advisory board re-approves of the trauma-informed principles previously adopted by the health system. The concept of cultural humility resonates deeply with them; they also advise that specific, widespread training on racism is needed to achieve an equitable experience for all patients and staff.*

Compassion, humility, and respect should be reflected throughout the trauma-informed healthcare system. Organizations embarking on trauma-informed transformation advocate for reducing organizational hierarchies, diversifying their staff, addressing trauma and secondary trauma for all staff, and implementing trauma-informed principles and practices including cultural humility and other practices that support inclusion and equity. A culture of respect and equity aids in the care of patients directly—patients who are particularly sensitive to judgment, for example, may notice when healthcare staff and co-workers treat one another well and feel that this trauma-informed healthcare environment is more psychologically safe. The insightful observations and ideas of diverse staff with important lived experience may inform and improve patient care. When compassionate, respectful, and equitable collaboration is the lived experience of the healthcare staff, the healthcare environment becomes a healing ecosystem for everyone.

*Understanding the influence of trauma on graduation rates and educational attainment, the Redwood Health System decides to partner with the local school district. Healthcare providers, teachers, and school administrators work together to begin a "trauma-informed schools" initiative. The school district adopts a policy based on the trauma-informed practice of asking, "What has happened to you?" whenever children behave in ways that might connote distress. When students are stressed, a more proactive, immediate response is taken. There are daily check-ins with students and a "peace" room where students can go to calm down and learn mindfulness skills. The school district examines their disciplinary practices and discovers large disparities in detentions and suspensions by race/ethnicity, gender, and disability status. Disciplinary action is completely revamped such that behavioral health support replaces suspension. The school also adopts a range of changes in their curriculum to reflect and celebrate the diverse cultural backgrounds of the students attending the schools. Over the next 4 years, graduation rates improve for all students, and disparities in graduation rates diminish.*

## *Cope*

**Cope** Emphasize coping skills, positive relationships, and interventions that build hope and resiliency. Inquire about practices that help the patient feel better. Provide evidence-based treatment for the sequelae of trauma including substance use and mental illness. Celebrate cultural practices that increase well-being and social connection.

*After witnessing Mr. Eric Johnson's reaction to her comments about trauma, Dr. Melissa Jones asks him to complete the PC-PTSD. His answers indicate that he may have PTSD, but he refuses to talk to a behavioral health clinician. Dr. Jones asks Mr. Johnson, "When you feel most stressed, what do you do to cope?" When Mr. Johnson says he drinks alcohol to deal with stress and fall asleep, Dr. Jones says, "It sounds like alcohol really helps you feel better. Tell me more about exactly how it makes you feel." "I can't go to sleep without drinking. Once I drink enough I stop thinking. I feel calmer. But then a few hours later I start to feel worse than I felt when I started drinking." Dr. Jones validates his experience, "I hear that alcohol really helps you feel calmer at first, but then you start to feel worse when it wears off." She asks him whether he can think of anything else in his life that helps him feel calm. He says, "Sometimes when I listen to music, I don't drink as much." Dr. Jones learns that even though Mr. Johnson listens to many different types of music, he only notices this calming effect when listening to R and B. Mr. Johnson likes Dr. Jones suggestion that he listen to R and B more often; he agrees he can do this for 20 min each morning and night. He declines an SSRI medication to treat the symptoms of PTSD but says he "will think about it." In the printed "after-visit summary", Dr. Jones writes, "You said that 'sometimes when I listen to music, I don't drink as* much.'" At his next visit, Dr. Jones, observes, "I am so happy to see that you are taking care of yourself by coming back for a second visit." Mr. Johnson once again declines an SSRI and referral to see behavioral health but agrees to look at the patient education materials about PTSD on the VA's National Center for PTSD website with her and download their PTSD Coach app.

Healing from trauma, while often a slow and challenging process, can occur through compassionate relationships that support the building of helpful coping techniques, confidence, self-esteem, resilience, and hope [80]. Once providers understand that coping skills that have adverse health and life consequences, like substance use, may have been attempts to survive trauma by achieving short-term positive effects like a reduction of anxiety and fear, they are able to be more helpful. Inquiring about the specific desirable mental and physical short-term effects of ultimately harmful coping techniques can provide the provider with important clues; the provider can ascertain which trauma symptoms are most distressing to the patient and what effects the patient most desires. These clues can assist the patient and provider in a search to find positive coping skills that have both short-term and long-term benefits.

Asking a patient, a question like "When you feel stressed, how do you cope?" is a simple and rapid way to elicit the patient's current coping practices, regardless of whether those practices have adverse effects. Especially when the patient is using a coping technique with adverse effects like substance use, cutting, over-eating, under-eating, binging on food, self-induced vomiting, gambling, or other techniques, it is important to explore the short-term benefits. For example, vomiting may induce a parasympathetic response that, in the short-term, markedly reduces anxiety. Substances may induce euphoria, eliminate intrusive thoughts, quell nightmares, reduce social phobia, or enable sexual activity. Exploring, without judgment, "What do you most like about smoking?" or "Can you describe to me exactly how cutting makes you feel?," can help the patient and provider gain a deeper understanding of the negative effects of trauma and the patient's most desired outcomes. Then, over time, as the provider demonstrates a non-judgmental attitude and trustworthy behavior, the provider and patient can explore other coping strategies that might achieve some of the same desired effects.

Purposefully exploring positive and strengths-based questioning can also give the healthcare provider clues about the patient's preferred individual and social strategies to build resilience. Healthcare providers can ask about a broad range of skills, behaviors, and interventions that build upon strength, resiliency, social connectedness, and hope. Healthcare providers can ask the patient questions like, "What are you doing or thinking when you have brief moments of feeling happy or calm?" "What thoughts or actions or people give you hope?" "What were you thinking or doing the last time you laughed?" "What do you think a best friend would say to you about this?" "Are faith or spirituality important to you?" "Can you think of something or someone you feel grateful for today?" "What do you do to take care of yourself or others?" "Can you describe someone in your past or current life who has been supportive to you?" "What do you think will help you heal?"

Healthcare providers can ask about self-care practices, exercise, music, art, religion or prayer or spirituality, caregiving for children or others or pets, nature, cooking and food, hobbies, volunteer or paid work, spending time with friends or loved ones, supportive people in one's community, helpful organizations or institutions, and more. These skills, behaviors, experiences, relationships, and interventions are the resiliency-building tools that the patient and provider can use to promote healing. Providers can engage patients in building positive self-regard and positive attachment to the healthcare system by acknowledging suffering while also inquiring about resiliency factors. Adding a "Solutions List" or "Preferred Coping List" in addition to a "Problem List" to our medical documentation can communicate these preferred healing tools to the healthcare team.

As discussed earlier, resiliency has been conceptualized in different ways with some proposing measurements of personal traits and others measurements of personal, relational, and contextual factors that buffer one from the negative effects of adversity. Resilience at the interpersonal and community level has been found to not just be associated with lower ACE scores but to mitigate the health effects of ACEs, even when controlling for socioeconomic status (SES) [13, 37]. In fact, having multiple relational resiliency factors (given opportunities to succeed, having supportive friends and a role model) was associated with a 2/3 reduction in the prevalence of poor childhood health (adjusted for SES) across all categories of ACE scores [37]. Reinforcing and building resilience occurs through helping patients who have experienced trauma and its negative sequelae experience positive coping strategies and through moments of healthy social connectedness with themselves and other supportive people and societal structures [81]. Over the long-term, through a process of reinforcing and building resilience, the patient can begin to re-frame the experience of victimization into a narrative of survival.

In order to focus on building positive coping techniques and resilience, the healthcare system must improve its ability to recognize and provide evidence-based treatment for the adverse and disabling mental health consequences of trauma. There are myriad mental health consequences of trauma, including depression, anxiety, PTSD, complex PTSD (cPTSD), and substance use. There is evidence that PTSD is under-diagnosed, under-treated, and ineffectively treated in healthcare systems [82, 83]. There are effective, evidence-based treatments for each of these mental health sequelae of trauma. For patients with PTSD and cPTSD, trauma-focused psychotherapies are the first line therapy. Trauma-focused cognitive behavioral therapy and exposure-based treatments, that is, having survivors repeatedly think about or re-tell their experiences in ways that ultimately allow one to appreciate oneself as a survivor rather than victim, are thought to be the most effective [84]. Child-parent psychotherapy in which a child and parent participate in dyadic therapy is effective even in children with a high burden of trauma [85]. Mindfulness meditation, yoga, and other somatic and creative therapies for the psychological sequelae of trauma all show promise in helping adults and children heal from trauma [62, 86–88]. A full discussion of trauma-focused treatment is beyond the scope of this chapter.

Patients with complex traumatic stress disorders, such as cPTSD, not only have the distressing symptoms of PTSD but also suffer from great difficulties in regulating their emotions, negative self-appraisal, and disrupted inter-personal relationships. When caring for patients with cPTSD, it is especially important for providers to practice calming techniques to assist with emotional regulation, remain closely attuned to power differentials, and model healthy and respectful relationship behaviors with clear boundaries. Promising therapies that promote healing for patients with cPTSD are being developed [89]. Ensuring that mental health services are trauma-informed and do not perpetuate oppressive, traumatic forces is critically important to promoting optimal healing [90]. Combining mental health treatment with traditional cultural healing practices, based on centuries of evidence of reported efficacy, may make mental health treatment more accessible and healing for patients [91]. Adapting evidence-based mental health therapies for different cultural groups is essential [91].

**Cope for providers**
*At the Redwood Health System, the providers and behavioral health clinicians report that they feel overwhelmed and disheartened by patients' traumatic experiences, especially when patients share visually graphic details about highly traumatic experiences. Everyone agrees that they need a more robust program to address secondary or vicarious traumatization.*

## Vicarious Traumatization

Healthcare providers as well as other professionals from police officers and emergency service personnel to social workers, child protective services workers, and hotline dispatchers frequently are exposed to the trauma suffered by others. Vicarious trauma (VT), or the exposure to the trauma experiences of others, is an occupational challenge for all of these professions [92]. It is considered inevitable that people exposed to the suffering of others will change—they may develop PTSD-like symptoms or become more afraid, cynical, or withdrawn; they may also be more grateful for what they have and appreciative of the resilience of those that they help.

Reactions and responses to vicarious trauma will invariably be different from person to person and from time to time [92]. Each individual working with victims of trauma, as does each patient, brings their own set of vulnerabilities and strengths to their work. Factors that may make providers more vulnerable to this occupational risk include: prior traumatic experiences; substance use or mental illness; social isolation; difficulty expressing feelings; lack of experience, preparation, orientation, training, and supervision in the work; frequency and intensity of exposure to trauma; and lack of an effective and supportive processes for discussing the traumatic exposures [93, 94].

Vicarious traumatization, secondary traumatic stress (STS), and compassion fatigue (CF), all describe negative reactions to exposure to trauma in others that range from emotional reactions very similar to PTSD to detachment and fatigue [94]. Responses that are more neutral occur when a person's own coping strategies, resilience, and support systems help them manage the changes in their worldview. Indeed, exposure to trauma can have positive effects. Vicarious resilience refers to the way that some people may be able to draw inspiration from the resilience they see in their patients [57]. Compassion satisfaction, or the sense of reward and meaning that comes from working with patients who have survived traumatic experiences, can also help protect against the more damaging consequences of exposure to trauma.

Trauma-informed systems of care, therefore, also strive to become vicarious trauma-informed by attending pro-actively and compassionately to the vicarious trauma of healthcare providers and staff. There are online toolkits for helping providers with vicarious trauma [95]. Healthcare systems can implement policies and programs to mitigate the negative reactions to exposure to trauma and support the positive reactions. For example, the supervision of clinicians, especially those with less experience, will include discussing vicarious trauma. Increasing opportunities for self-care through flexible work schedules, reasonable workloads and work hours, small breaks, time and support for individual and group reflection, and accessible therapeutic support are examples of steps to take in making an organization vicarious trauma-informed. Practice of the 4 Cs synergistically benefits staff as well as patients. Creating a nurturing culture of appreciation and inspiration for patients and staff bolsters compassion satisfaction, curtails isolation, and builds a shared sense of hope for healing from trauma.

*Mr. Eric Johnson, who lives in a neighborhood that was previously a community with mostly African American/Black residents but is rapidly becoming gentrified and is now predominantly populated with white residents, alludes to feeling very worried that he might be evicted. Dr. Melissa Jones asks him whether he is behind on rent. Mr. Johnson looks slightly offended and proudly explains that he has never been late with a single rent payment in his entire life. Dr. Jones, who identifies as white but is acutely aware of the pervasiveness of racism and discrimination, asks Mr. Johnson, who identifies as African American, whether he thinks he is being treated unfairly in some way by his landlord. Mr. Johnson, who has found Dr. Jones to be extremely respectful and compassionate, tells her that the new owner/landlord of his building is harassing all of the residents who live in rent-controlled units, but especially the residents who are African American. Dr. Jones tells Mr. Johnson that she is extremely saddened by but not at all surprised by his experience; she describes the new Redwood Health System medical-legal partnership program and tells him that the lawyer running the program is very skilled in handling cases related to discrimination. Mr. Johnson agrees to see the lawyer.*

Optimizing healing and building resilience necessitates providing essential structural social supports like food, housing, employment, financial benefits, legal assistance, immigration assistance, and advocacy to address various forms of discrimination and oppression. It is important to ask ourselves how we can collaborate with advocacy, social services, legal services, and other resources without re-traumatizing our patients. Recognizing that some societal institutions like law enforcement may be major sources of trauma for minority communities [9, 96] and that medicine has participated in traumatic racist and oppressive practices [97–99] is important in providing trauma-informed care. Developing partnerships with individuals and organizations that are trauma-informed and equity-promoting also prevents re-traumatization and increases trust. Acknowledging and naming the trauma that results from discrimination and oppression and actively engaging in advocating for justice for patients and communities is an essential trauma-informed practice.

Recognizing that stressors, such as food or housing insecurity, can be adverse experiences of their own, trauma-informed practices also need to have deep knowledge of the resources in the community to make individualized referrals. Bolstering resilience for one member of the family may not be sufficient; the entire family may need support. Of course, barriers to accessing services, whether due to logistics such as transportation, coverage, or lack of social support, also need to be assessed and mitigated. Providing universal education about resources and offering these resources without requiring full disclosure or recitation of one's traumatic experiences reduces re-traumatization. Embedding "patient navigators" who actively facilitate access to these structural supports in the healthcare setting is more effective than routine care [49, 50]. Co-locating access to essential structural supports in the healthcare setting whenever possible is likely even more effective than facilitating off-site referrals [100].

Medical-legal partnerships, collaborative programs with legal aid professionals embedded in healthcare settings, can assist healthcare providers in addressing some of these barriers and other social inequities that undermine health and resilience. These partnerships have been shown to improve patients' ability to obtain healthcare coverage, debt relief, and avoid utility shutoffs, as well as reduce hospital admissions, readmissions, emergency department use, and patient stress [101]. Physicians who work with legal partners are more likely to discuss the unmet social needs of their patients. Screening tools to assist in legal need assessment also exist, such as the I-HELP framework for identifying unmet legal needs—*I*ncome and insurance (food stamp eligibility, benefits, etc.), *H*ousing and utilities (eviction prevention, housing conditions), *E*ducation and *E*mployment (accommodations for disease/disability/ getting IEPs), *L*egal status (incarceration issues; immigration), and *P*ersonal and family (IPV, child support, payee, estate planning) [102].

## Prevention: Reducing Trauma to Achieve Health Equity

*The Redwood Health System restructures their community benefits program to partner more effectively with community-based organizations, hires new "navigators" from community-based organizations to work on community engagement initiatives, and commits to functioning as an anchor institution that supports social and health equity. The CEO initiates a metric-driven process to monitor their hiring of diverse members of the local community, sourcing of supplies from locally and minority-owned businesses, housing subsidies for employees, and more. One of the first community navigators hired by the Redwood Health System is Ms. Sullivan. She has now graduated from community college with a degree in early childhood education. As a community navigator, she provides training and resources on the intergenerational effects of trauma and resiliency-based parenting practices. She connects patients and community members with various evidence-based programs to prevent child abuse like the Nurse-Family Partnership program and a pioneering parent/caregiver-child urban gardening program that is being supported and evaluated by the Redwood Health System. Ms. Sullivan's own children, who have benefited from child-focused trauma therapy, are thriving.*

Collaboration in promoting resilience and healing should also extend into the community. This may mean working with community organizations to support an individual patient or family in multifaceted ways. On the other hand, collaboration with community can also mean extending the scope of the health system's activities to partnering with the community as a whole on broad issues of trauma prevention and health promotion. This might involve working with schools or churches on health education programs or by participating in programs of community development that address root causes of trauma. The Wraparound Project at the University of California, San Francisco, for example, works with those exposed to gun violence [103]. Founded by a trauma surgeon in response to the epidemic of young minority men being injured and killed by gun violence, it provides not just treatment of physical wounds and behavioral and psychiatric support but substance use treatment, educational support, vocational training, housing assistance, and tattoo removal. It partners with schools, churches, and community violence prevention organizations not only to prevent recidivism in the patients enrolled in the program but also to prevent violence in the community at large.

*The Redwood Health System's commitment to equity grows each year. They have developed a robust institutional diversity, inclusion, and equity program in the health system. They are making progress in diversifying their staff, and staff satisfaction scores are increasing. Their employees feel proud to work for an organization that cares about their well-being and that of their surrounding community. Their community engagement and anchor institution initiatives are growing. They begin to advocate for policy changes to promote equity. The Redwood Health System advocates locally for a living wage initiative, affordable housing, and a Sanctuary City policy and, nationally, for the preservation and strengthening of the Affordable Care Act.*

Ideally, trauma-informed care will prompt examination of all of the ways in which injustice and inequity cause and perpetuate trauma and its associated health disparities [104, 105]. Healthcare systems and staff can address the discrimination and oppression that cause trauma through fostering diversity, inclusion, and equity within their own organizations. Healthcare systems and staff, who see how the structural roots of trauma are based in oppression, look beyond the walls of the clinic or hospital [98]. They understand that access to employment that pays a living wage and education that promotes social mobility, especially in locations with large income and wealth disparities, markedly reduces trauma. They know that sufficient income and the means to secure stable housing, healthy food, affordable transportation, access to nature [106], recreation, cultural resources, and other social supports reduce trauma and promote resilience. They commit to dismantling discriminatory policies and programs that have resulted in social and health inequities. Trauma-informed healthcare systems and staff advocate for equity for individuals, families, and communities, especially for those who are most marginalized and under-resourced, to generate shared resilience and communal healing.

## Key Concepts

- Trauma is a nearly universal human experience but is more common in vulnerable populations.
- Childhood trauma results in later adulthood high-risk behaviors and disease.
- Individual, family, community and societal risk and protective factors and resiliency affects the prevalence and experience of all types of violence and trauma.
- Trauma-informed care holds promise for improving health outcomes and helping to break the cycle of intergenerational transmission of trauma.
- Trauma-informed systems change is a process that leads to equity.

## References

1. Kilpatrick DG, Resnick HS, Milanak ME, Miller MW, Keyes KM, Friedman MJ. National estimates of exposure to traumatic events and PTSD prevalence using DSM-IV and DSM-5 criteria. J Trauma Stress. 2013;26(5):537–47.
2. Raja S, Hasnain M, Hoersch M, Gove-Yin S, Rajagopalan C. Trauma informed care in medicine: current knowledge and future research directions. Fam Community Health. 2015;38(3):216–26.
3. Gallo-Silver L, Anderson CM, Romo J. Best clinical practices for male adult survivors of childhood sexual abuse: "do no harm". Perm J. 2014;18(3):82–7.
4. Raja S, Hoersch M, Rajagopalan CF, Chang P. Treating patients with traumatic life experiences: providing trauma-informed care. J Am Dent Assoc. 2014;145(3):238–45.
5. National Center for Trauma-Informed Care and Alternatives to Seclusion and Restraint (NCTIC). Substance Abuse and Mental Health Services Administration. About NCTIC 2017, September 15 (Updated). Accessed 30 June 2018. Available from: https://www.samhsa.gov/nctic.
6. Courtois CA, Ford JD, editors. Treating complex traumatic stress disorders: an evidence-based guide. New York: The Guilford Press; 2009.
7. Gone JP. Redressing first nations historical trauma: theorizing mechanisms for indigenous culture as mental health treatment. Transcult Psychiatry. 2013;50(5):683–706.
8. Goodkind JR, Hess JM, Gorman B, Parker DP. "We're still in a struggle": diné resilience, survival, historical trauma, and healing. Qual Health Res. 2012;22(8):1019–36.
9. Bor J, Venkataramani AS, Williams DR, Tsai AC. Police killings and their spillover effects on the mental health of black Americans: a population-based, quasi-experimental study. Lancet. 2018;392:302.

10. Substance Abuse and Mental Health Services Administration (SAMHSA). Trauma resilience resources. Accessed 31 July 2018. Available from: https://www.samhsa.gov/capt/tools-learning-resources/trauma-resilience-resources.
11. Traub F, Boynton-Jarrett R. Modifiable resilience factors to childhood adversity for clinical pediatric practice. Pediatrics. 2017;139(5):e20162569.
12. Heise L. What works to prevent partner violence? An evidence overview. London: STRIVE, London School of Hygiene and Tropical Medicine; 2011.
13. Bellis MA, Hardcastle K, Ford K, Hughes K, Ashton K, Quigg Z, et al. Does continuous trusted adult support in childhood impart life-course resilience against adverse childhood experiences – a retrospective study on adult health-harming behaviours and mental well-being. BMC Psychiatry. 2017;17:110.
14. Sapienza JK, Masten AS. Understanding and promoting resilience in children and youth. Curr Opin Psychiatry. 2011;24(4):267–73.
15. Vanderbilt-Adriance E, Shaw DS. Protective factors and the development of resilience in the context of neighborhood disadvantage. J Abnorm Child Psychol. 2008;36(6):887–901.
16. Harvard University Center on the Developing Child. Resilience Cambridge, MA; 2018. Accessed 31 July 2018. Available from: https://developingchild.harvard.edu/science/key-concepts/resilience/.
17. National Scientific Council on the Developing Child. 2015. Supportive Relationships and Active Skill-Building Strengthen the Foundations of Resilience: Working Paper 13. Accessed 1 Aug 2018. Available from: http://www.developingchild.harvard.edu.
18. Jaffee SR, Bowes L, Ouellet-Morin I, Fisher HL, Moffitt TE, Merrick MT, et al. Safe, stable, nurturing relationships break the intergenerational cycle of abuse: a prospective nationally representative cohort of children in the United Kingdom. J Adolesc Health. 2013;53(4, Supplement):S4–S10.
19. National Center for Injury Prevention and Control, Centers for Disease Control and Prevention. Child maltreatment: risk and protective factors. Atlanta, GA; 2014.
20. Hochman A. Curiosity and reciprocity: engaging community in the ACE and resilience movement. Aces Too High News [Internet]. 2017, August 8. Accessed 1 Aug 2018. Available from: https://acestoohigh.com/2017/08/08/curiosity-and-reciprocity-engaging-community-in-the-ace-and-resilience-movement/.
21. Felitti V, Anda R, Nordenberg D. Relationship of childhood abuse and household dysfunction to many of the leading causes of death in adults. The Adverse Childhood Experiences (ACE) Study. Am J Prev Med. 1998;14:245–58.
22. Center for Youth Wellness. The Center for Youth Wellness Hidden Crisis Report. San Francisco, CA; 2014. Available from: https://centerforyouthwellness.org/wp-content/themes/cyw/build/img/building-a-movement/hidden-crisis.pdf.
23. Centers for Disease Control and Prevention (CDC). Adverse childhood experiences reported by adults — five states, 2009. Morb Mortal Wkly Rep. 2010;59(49):1609–13.
24. Sacks V, Murphey D. The prevalence of adverse childhood experiences, nationally, by state, and by race or ethnicity. Child Trends [Internet]. 2018, February 20. Accessed 31 July 2018. Available from: https://www.childtrends.org/publications/prevalence-adverse-childhood-experiences-nationally-state-race-ethnicity.
25. Cronholm PF, Forke CM, Wade R, Bair-Merritt MH, Davis M, Harkins-Schwarz M, et al. Adverse childhood experiences: expanding the concept of adversity. Am J Prev Med. 2015;49(3):354–61.
26. United States Government Accountability Office (GAO). Report to congressional requesters: K-12 EDUCATION discipline disparities for black students, boys, and students with disabilities Washington, DC; 2018, March [GAO-18-258]: Available from: https://www.gao.gov/assets/700/690828.pdf.
27. McIntosh KG, Erik J, Horner RH, Smolkowski K. Education not incarceration: a conceptual model for reducing racial and ethnic disproportionality in school discipline. J Appl Res Child: Inf Policy Child Risk. 2014;5(2):1–23.
28. Skiba RJ, Arredondo MI, Williams NT. More than a metaphor: the contribution of exclusionary discipline to a school-to-prison pipeline. Equity Excell Educ. 2014;47(4):546–64.

29. Kelly VG, Merrill GS, Shumway M, Alvidrez J, Boccellari A. Outreach, engagement, and practical assistance: essential aspects of PTSD care for urban victims of violent crime. Trauma Violence Abuse. 2010;11(3):144–56.
30. Institute of Safe Families and the Public Health Management Corporation. Findings from the Philadelphia urban ACE study. Philadelphia; 2013. Available at: https://www.rwjf.org/en/library/research/2013/09/findings-from-the-philadelphia-urban-ace-survey.html.
31. World Health Organization. Adverse childhood experiences international questionnaire. In: Adverse childhood experiences international questionnaire (ACE-IQ). [website]: Geneva: WHO; 2018. Accessed 2 March 2019. Available at https://www.who.int/violence_injury_prevention/violence/activities/adverse_childhood_experiences/en/.
32. Johnson SB, Riley AW, Granger DA, Riis J. The science of early life toxic stress for pediatric practice and advocacy. Pediatrics. 2013;131(2):319–27.
33. Dong M, Giles W, Felitti V. Insights into causal pathways for ischemic heart disease: adverse childhood experiences study. Circulation. 2004;110:1761–6.
34. Bellis MA, Hughes K, Leckenby N, Hardcastle KA, Perkins C, Lowey H. Measuring mortality and the burden of adult disease associated with adverse childhood experiences in England: a national survey. J Public Health (Oxf). 2015;37(3):445–54.
35. Kelly-Irving M, Lepage B, Dedieu D, Bartley M, Blane D, Grosclaude P, et al. Adverse childhood experiences and premature all-cause mortality. Eur J Epidemiol. 2013;28(9):721–34.
36. Giovanelli A, Reynolds AJ, Mondi CF, Ou SR. Adverse childhood experiences and adult well-being in a low-income, urban cohort. Pediatrics. 2016;137(4):e20154016.
37. Bellis MA, Hughes K, Ford K, Hardcastle KA, Sharp CA, Wood S, et al. Adverse childhood experiences and sources of childhood resilience: a retrospective study of their combined relationships with child health and educational attendance. BMC Public Health. 2018; 18:792.
38. Substance Abuse and Mental health Services Administration (SAMHSA). Definitions. SAMHSA News [Internet]. 2014; 22(2). Accessed 1 August 2018. Available from: https://www.samhsa.gov/samhsaNewsLetter/Volume_22_Number_2/trauma_tip/key_terms.html.
39. Morrissey JP, Jackson EW, Ellis AR, Amaro H, Brown VB, Najavits LM. Twelve-month outcomes of trauma-informed interventions for women with co-occurring disorders. Psychiatr Serv. 2005;56(10):1213–22.
40. Suarez E, Jackson DS, Slavin LA, Michels MS, McGeehan KM. Project Kealahou: improving Hawai'i's system of care for at-risk girls and young women through gender-responsive, trauma-informed care. Hawai'i J Med Public Health. 2014;73(12):387–92.
41. Substance Abuse and Mental Health Services Administration. SAMHSA's concept of trauma and guidance for a trauma-informed approach. Rockville, MD: Substance Abuse and Mental Health Services Administration; 2014. Contract No: HHS Publication No. (SMA) xx-xxxx. Available at: http://www.traumainformedcareproject.org/resources/SAMHSA%20TIC.pdf.
42. Tervalon M, Murray-García J. Cultural humility versus cultural competence: a critical distinction in defining physician training outcomes in multicultural education. J Health Care Poor Underserved. 1998;9(2):117–25.
43. Machtinger EL, Cuca YP, Khanna N, Rose CD, Kimberg LS. From treatment to healing: the promise of trauma-informed primary care. Womens Health Issues. 2015;25(3):193–7.
44. Brown VB, Harris M, Fallot R. Moving toward trauma-informed practice in addiction treatment: a collaborative model of agency assessment. J Psychoactive Drugs. 2013;45(5):386–93.
45. Bloom SL. The sanctuary model. Available from: http://www.sanctuaryweb.com/.
46. Machtinger E, Cuca YP, Khanna N, Rose CD, Kimberg LS. From treatment to healing: the promise of trauma-informed primary care. Womens Health Issues. 2015;25(3):193–7.
47. Loomis B, Epstein K, Dauria E, Dolce L. Implementing a trauma-informed public health system in San Francisco, California. Health Educ Behav. 2018;00(0):1–9.
48. Gone JP. A community-based treatment for native American historical trauma: prospects for evidence-based practice. Spiritual Clin Pract. 2013;1(S):78–94.
49. Natale-Pereira A, Enard KR, Nevarez L, Jones LA. The role of patient navigators in eliminating health disparities. Cancer. 2011;117(15 Suppl):3543–52.

50. Catholic Health Initiatives, Oncology Service Line, Navigation Program Resource Guide: Best Practices for Patient Navigation Programs, 2013. Accessed 20 Dec 2018. Available at: https://mdpnn.files.wordpress.com/2013/04/chi-navigation-program-resource-guide-_final-012013_.pdf.
51. Canham SL, Davidson S, Custodio K, et al. Health supports needed for homeless persons transitioning from hospitals. Health Soc Care Community. 2018;00:1–15.
52. Purtle J, Cheney R, Wiebe DJ, Dicker R. Scared safe? Abandoning the use of fear in urban violence prevention programmes. Inj Prev. 2015;21(2):140–1.
53. Saakvitne KW, Pearlman LA. Transforming the pain: a workbook on vicarious traumatization. New York: W. W. Norton and Company; 1996.
54. Kimberg L. Trauma and trauma-informed care In: King TE, Wheeler MB, editors. Medical management of vulnerable and underserved patients: principles, practice, and populations, 2e. New York: McGraw-Hill; 2016.
55. Machtinger EL, Davis KB, Kimberg LS, Khanna N, Cuca YP, Dawson-Rose C, et al. From treatment to healing: inquiry and response to recent and past trauma in adult health care. Womens Health Issues. 2018.
56. Reed RG, Barnard K, Butler EA. Distinguishing emotional co-regulation from co-dysregulation: an investigation of emotional dynamics and body-weight in romantic couples. Emotion (Washington, DC). 2015;15(1):45–60.
57. Isobel S, Angus-Leppan G. Neuro-reciprocity and vicarious trauma in psychiatrists. Australas Psychiatry. 2018;00(0):1–3.
58. Leitch L. Action steps using ACEs and trauma-informed care: a resilience model. Health Justice. 2017;5(5):1–10.
59. Bakken H, Kimberg L. Trauma-informed primary care: enhancing intergenerational resilience. Presentation at Futures without Violence, National Conference on Health and Domestic Violence, 2017.
60. Bakken EH.Trauma-informed care: 4C's in pediatric practice. Personal Communication, 2017.
61. Marsac M, Kassam-Adams N, Hildenbrand A, Nicholls E, Winston F, Leff S, Fein J. Implementing a trauma-informed approach in pediatric health care networks. JAMA Pediatr. 2016;170(1):70.
62. Bethell C, Gombojav N, Solloway M, Wissow L. Adverse childhood experiences, resilience and mindfulness-based approaches: common denominator issues for children with emotional, mental, or behavioral problems. Child AdolescPsychiatr Clin N Am. 2016;25(2):139–56.
63. Committee on Community-Based Solutions to Promote Health Equity in the United States. The root causes of health inequity. 2017 Jan 11. In: Communities in action: pathways to health equity [Internet]. Washington, DC: National Academies Press (US). Available from:https://www.ncbi.nlm.nih.gov/books/NBK425845/.
64. UCSF Center for Community Engagement. Our principles 2018. Available from: https://partnerships.ucsf.edu/our-principles.
65. Miller E, Decker MR, McCauley HL, Tancredi DJ, Levenson RR, Waldman J, et al. A family planning clinic partner violence intervention to reduce risk associated with reproductive coercion. Contraception. 2011;83(3):274–80.
66. O'Doherty L, Hegarty K, Ramsay J, Davidson LL, Feder G, Taft A. Screening women for intimate partner violence in healthcare settings. Cochrane Database Syst Rev. 2015;(7)
67. Gerbert B, Caspers N, Bronstone A, Moe J, Abercrombie P. A qualitative analysis of how physicians with expertise in domestic violence approach the identification of victims. Ann Intern Med. 1999;131(8):578–84.
68. Feder G, Hutson M, Ramsay J, Taket A. Women exposed to intimate partner violence: expectations and experiences when they encounter health care professionals: a meta-analysis of qualitative studies. Arch Intern Med. 2006;166(1):22–37.
69. Futures without Violence, The Healthcare Response to IPV, Presentation. Available from: https://www.ihs.gov/california/tasks/sites/default/assets/File/GPRA/BP2018-HealthResponsestoIntimateViolence_Vander-Tuig.pdf.
70. Curry SJ, Krist AH, Owens DK, Barry MJ, Caughey AB, Davidson KW, et al. Screening for intimate partner violence, elder abuse, and abuse of vulnerable adults: US preventive services task force final recommendation statement. JAMA. 2018;320(16):1678–87.

71. Goldstein E, Athale N, Sciolla AF, Catz SL. Patient preferences for discussing childhood trauma in primary care. Perm J. 2017;21:16–055.
72. Afifi TO. Continuing conversations: debates about adverse childhood experiences (ACEs) screening. Child Abuse Negl. 2018;85:172–3.
73. Bethell CD, Carle A, Hudziak J, Gombojav N, Powers K, Wade R, et al. Methods to assess adverse childhood experiences of children and families: toward approaches to promote child well-being in policy and practice. Acad Pediatr. 2017;17(7 Suppl):S51–69.
74. Liu H, Prause N, Wyatt GE, Williams JK, Chin D, Davis T, et al. Development of a composite trauma exposure risk index. Psychol Assess. 2015;27(3):965–74.
75. Street AE, Gerber MR. Using lessons from VA to improve care for women with mental health and trauma histories, Part II. Washington, DC; 2014, October 1. Accessed 20 Dec 2018. Available from: https://www.hsrd.research.va.gov/for_researchers/cyber_seminars/archives/video_archive.cfm?SessionID=900.
76. Flanagan T, Alabaster A, McCaw B, Stoller N, Watson C, Young-Wolff KC. Feasibility and acceptability of screening for adverse childhood experiences in prenatal care. J Women's Health. 2018;27(7):903–11.
77. Substance Abuse and Mental Health Services Administration (SAMHSA). Understanding the impact of trauma in trauma-informed care in behavioral health services. Treatment improvement protocol (TIP) series, no. 57. Rockville, MD; 2014. Available from: https://www.ncbi.nlm.nih.gov/books/NBK207191/.
78. SAMHSA. Trauma-informed care in behavioral health services, Part 3: a review of the literature. Treatment improvement protocol (TIP) series 57. Rockville, MD: USDepartment of Health and Human Services, Substance Abuse and Mental Health Services Administration; 2013.
79. Babaria P, McCaw B, Kimberg L. Intimate partner violence. In: King Jr TE, Wheeler MB, editors. Medical management of vulnerable and underserved patients: principles, practice, and populations. New York: McGraw Hill Lange series; 2016.
80. Sege RD, Harper Browne C. Responding to ACEs with HOPE: health outcomes from positive experiences. Acad Pediatr. 2017;17(7, Supplement):S79–85.
81. Bethell CD, Solloway MR, Guinosso S, Hassink S, Srivastav A, Ford D, et al. Prioritizing possibilities for child and family health: an agenda to address adverse childhood experiences and foster the social and emotional roots of well-being in pediatrics. Acad Pediatr. 2017;17(7,. Supplement):S36–50.
82. Wang PS, Berglund P, Olfson M, Pincus HA, Wells KB, Kessler RC. Failure and delay in initial treatment contact after first onset of mental disorders in the national comorbidity survey replication. Arch Gen Psychiatry. 2005;62(6):603–13.
83. Hepner KA, Roth CP, Sloss EM, Paddock SM, Iyiewuare PO, Timmer MJ, et al. Quality of care for PTSD and depression in the military health system: final report. Rand Health Q. 2018;7(3):4.
84. Institute of Medicine. Treatment of posttraumatic stress disorder: an assessment of the evidence. Washington, DC: National Academies Press; 2008. Accessed 20 Dec 2018 at: https://www.nap.edu/catalog/11955/treatment-of-posttraumatic-stress-disorder-an-assessment-of-the-evidence.
85. Ippen CG, Harris WW, Van Horn P, Lieberman AF. Traumatic and stressful events in early childhood: can treatment help those at highest risk? Child Abuse Negl. 2011;35(7):504–13.
86. Boyd JE, Lanius RA, McKinnon MC. Mindfulness-based treatments for posttraumatic stress disorder: a review of the treatment literature and neurobiological evidence. J Psychiatry Neurosci: JPN. 2018;43(1):7–25.
87. Van der Kolk BA. The body keeps the score: brain, mind, and body in the healing of trauma. New York: The Penguin Group; 2014.
88. Machtinger EL, Lavin SM, Hilliard S, Jones R, Haberer JE, Capito K, Dawson-Rose C. An expressive therapy group disclosure intervention for women living with HIV improves social support, self-efficacy, and the safety and quality of relationships: a qualitative analysis. J Assoc Nurses AIDS Care. 2015;26(2):187–98.
89. Cloitre M, Courtois CA, Charuvastra A, Carapezza R, Stolbach BC, Green BL. Treatment of complex PTSD: results of the ISTSS expert clinician survey on best practices. J Trauma Stress. 2011;24(6):615–27.

90. Corneau S, Stergiopoulos V. More than being against it: anti-racism and anti-oppression in mental health services. Transcult Psychiatry. 2012;49(2):261–82.
91. Bernal G, Adames C. Cultural adaptations: conceptual, ethical, contextual, and methodological issues for working with ethnocultural and majority-world populations. Prev Sci. 2017;18(6):681–8.
92. Molnar BE, Sprang G, Killian KD, Gottfried R, Emery V, Bride BE. Advancing science and practice for vicarious traumatization/secondary traumatic stress: a research agenda. Traumatology. 2017;23(2):129–42.
93. Coles J, Dartnall E, Astbury J. "Preventing the pain" when working with family and sexual violence in primary care. Int J Family Med. 2013;2013:198578.
94. Nimmo A, Huggard P. A systematic review of the measurement of compassion fatigue, vicarious trauma, and secondary traumatic stress in physicians. Australas J Disaster Trauma Stud. 2013;1:37–44.
95. International Society for Traumatic Stress Studies (ISTSS). Self-care for providers. Terrace, IL; 2018. Accessed 20 Dec 2018. Available from: http://www.istss.org/treating-trauma/self-care-for-providers.aspx.
96. Mesic A, Franklin L, Cansever A, Potter F, Sharma A, Knopov A, et al. The relationship between structural racism and black-white disparities in fatal police shootings at the state level. J Natl Med Assoc. 2018;110(2):106–16.
97. Charles D, Himmelstein K, Keenan W, Barcelo N, White Coats for Black Lives National Working Group. White coats for black lives: medical students responding to racism and police brutality. J Urban Health. 2015;92(6):1007–10.
98. Bassett MT. #BlackLivesMatter — a challenge to the medical and public health communities. N Engl J Med. 2015;372(12):1085–7.
99. Washingon HA. Medical apartheid: the dark history of medical experimentation on black Americans from colonial times to the present. New York: Harlem Moon; 2006.
100. Garg A, Jack B, Zuckerman B. Addressing the social determinants of health within the patient-centered medical home. JAMA. 2013;309(19):2001.
101. Regenstein M, Trott J, Williamson A, Theiss J. Addressing social determinants of health through medical-legal partnerships. Health Aff (Millwood). 2018;37(3):378–85.
102. National Center for Medical-Legal Partnership. New MLP legal needs screening tool available for download. Washington, DC; 2015, October 14. Available from: http://medical-legal-partnership.org/screening-tool/.
103. UCSF San Francisco Wraparound Project. Stopping the revolving door of violent injuries 2018. Accessed 20 Dec 2018. Available from: https://violenceprevention.surgery.ucsf.edu/.
104. Gee GC, Walsemann KM, Brondolo E. A life course perspective on how racism may be related to health inequities. Am J Public Health. 2012;102(5):967–74.
105. Goosby BJ, Heidbrink C. The transgenerational consequences of discrimination on African-American health outcomes. Sociol Compass. 2013;7(8):630–43.
106. South EC, Hohl BC, Kondo MC, MacDonald JM, Branas CC. Effect of greening vacant land on mental health of community-dwelling adults: a cluster randomized trial. JAMA Netw Open. 2018;1(3):e180298.

# Part II
# Special Populations

# Chapter 3
# Cultural Humility in Trauma-Informed Care

**Joseph Vinson, Ariel Majidi, and Maura George**

## Why This Topic?

With an increasingly diverse patient population, there comes the challenge of continuing to provide outstanding healthcare despite cultural barriers [1]. These barriers can be especially problematic for trauma-informed care given the complexity of traumatic experiences that diverse communities face. It has been suggested that cultural factors can affect:

- How traumas are experienced.
- The meaning assigned to the trauma.
- How symptoms are expressed.
- Whether certain symptoms or behaviors are considered abnormal.
- Willingness to seek help from a mental health provider.
- Willingness to seek help inside and/or outside of one's culture.
- Response to treatment.
- Treatment outcome.
- Sources of strength, resilience, and coping strategies.

Studies suggest that there are health disparities, structural inequalities, and poorer quality of healthcare and outcomes among people from minority cultural and lin-

---

J. Vinson
Department of Psychiatry and Behavioral Sciences, Emory University School of Medicine, Atlanta, GA, USA

A. Majidi
Cambridge Health Alliance, Harvard Medical School, Cambridge, MA, USA

M. George (✉)
Division of General Medicine, Emory University, Atlanta, GA, USA
e-mail: maura.george@emory.edu

guistic backgrounds [2]. These healthcare disparities have led governing bodies, policymakers, and educators to call for improved cultural competence as a potential remedy, and it has now become a key component of standards and accreditation processes for healthcare systems. A large review of the outcomes of cultural competence education found a "positive, albeit low-quality evidence, showing improvements in the involvement of CALD (culturally and linguistically diverse) patients [2]." Another review concluded that "the evidence base is relatively weak, and there continues to be uncertainty in the field [3]." Some of this uncertainty may be due to a lack of consistency in how the terms and concepts are used and understood as well as the heterogeneity of outcomes chosen.

With that in mind, we prefer to use the most commonly cited definition of cultural competence developed by Cross et al.: "Cultural and linguistic competence is a set of congruent behaviours, attitudes, and policies that come together in a system, agency, or among professionals that enables effective work in cross-cultural situations [4]." In essence, cultural competence involves development of attitudes, knowledge, and skills.

## Cultural Humility

More recently, many have begun to argue that the idea of cultural competence and its implementation may be flawed [5, 6]. For example, it may be a false assumption that someone can learn a set of skills or learn about cultures and become competent as an end point. Likewise, it may incorrectly view culture as static and the end points as fixed. A culturally competent perspective regards cultural factors as discrete concepts to be learned in addition to one's own culture, rather than instructing individuals of a dominant group to be mindful or think outside of their own identity.

The concept of "cultural humility" is a proposed alternative. Generally attributed to Tervalon and Murray-Garcia [7, 8], the concept was described by them as incorporating "a lifelong commitment to self-evaluation and critique, to redressing the power imbalances in the physician-patient dynamic, and to developing mutually beneficial and non-paternalistic partnerships with communities on behalf of individuals and defined populations." It has been described in many ways in recent years but can be conceived of as having several components [9]:

- Openness.
- Self-awareness and self-critique.
- Egolessness.
- Supportive interactions.
- Lifelong learning.

Whereas cultural competence is often critiqued as being static, cultural humility has a more dynamic view of culture and has dynamic end points as well. Instead, it can be thought of as a transformation of perspective, orientation, or way of thinking and being. Cultural humility has been less well-studied and has not been adopted by most governing bodies. Nonetheless, there is some data that higher perceptions of organizational cultural humility were associated with higher levels of general perceptions of hospital safety, as well as more positive ratings on nonpunitive response to error (i.e., mistakes of staff are not held against them), handoffs and transitions, and organizational learning [10]. One could argue that the concept of cultural humility is helpful in theory but that it faces challenges with implementation and outcomes assessment. Perhaps it is best to think of competence and humility as each having a role complementing the other.

## Populations of Interest

One of the first steps in providing culturally humble care is to reject the monolith of a "migrant" or "foreign" patient. There are a variety of experiences of human migration, each associated with different obstacles, implications for health, and exposures to traumatic events. It is especially important to be perceptive to the type of migration story the patient carries or, if he or she is a second-generation migrant, the story which the family carries. Also, understanding the differences in the legal status and narrative of different migrant groups can be a helpful step in providing culturally humble and trauma-informed care. Here, the groups discussed include refugees, asylum seekers, and economic migrants. Other migratory groups not discussed include victims of trafficking and internally displaced peoples.

### *Refugees*

According to the United Nations High Commissioner for Refugees, a refugee is "someone who has been forced to flee his or her country because of persecution, war, or violence [11, 12]. A refugee has a well-founded fear of persecution for reasons of race, religion, nationality, political opinion or membership in a particular social group. Most likely, they cannot return home or are afraid to do so." They are often forced out of their country of origin suddenly and without prior preparation. In 2016 alone, 65.6 million individuals were forcibly displaced worldwide, 22.5 million were considered refugees. This constitutes the highest levels of displacement on record (UNHCR website) [12]. More than half of the refugees came from just three countries: Syria, Afghanistan, and South Sudan. Other top countries of origin as of 2016 include Somalia, Sudan, Democratic Republic of the Congo, Central African Republic, Myanmar, Eritrea, and Burundi [13, 14]. The largest refugee resettlement programs are found in the United States, Canada, Australia, United Kingdom, Norway, and Sweden. Still less than 1% of refugees are ever resettled, and 50% fewer refugees were resettled in 2017 compared to 2016.

## *Asylum-Seekers*

Asylum-seekers are internationally displaced people awaiting legal determination of refugee status. In the case of a negative decision, they may be expelled, unless permission to stay is provided on humanitarian or other related grounds [15]. By the end of 2016, there were 2.8 million asylum-seekers [13, 16]. Germany is the top recipient of applications for asylum, followed by the United States and Italy.

## *Migrant, Immigrant, Emigrant*

Other terms one might encounter include migrant, immigrant, and emigrant. There is some disagreement about how to use the term "migrant". The United Nations defines "migrant" as an individual who has resided in a foreign country for more than 1 year irrespective of the causes, voluntary or involuntary, and the means used to migrate. However, it is often understood as describing cases where the decision to migrate was taken freely by the individual without intervention of an external compelling factor. Economic migrants include people who attempt to enter a country without legal permission and/or leave their country of origin for the purpose of employment. Other similar terms include "migrant worker" or "frontier worker". An immigrant is simply one who moves into a country for the purpose of settlement (from the perspective of the destination country). An emigrant is one who departs or exits from one country with a view to settling in another (from the perspective of the country of origin) [15].

## Traumatic Experiences and Phases of Displacement

Trauma can occur at any point in the displacement experience. The first or acute phase of displacement happens in the country of origin. Often the primary event driving refugees from their home countries is war, which can involve a variety of traumatic experiences including imprisonment, combat atrocities, separation from and even death of family members, the destruction of possessions, and physical and psychological torture [17]. Refugees may be put in such austere environments that a normal emotional response to traumatic events is suppressed.

The second or transition phase happens between initial displacement and settlement. This may include time in refugee camps, countries of first asylum, and frequent migration between locations. The process of leaving one's home country can be perilous and involve the sudden loss of treasured familial and social relations as well as material possessions. The process of bereavement may not be expressed due to rapidly changing environments requiring constant readjustment. Often, only basic needs are met in a refugee camp, and conditions may be dangerous and restrictive, similar to that of a prison environment. Additionally, asylum-seekers may stay in this phase indefinitely, and this state of "limbo" can be a risk factor for developing psychiatric problems [18].

The third or chronic phase, which includes the so called "after-effects" and "recovery" phases, begins with resettlement in the destination country. In this stage, refugees often experience a loss of power as they struggle to acquire new language skills, lose previous professional or social identities, and enter a new cultural value system. This can exacerbate chronic anxiety, stress, and depression and at times results in poor coping mechanisms such as substance use. Also, sometimes the survivalist nature honed during the acute and transition phases may conflict with the ego or one's sense of self, which can lead to mental health problems [17].

Economic migrants and undocumented immigrants also face challenges which can prove to be traumatic. For example, crossing a border illegally carries a great deal of risk, including the physical dangers associated with precarious routes of entry and the use of mediating parties (e.g., smugglers) [17]. Once in the host country, the economic migrant faces a constant threat of deportation, and contact with any type of authority or official (legal, health, etc.) may trigger a fear of deportation. Migrants without legal documentation are often unable to access social services, including health insurance, or have the basic rights given to legal immigrants [17, 18].

## Recommendations for Healthcare Delivery

A good starting place for delivering culturally competent and humble care is the National Culturally and Linguistically Appropriate Services (CLAS) Standards [19, 20]. This set of 15 recommendations developed by the US Department of Health and Human Services aims to advance health equity, improve quality, and help eliminate disparities. Centers for Medicare and Medicaid Services has also developed a toolkit to help with their implementation (https://www.cms.gov/About-CMS/Agency-Information/OMH/Downloads/CLAS-Toolkit-12-7-16.pdf). The standards are as follows:

**Principal Standard**

1. Provide effective, equitable, understandable, and respectful quality care and services that are responsive to diverse cultural health beliefs and practices, preferred languages, health literacy, and other communication needs.

**Governance, Leadership, and Workforce**

2. Advance and sustain organizational governance and leadership that promotes CLAS and health equity through policy, practices, and allocated resources.
3. Recruit, promote, and support a culturally and linguistically diverse governance, leadership, and workforce that are responsive to the population in the service area.

4. Educate and train governance, leadership, and workforce in culturally and linguistically appropriate policies and practices on an ongoing basis.

**Communication and Language Assistance**

5. Offer language assistance to individuals who have limited English proficiency and/or other communication needs, at no cost to them, to facilitate timely access to all health care and services.
6. Inform all individuals of the availability of language assistance services clearly and in their preferred language, verbally and in writing.
7. Ensure the competence of individuals providing language assistance, recognizing that the use of untrained individuals and/or minors as interpreters should be avoided.
8. Provide easy-to-understand print and multimedia materials and signage in the languages commonly used by the populations in the service area.

**Engagement, Continuous Improvement, and Accountability**

9. Establish culturally and linguistically appropriate goals, policies, and management accountability, and infuse them throughout the organization's planning and operations.
10. Conduct ongoing assessments of the organization's CLAS-related activities and integrate CLAS-related measures into measurement and continuous quality improvement activities.
11. Collect and maintain accurate and reliable demographic data to monitor and evaluate the impact of CLAS on health equity and outcomes and to inform service delivery.
12. Conduct regular assessments of community health assets and needs and use the results to plan and implement services that respond to the cultural and linguistic diversity of populations in the service area.
13. Partner with the community to design, implement, and evaluate policies, practices, and services to ensure cultural and linguistic appropriateness.
14. Create conflict and grievance resolution processes that are culturally and linguistically appropriate to identify, prevent, and resolve conflicts or complaints.
15. Communicate the organization's progress in implementing and sustaining CLAS to all stakeholders, constituents, and the general public.

The Substance Abuse and Mental Health Services Administration (SAMHSA) also put forth some helpful principles for delivering culturally sensitive care in their Treatment Improvement Protocol on trauma-informed care [21]:

- Recognize the importance of culture and respect diversity.
- Maintain a current profile of the cultural composition of the community.
- Recruit workers who are representative of the community or service area.
- Provide ongoing cultural competence training to staff.
- Ensure that services are accessible, appropriate, and equitable.

- Recognize the role of help-seeking behaviors, traditions, and natural support networks.
- Involve community leaders and organizations representing diverse cultural groups as "cultural brokers".
- Ensure that services and information are culturally and linguistically responsive.
- Assess and evaluate the program's level of cultural responsiveness.

It is necessary to provide easily accessible language interpretation free of charge to the patient in all clinical settings in order to maintain a collaborative provider-client relationship. In fact, federal law mandates that healthcare settings which accept Medicare/Medicaid "shall take reasonable steps to provide meaningful access to each individual with limited English proficiency eligible to be served or likely to be encountered in its health programs and activities" (Section 1557 of the Affordable Care Act: 45 C.F.R. Part 92, https://www.hhs.gov/civil-rights/for-providers/clearance-medicare-providers/technical-assistance/limited-english-proficiency/index.html) [22]. Considering the nuances of nonverbal communication, live interpreters are preferable to phone interpreters whenever possible. Also, specially trained interpreters are preferable to family members or friends due to concerns about confidentiality as well as relationship complexities. It should be noted that occasionally a patient will be uncomfortable sharing with an interpreter if there might be social overlap (e.g., a small community wherein the interpreters and patients have mutual acquaintances). In these difficult cases, it is important to reflect on the goals of respecting privacy while also gaining essential information. It may also be helpful to speak with the patient, family, and interpreter separately (before and/or after the interview) if possible to gain a better understanding of the culture and the privacy concerns.

It has also been pointed out that healthcare organizations should not make the mistake of assuming that because providers share some component of culture (e.g., ethnicity, country of origin, etc.) with a patient, that cultural competency will naturally emerge. There may be significant differences in socioeconomic class, religion, or beliefs about illness and treatment [23]. Furthermore, even if nearly every component of culture is shared, one is not exhibiting true cultural humility until the orientation/attitude toward oneself and others is put into action as described earlier.

Another strategy which may be helpful is the use of cultural brokers. The concept of cultural brokerage arose out of the field of anthropology in the 1950s and 1960s when it was noted that negotiators or middlemen seemed to emerge to help resolve conflict between certain cultures or societies. In its application to the healthcare field, it has come to mean "the act of bridging, linking, or mediating between groups or persons of differing cultural backgrounds for the purpose of reducing conflict or producing change" [24]. The attributes of a cultural broker can be highly variable, but they are generally thought to function as liaison, cultural guide, mediator, and catalyst for change. Almost anyone can act as a cultural broker as long as they have adequate understanding of the parties involved and the issue(s) at hand, the trust and respect of the parties, and good communication skills. For example, cultural brokers could include interpreters, healthcare providers, lay health workers, clergy, or other community members and may be found in healthcare organizations, faith-based organizations, government offices, and many other settings. Georgetown University's National Center for Cultural Competence created a guide to assist health care organizations in planning, implementing, and sustaining cultural broker programs (https://nccc.georgetown.edu/documents/Cultural_Broker_Guide_English.pdf) [25].

## Conclusion

In this chapter, we discussed how cultural factors shape the way people experience, express, and recover from trauma. The concepts of "cultural competency" and "cultural humility" can both be helpful frameworks (one more objective, one more subjective, respectively). It is helpful and important for providers to understand some basic concepts about culture and about specific groups (e.g., refugees, immigrants, or specific subcultures). With that in mind, it is arguably more important to maintain an attitude of humility and curiosity. Any encounter has the potential to be a cross-cultural encounter, and should be conceived of as such. Organizations and providers are encouraged to apply both trauma-sensitive and culturally sensitive lenses when approaching each patient encounter to work toward the ultimate goals of social justice and relief of suffering.

## References

1. Brown L. Cultural competence in trauma therapy: beyond the flashback. Washington, DC: American Psychological Association; 2008.
2. Horvat L, Horey D, Romios P, Kis-Rigo J. Cultural competence education for health professionals. Cochrane Database Syst Rev. 2014;(5):CD009405.
3. Truong M, Paradies Y, Priest N. Interventions to improve cultural competency in healthcare: a systematic review of reviews. BMC Health Serv Res. 2014;14:99.
4. Cross TL, Bazron BJ, Dennis KW, Isaacs MR. Towards a culturally competent system of care. Washington, DC: Georgetown University Child Development Center; 1989.
5. Kumaş-Tan Z, Beagan B, Loppie C, MacLeod A, Frank B. Measures of cultural competence: examining hidden assumptions. Acad Med. 2007;82(6):548–57.
6. Kumagai AK, Lypson ML. Beyond cultural competence: critical consciousness, social justice, and multicultural education. Acad Med. 2009;84(6):782–7.
7. Tervalon M, Murray-García J. Cultural humility versus cultural competence: a critical distinction in defining physician training outcomes in multicultural education. J Health Care Poor Underserved. 1998;9(2):117–25.
8. Murray-García J, Tervalon M. The concept of cultural humility. Health Aff (Millwood). 2014;33(7):1303.
9. Foronda C, Baptiste DL, Reinholdt MM, Ousman K. Cultural humility: a concept analysis. J Transcult Nurs. 2016;27(3):210–7.
10. Hook JN, Boan D, Davis DE, Aten JD, Ruiz JM, Maryon T. Cultural humility and hospital safety culture. J Clin Psychol Med Settings. 2016;23(4):402–9.

11. United Nations High Commissioner for Refugees (UNHCR). Protecting refugees: questions and answers. 2002, February 1. Available from: http://www.unhcr.org/afr/publications/brochures/3b779dfe2/protecting-refugees-questions-answers.html.
12. Division of International Protection/United Nations High Commissioner for Refugees. UNHCR resettlement handbook. 2011. Available from: http://www.unhcr.org/46f7c0ee2.pdf.
13. McAuliffe M, Ruhs M. Making sense of migration in an increasingly interconected world. 2017. In: World migration report 2018 [Internet]. Geneva, Switzerland: International Organization for Migration (IOM), Accessed 29 July 2018. Available from: https://publications.iom.int/system/files/pdf/wmr_2018_en_chapter1.pdf.
14. United Nations High Commission for Refugees. UNHCR global trends report: forced displacement in 2016. Accessed 29 July 2018. Available from: http://www.unhcr.org/5943e8a34.pdf.
15. Perruchoud R, Redpath-Cross J. Glossary on migration: International Organization for Migration; 2011, 2nd. Available from: https://publications.iom.int/system/files/pdf/iml25_1.pdf.
16. United Nations High Commission for Refugees. UNHCR global trends report 2016. 2016. Available from: http://www.unhcr.org/5943e8a34.pdf.
17. Kemp C, Rasbridge L. Refugee and immigrant health: a handbook for health professionals. Cambridge, UK: Cambridge University Press; 2004.
18. Bhugra D, Gupta S, Schouler-Ocak M, Graeff-Calliess I, Deakin NA, Qureshi A, et al. EPA guidance mental health care of migrants. Eur Psychiatry. 2014;29(2):107–15.
19. Office of Minority Health/US Department of Health and Human Services. Nationally Culturally and Linguistically Appropriate Services Standards (CLAS). 2013. Available from: https://www.thinkculturalhealth.hhs.gov/clas/standards.
20. National Committee for Quality Assurance. A practical guide to implementing the national CLAS standards: for racial, ethnic and linguistic minorities, people with disabilities and sexual and gender minorities. December 2016. Accessed 2 March 2019. Available from: https://www.cms.gov/About-CMS/Agency-Information/OMH/Downloads/CLAS-Toolkit-12-7-16.pdf.
21. Substance Abuse and Mental Health Services Administration. Improving Cultural Competence. Treatment Improvement Protocol (TIP) Series No. 59. HHS Publication No. (SMA) 14-4849. Rockville, MD: Substance Abuse and Mental Health Services Administration, 2014. Accessed 2 March 2019. Available from: https://samhsa.gov/system/files/sma14-4849.pdf.
22. Affordable Care Act, Pub. L. No. 45 C.F.R. Part 92, § 92.201 (2010).
23. Ardino V. Trauma-informed care: is cultural competence a viable solution for efficient policy strategies? Clin Neuropyschiatry. 2014;11(1):45–51.
24. Jezewski MA. Culture brokering in migrant farmworker health care. West J Nurs Res. 1990;12(4):497–513.
25. National Center for Cultural Competence/Georgetown University Center for Child and Human Development. Bridging the cultural divide in health care settings: the essential role of cultural broker programs. Washington, DC: Georgetown University Medical Center; 2004. Accessed 29 July 2018. Available from: https://nccc.georgetown.edu/documents/Cultural_Broker_Guide_English.pdf.

## Selected Additional Readings

Cleaver SR, Carvajal JK, Sheppard PS. Cultural humility: a way of thinking to inform practice globally. Physiother Can. 2016;68(1):1–4.
Fahlberg B, Foronda C, Baptiste D. Cultural humility: the key to patient/family partnerships for making difficult decisions. Nursing. 2016 Sep;46(9):14–6.
Henderson S, Horne M, Hills R, Kendall E. Cultural competence in healthcare in the community: a concept analysis. Health Soc Care Community 4 ed. 2018;10(2):3.
Hook JN, Davis DE, Owen J, Worthington EL, Utsey SO. Cultural humility: measuring openness to culturally diverse clients. J Couns Psychol. 2013;60(3):353–66.

Hunt LM. Beyond cultural competence: applying humility in clinical settings. In: King NMP, Strauss RP, Churchill LR, Estroff SE, Henderson GE, Oberlander J, editors. The social medicine reader: Vol. 2. Social and cultural contributions to health, difference, and inequality. 2nd ed. Durham: Duke University Press; 2005. p. 133–7.

Isaacson M. Clarifying concepts: cultural humility or competency. J Prof Nurs. 2014;30(3):251–8.

McKesey J, Berger TG, Lim HW, McMichael AJ, Torres A, Pandya AG. Cultural competence for the 21st century dermatologist practicing in the United States. J Am Acad Dermatol. 2017;77(6):1159–69.

Metzl JM, Hansen H. Structural competency: theorizing a new medical engagement with stigma and inequality. Soc Sci Med. 2014;103:126–33.

Paparella-Pitzel S, Eubanks R, Kaplan SL. Comparison of teaching strategies for cultural humility in physical therapy. J Allied Health. 2016;45(2):139–46.

Prasad SJ, Nair P, Gadhvi K, Barai I, Danish HS, Philip AB. Cultural humility: treating the patient, not the illness. Med Educ Online. 2016;21:30908.

Vidaeff AC, Kerrigan AJ, Monga M. Cross-cultural barriers to health care. South Med J. 2015;108(1):1–4.

Woods-Jaeger BA, Kava CM, Akiba CF, Lucid L, Dorsey S. The art and skill of delivering culturally responsive trauma-focused cognitive behavioral therapy in Tanzania and Kenya. Psychol Trauma. 2017;9(2):230–8.

Yeager KA, Bauer-Wu S. Cultural humility: essential foundation for clinical researchers. Appl Nurs Res. 2013;26(4):251–6.

# Chapter 4
# Trauma-Informed Care: A Focus on African American Men

**Marshall Fleurant**

## Introduction: Prevalence of Trauma

*Mr. J was a tall African American male who presented to my evening clinic complaining of headaches. He came preferentially to evening clinic because "less people were around". Upon our first visit, he wore dark glasses, a leather jacket, and a Kangol hat. He came with his wife, who wore a neat dress and a light jacket. His headaches described as "sharp"," severe" and "blinding", even affecting his eyes. They were chronic over four years and have been getting worse, mainly affecting the back of his head. On examination, Mr. J removed his sunglasses and hat to reveal an old large surgical scar in the back of his head that ends at the nape of his neck. At the base of the scar was a hardened nodule/object. Upon palpation, the patient flinched. He then mentioned "It's a bullet doc" ....*

Trauma from either physical violence or a stressful event forever shapes the lives of those who experience it. Nearly 36% of women and 29% of men experience interpersonal violence [1]. Violence, one precipitant of trauma, is particularly prevalent in the United States. For African Americans compared to other male populations, especially those in certain communities, trauma and violence are widespread. African Americans have the highest rates of death from fatal injuries and suffer the highest number of nonfatal injuries among all minority groups (see Tables 4.1 and 4.2). The Centers for Disease Control and Prevention (CDC) and National Center for Injury Prevention and Control use tools such as the Web-based Injury Statistics Query and Reporting System (WISQARS) [2] to capture information on injuries and death by variables such as race and age. From this resource it is noted that in the general population, 7.77% of nonfatal injuries are related to violence, but for African

---

M. Fleurant (✉)
Emory University School of Medicine, Atlanta, GA, USA
e-mail: marshall.fleurant@emory.edu

**Table 4.1** Nonfatal violence estimates

| Gender | Race | Violence | Injuries | Population[a] | Proportion[b] |
|---|---|---|---|---|---|
| Both | N/A | 3,971,773 | 51,145,229 | 518,230,121 | 0.078 |
| Male | N/A | 2,278,948 | 26,831,581 | 252,835,346 | 0.085 |
| Male | W | 892,183 | 13,341,368 | 164,903,743 | 0.067 |
| Male | B | 469,571 | 2,984,694 | 32,384,146 | 0.157 |

Citation: Centers for Disease Control and Prevention. Web-Based Injury Statistics Query and Reporting System (WISQARS) [online].2003. National Center for Injury Prevention. www.cdc.gov/injury/wisqars

Note: Both: both sexes, violence: nonfatal injury count related to assault, legal intervention, self-harm; injuries: all injuries including violence-related injuries and accidents
[a]estimates from the population estimates program of the US Census Bureau
[b]nonfatal violence-related injuries/all nonfatal injuries

**Table 4.2** Fatal deaths from violence estimates

| Gender | Race | AADR | Violence | Deaths | Population | Homicide % | H/V |
|---|---|---|---|---|---|---|---|
| Both | N/A | 81.88 | 124,689 | 436,636 | 522,049,854 | 8.10% | 28.30% |
| Male | N/A | 117.72 | 97,902 | 296,168 | 254,756,127 | 9.70% | 29.30% |
| Male | W | 126.45 | 63,176 | 209,893 | 165,338,186 | 3.30% | 10.80% |
| Male | B | 139.62 | 20,279 | 43,142 | 30,770,913 | 37.20% | 79.80% |

Citation: Centers for Disease Control and Prevention, National Center for Injury Prevention and Control, Web Based Injury Statistics Query and Reporting System(WISQARS). 2017. www.cdc.gov/injuries/wisqars

Both – both sexes, N/A not applicable, AADR age adjusted death rate/100,000 from all intents (all intents = violence-related deaths, unintentional deaths, suicide, undetermined), #Violence number of deaths related to violence, #Deaths number of deaths related to all intents, population US Census Bureau population estimates, homicide percentage proportion of deaths related to homicide, H/V proportion of violence deaths related to homicide

American men, 15.77% of nonfatal injuries are related to violence (Centers for Disease Control and Prevention) [3] (Table 4.2).

Trauma is ubiquitous and may result from violence, neglect, emotional pain, stress, accidents or natural disasters. Victims of violence experience a broad constellation of emotions and physiological responses that go well beyond physical injury. Trauma exerts health effects through a complicated web of behavioral patterns, physiological alterations, and psychological sequela. Trauma-informed care (TIC) is an approach that is sensitive to patients' traumatic experiences, and is a worthwhile framework to apply to the care of trauma-afflicted African American males. In this chapter, we will take a focused look at the African American population, particularly men in urban communities, and explore the basic epidemiology of violence and trauma affecting this population and potential etiologies for these. We will consider strategies for providing medical care to this community, highlighting successful programs along the way. To provide context, we will briefly review the prevalence and effects of trauma, on the general population in the United States, particularly posttraumatic stress disorder (PTSD), and explore how men are affected by trauma and PTSD compared to women. This will provide context to explore the possibilities of TIC for African Americans, particularly men, and help thoughtfully inform the field and guide the implementation of TIC in healthcare settings and systems that serve men of color.

## Trauma, PTSD, and the General Population

Early signs of trauma can manifest as soon as 2 days following an event and are characterized by fear, anxiety, helplessness, distressing memories, and even a loss of functioning. If symptoms last longer than 30 days, these patients may begin to fit the diagnostic criteria for PTSD. Loss of functioning can be particularly crippling and manifests as patients having difficulty, or having worse performance when, returning to work, poor coping mechanisms, and decreased ability to perform activities of daily living [4, 5]. In addition, studies have demonstrated a clear connection between trauma and physical health that goes beyond just direct injury. Adults who have experienced four or more traumatic events during childhood have higher odds of medical disease such as diabetes (odds ratio [O.R] 1.6), ischemic heart disease (O.R. 2.2), and cancer (O.R. 1.9) [6]. Patients with PTSD also suffer from a higher number of medical conditions compared to similar patients without the diagnosis; lumbrospinal disorders, joint disorders, skin disorders, headache, and sleep disturbances are among the most common [7]. Comorbid conditions such as anxiety and depression can manifest in new psychiatric diagnoses for the patient or may become persistent conditions lasting for months to years [4].

## Men and Trauma

*On our first visit Mr. J barely spoke, so the majority of his history came from his wife. She stated that he has had headaches since his "accident" She stated that they have been to a lot of doctors and that no one really gives him a chance. He truly has a lot of pain and it has gotten to the point that it is affecting their relationship. She asked, "If you can help us with at least some of the medicine . . . until we can figure out what's going on." The patient burst out, "Look, I don't want no problems . . . just give me my pills and I'll leave." I paused and requested that we continue. He proceeded to jump off the examination table and headed toward the door.*

In men, the patterns of trauma exposure and responses to trauma differ from those of women. Theories of masculinity posit that in response to societal norms, men may avoid help-seeking behavior by maintaining a desire to have control in situations—for example, by displaying toughness, remaining stoic, and coping autonomously. It is important to note that not all men behave the same. Theoretically, for the individual male, help-seeking behavior is thought to be a function of a man's personal endorsement of masculine gender role norms, perceived characteristics of possible helpers, and characteristics of the social group to which that man belongs, as well as the perceived potential for loss of control [8–10]. Alternatively men are more likely to engage in help-seeking behavior if they have the opportunity to reciprocate, like paying back a loan or offering to repair an item after borrowing a tool [11]. Men also interact with the healthcare system differently from women. Studies have reported, in general, that men make fewer ambulatory visits compared to women (258 physician office visits per 100 males vs. 342 physician office visits per 100 females) [12, 13]. When men seek help, they ask fewer questions than women [11].

Male exposure to trauma also differs. Men are exposed to a higher prevalence of physical attacks than women [14]. Homicide rates for men are four times that of women (9.8/100,000 vs. 2.2/100,000) [3]. Interpersonal violence, normally seen as primarily affecting women, still affects 28.5% of men [15]; these numbers are likely underestimates. It is thought that underreporting may be due to male tendencies to remain relatively silent due to fear of being portrayed as cowardly or powerless [16]. One report noted that fewer than 32% of male intimate partner violence victims spoke to the police about being victimized and only 15% made an official report [15]. These factors may be amplified for men of color whose experience stemming from prejudice, racism, inequality, and perceptions of racial norms and expectations may mediate or even amplify how they respond to trauma.

## Trauma and Men of Color

*In a follow-up visit Mr. J came alone and decided to discuss the circumstances of his accident. He stated that him [sic] and his friend were driving a nice car at the time. He commented that others in his neighborhood were 'jealous' because him [sic] and his friend were 'flossing' (meaning he had nice material possessions relative to others in the surrounding neighborhood or peer group). Two men ran up to his vehicle, shot him and his friend 'execution' style and ran. His friend didn't make it. Mr. J was in the hospital for over a month; he stated that he was "messed up" for a while after that. He still thinks about it to this day and has occasional nightmares.*

Minority populations, particularly the African American community, have a complex relationship with health care due to historical, social, and economic issues that greatly affect the receipt of medical care and treatment by providers. In this chapter, we will explore African American experiences with trauma and PTSD and compare these to those of the general population by reviewing differences in the epidemiology of trauma and violence. Next, the chapter considers the sociological issues affecting Black males, their receipt of mental health care, and the role of TIC in this population.

## Epidemiology of Violence and Trauma Among Black Men

Despite comprising only 5% of the American population, African American males suffer the highest death rates. The overall crude death rate[1] for African American males between 2015 and 2016 was 140.18 per 100,000, compared to overall crude death rates among all males which was 116.26 per 100,000. Rates remain elevated even when adjusting for age (Table 4.2). Death rates from homicide are particularly striking. In 2010, the overall crude homicide rate was 4.8 deaths per 100,000, and for African Americans it was 15.2 deaths per 100,000, accounting for almost half (49.7%) of US homicide deaths [17]. For African American males, homicide accounts for 37.2% of fatal injuries, whereas homicide accounts for 3.3% of fatal injuries among European American males (see Table 4.2) [3]. This is particularly evident among young African American males. Estimates vary, but for those between ages 15 and 25, homicide is the leading cause of death [3, 18]. Overall, African American males are more likely to experience trauma [19] and homicide from gun violence [20].

These rates may be compounded by a relatively high prevalence of Adverse Childhood Experiences (ACEs) among African American males. In a study of 191 hospitalized violently injured predominantly African American men in their 20s, researchers noted a high prevalence of ACEs. Although only 44 opted to participate, all participants who completed ACE questionnaires had at least 1 ACE, and 81% ($n = 26$) had two or more ACEs [21]. In certain urban settings, the probable lifetime rates of PTSD range between 15% and 23% [21]. In one study looking at 738 African American patients at an urban hospital center, 501 (67.8%) endorsed having experienced at least one traumatic event. Of this population, 91 (12%) were noted to have PTSD, 30.6% of these patients were male [22].

Unfortunately, those who do experience injury or trauma are at greater risk of increased future morbidity. Re-injury rates have been estimated to be as high as 45% and mortality rates as high as 20% at 5-year follow-up [21, 23]. These unfortunate statistics remind us that not only is the African American population vulnerable to violent injury, they remain persistently at risk for recurrent injury, underscoring the need for a trauma-informed approach to care.

Risk factors for under-identification of PTSD include younger age, male gender, and being African American [22]. Under-diagnosis of PTSD is common for this population. To appropriately discuss TIC among African American males, it is important to consider the historical, social, and structural factors that promote differences in exposures especially those that are associated with race.

---

[1] The crude death rate is the overall number of deaths for a particular population divided by the total number of people in that population. These crude death rates reflect the total number of injury-related death rates.

## Race and Racism

Race, in itself, is a very imprecise measure as a category, but it is used as a proxy for a combination of measures including social class, culture, and biological make-up. The use of race as a categorical measure has some weaknesses; as a purely biological construct for classifying individuals, race fails. Science has shown that genetic variation within race may actually be greater than that between races, and genetic composition among individuals is not static; it changes and evolves over time, influenced by natural selection, mutation and genetic exchange between populations, and environmental adoption. Race is also an imperfect identifier, one's self-perceived race may differ from an observer's perception. For example, a light-skinned African American may be seen as Black within the United States, but in a country like Brazil, that person may be considered quadroon or mulatto, instantly changing this person's social classification or identification [24–26]. So why is race used so frequently to categorize populations? In particular, what relevance does it have to health and receipt of health care? In the United States, race may be better used as a measure of social exposure to racism or to capture social classification. For this reason, racial categories have shown some consistency in predicting variations in health status [24, 27]. The historical legacy of phenomena such as prejudice and racism is critically important in understanding challenges faced by minority populations and men of color.

As described by Jones et al., [25] racism has three broad manifestations: institutional racism, personally mediated racism, and internalized racism. Institutional racism is defined as differential access to goods, services, power, and opportunities that has been codified into our customs, practices, and law. Personally mediated racism, or discrimination, is the differential assumption about the abilities, motives, and intentions of others based on race. It can be intentional or unintentional and may manifest as a lack of respect, suspicion, and dehumanization. Finally, internalized racism is acceptance by members of a stigmatized race of negative messages about their intrinsic worth and abilities. Internalized racism manifests itself as helplessness, hopelessness, and self-devaluation [28]. A greater understanding of race and racism as a social norm and/or construct helps us understand how this phenomenon diffuses through individual, institutional, and community levels—particularly for African American males [29].

## Personally Mediated Racism

Society as a whole has made great progress in addressing personally mediated racism [28] and discrimination. It is socially unacceptable and unlawful in medical institutions to be denied treatment based solely on race. Individuals in many areas of the country risk social exclusion if they commit blatant acts of prejudice, and federal investigators may be involved if individuals are caught in the practice [30].

Although individual acts of personally mediated racism still exist, progress in reducing this critical issue has greatly lessened some barriers to care for African Americans and increased trust between non-race concordant patients and providers. Nonetheless, implicit bias remains widespread in healthcare settings [31, 32].

## Institutional Racism: Inequity and Social Determinants of Health

We tend to look at institutional racism through the lens of inequity. According to Phelan et al.'s [33] theory of fundamental causes, individuals and groups tend to deploy resources to avoid risk and adopt protective strategies, such as social connections, money, or power to avoid harm. They distribute these resources in a flexible manner that allows inequities to persist even under conditions where we would expect them to diminish or extinguish; this results in an inverse relationship between socioeconomic status (SES) and disease. Inequity has four essential features: (a) it impacts multiple disease outcomes; (b) it interacts with disease through multiple risk factors; (c) it determines access to resources; and (d) the association between disease and health is reproduced over time by an intervening mechanism [33, 34]. Historically, underserved populations have been unable to deploy sufficient resources to provide themselves with a significant level of protection from the sequela of inequity such as poor housing, limited representation in government, or inadequate wealth. When this theory is applied to the receipt of mental health care by minority populations, access is limited by geographic separation; mental health providers tend to be located in more affluent neighborhoods [35]. African Americans are also less likely to be referred to behavioral health providers and may also be less willing to seek behavioral health care due to social stigma, less perceived need, or deficits in patient-provider trust [36–38].

Disparities and inequity are terms that have often been used interchangeably. Health disparities result from ongoing interactions among factors in the healthcare environment: healthcare organizations, communities, providers, and persons in the course of the treatment-seeking process [29]. As a core element of treatment for mental health conditions such as PTSD, depression, or anxiety, counseling is necessary; persistence in treatment is defined as the ability to stick to a treatment schedule for a minimum duration of time or visits, typically eight visits [39]. Researchers looking at racial concordance suggest a lack of mental health providers of color as a potential reason for low treatment persistence among some minority patients. However, even nonminority patients struggle to persist in PTSD-related counseling and may discontinue treatment prematurely.

In one Veterans Administration study of 1813 patients who initiated psychotherapy, only 13% ($n = 228$) persisted in therapy for eight sessions [39]. White Veterans were more likely to persist in treatment than African American or Latino patients. In addition, African Americans were more likely to discontinue treatment if they perceived that they did not receive adequate care for side effects of pharmacotherapy. All groups were more likely to stay in treatment if the patient perceived that the treatment was effective, they could easily ask questions, and they were linked with providers who listened [39]. These data suggest that provider contributions to therapeutic retention are critical.

Even if past events have long been forgotten, everyday experiences that maintain historical structure and inequity can impact the manner in which patients receive care. For example, historical events such as the infamous Tuskegee experiment have influenced the way Americans interact with the healthcare system in a broad way [40]. Many African Americans may not be aware of the actual events of the Tuskegee experiment, yet are more likely to distrust the medical care system mainly because of what is known as everyday racism (*small daily experiences with prejudice*) or microaggressions [41].

## Intrinsic Racism

Individual-level factors that affect African American males' use of health care or health help-seeking are rarely discussed. At the individual level, African American male health-seeking behavior may be influenced by additional racial dynamics described as race identity (or racial centrality), race-related stress effects, and John Henryism. As defined by Powell et al., [12] race identity, or race centrality, is the qualitative meaning that individuals attribute to their membership in a racial group. It is the importance of race to a person's identity. Race-related stress events or discrimination are microaggressions that negatively impact African Americans' everyday experiences. John Henryism is the self-perception that individuals can overcome demands with persistence and hard work. It suggests that under adverse social and economic conditions, high-effort coping styles that reflect hard work and determination may contribute to, for example, elevated blood pressure [42]. It can promote unmitigated self-reliance with a sense that seeking treatment denotes weakness or a character flaw.

These dynamics can contribute to barriers to health-seeking, particularly those that impact access to mental health. Among African American males, self-reported racial discrimination is associated with poorer mental health outcomes including greater risks for depression, anxiety, substance abuse, and global psychological distress. Race-related stresses threaten sense of control. African American men report experiencing race-related stress disproportionally more than African American women [12].

Reactance theory states that individuals are more likely to resist help-seeking when they confront life events that diminish their sense of control, threaten their freedom, and induce negative psychological states. According to Powell et al., [12] in a study on masculinity and race, using reactance theory as a theoretical base, the authors found significant associations between self-perceived racial identity, discrimination, and health help-seeking. African American men who place a high level of importance on masculinity norms (male social identities such as emotional stoicism, toughness, and autonomous coping strategies), and had frequent race-related stress, displayed higher barriers to seeking care. Alternatively, those with greater race centrality reported a greater sense of control and lower depressed mood scores. Depressed mood was found to mediate the relationship between masculinity and seeking care, as men with depressed mood reported greater barriers to health help-seeking. The researchers did not find a relationship between barriers to health help-seeking and John Henryism, but commented that John Henryism can act as a double-edged sword; it may lead to unintentional decreased health help-seeking in the face of health threats [12]. For healthcare providers, understanding these dynamics at play may be powerful tools to overcome barriers to care and build strong therapeutic relationships with Black male patients.

## Neighborhood Effects

*Mr. J still lives in the same neighborhood as before. Violence has calmed since he was shot years ago. He states he doesn't feel threatened because his perpetrators are not around anymore, and he has a different peer group. He spends most of the time either with his wife or with a couple of close friends and doesn't really go out anymore.*

To what extent does the context of one's environment, particularly neighborhood effects, influence patterns of healthcare consumption or health outcomes? Are neighborhood effects simply attributable to the characteristics of individuals that live there or is there something more? There is evidence to suggest that neighborhoods have an independent effect on health [43]. African American males are not genetically predisposed to poorer outcomes, and their significant health disadvantage may be attributable to social ecological exposures. For example, researchers in a study of coronary heart disease (CHD) reported that African Americans tend to live in more disadvantaged neighborhoods, even when they are among the highest socioeconomic groups [44].

Studies have demonstrated that family violence is more likely to occur in poor, disadvantaged neighborhoods than in advantaged neighborhoods [45, 46]. When economically secure couples live in advantaged neighborhoods, the proportion of both partners reporting interpersonal violence is 2%; similarly economically secure couples in disadvantaged neighborhoods report interpersonal violence at 9.5%, a statistically significant difference [45]. Individuals residing in socially and economically disadvantaged neighborhoods report more stressful life experiences, such areas where neighborhood violence disrupts social networks are associated with self-reported PTSD symptoms [46, 47]. Residents of disadvantaged neighborhoods are often more socially isolated from one another and may not rely as much on their neighbors to help them [45, 46]. Such phenomena may engender neighborhood norms such as the belief that people are expected to mind their own business or stay out of others' personal affairs; it can make it difficult and uncomfortable for persons to form alliances not only with neighbors but also with healthcare providers.

## Empowering Men of Color: Interventions

*In the past two years Mr. J had two different physicians. His first doctor "never did nothing for his headache" and his last doctor he "disagreed with". Over the next two visits, Mr. J came with his wife to the evening clinic. We agreed on a course of tramadol and ibuprofen for pain. We had at least one conversation over the phone where we reviewed his medical records.*

*Over several visits, we were able to arrange for removal of this bullet secondary to its relatively superficial position. Mr. J was pleasantly surprised as 'no doctor ever did anything for him'. Mr. J eventually agreed to take antidepressants, but he continued to refuse psychotherapy, his pain regimen has remained the same. He continues to make regular primary care visits at least twice a year.*

## Culturally Focused Interventions

There are few, if any, culturally tailored interventions focused on trauma-informed care and particularly geared toward men of color. Culturally tailored interventions must be sensitive to stigmatization of mental health care among some minority communities. Historical legacies between the healthcare institution and community should be explored, inherent strengths of the community should be capitalized on (such as extended family networks), and an appreciation for the meaning and significance of racial identity to an individual's sense of self should be cultivated [37, 48, 49].

Examples of interventions showing cultural sensitivity exist. In a randomized trial of a health promotion program that focused on hypertension based in Black barbershops, intervention barbershops employed African American barbers to continuously offer blood pressure checks, tailored sex-specific health messaging, and modeling healthy behaviors, while control barbershops received culturally adapted reading materials alone to influence blood pressure control. Researchers found that patients in both the intervention and control groups who received culturally adapted reading materials experienced improvements in hypertension control. However, the intervention barbershops had an even greater improvement in blood pressure control with an absolute group difference of 8.8% (CI 0.8–16.9%, $p = 0.04$) [50]. The barbers took on the role of influential peers who provided an atmosphere where it was normative to discuss blood pressure problems. As a well-regarded cultural institution for African American men, barbershops served as an environment where the social group provided motivation to seek blood pressure control. Culturally sensitive interventions may be a successful motivator for African American men needing mental health care.

We have examples of success among African American women. In a study testing culturally tailored cognitive behavioral therapy (CBT) vs standard CBT among African American women, researchers found that participants in the culturally tailored CBT intervention had greater declines in depression levels than those in standard CBT [49, 51]. Similar interventions can be tailored toward African American men.

In terms of trauma, Hospital Violence Intervention Programs (HVIPs) have helped coordinate medical care, manage symptoms of PTSD, and engage victims to resist pressure to retaliate against their perpetrators, potentially reducing the cycle of violence [52]. HVIPs treat victims of violence through a combination of community-based organizations, brief in-hospital interventions, counseling, and targeted services to reduce risk factors for re-injury [52]. Early studies of HVIPs have shown they have potential to reduce hospital admissions, arrests, and convictions for violent crime and also increase employment [23]. These programs also offer means to identify patients with PTSD and their need for social services. These programs can help overcome barriers to accessing mental health services early in the course of trauma and possibly lessen perceived stigma.

## Interventions

Single-component interventions that focus on individuals alone or education alone may not be sufficient to address the difficulty in treating trauma-affected individuals. In mental health, such treatments may have some efficacy in mild to moderate depression but appear inadequate in more severe depression or more complicated psychiatric conditions [49]. Multicomponent interventions involving organization-wide or system-wide programs have demonstrated an ability to reduce disparities between non-Hispanic Whites and minorities. Interventions that target a combination of multiple health providers, health systems, and even several health systems seem to show the most promise.

Multicomponent interventions have been demonstrated to reduce disparities between non-Hispanic White Americans and minorities in randomized control trials. The core component of these interventions appears to be active case management, a trained nurse, layperson, or social worker who may be effective across the life course [49]. Active case management may work by helping patients navigate the healthcare system and by providing help securing insurance coverage. These multicomponent interventions have been shown to be effective in treating depression in certain minority populations, but studies with younger male African American populations are needed.

The IMPACT study [54] found that a program focused on coordination of mental health services through primary care led to increases in the use of psychotherapy and antidepressant medication and reduced health-related functional impairment among older African American males. Although extensive cultural adaptations were not part of the intervention, depression care managers worked actively to engage patients, while providing real-time assistance to facilitate use of services, and responded to patient treatment needs and preferences. Like younger men, older patients are wary of mental health services. Forming linkages and relationships with professional healthcare services can facilitate mental health treatment for African American men.

Finally, the Center for Nonviolence and Social Justice at Drexel University in its *Healing the Hurt: Trauma-Informed Approaches to the Health of Boys and Young Men of Color* detailed some specific recommendations for implementing TIC in this population [53]:

1. Healthcare providers and teams serving men of color should be trained in trauma and supported with follow-up professional development. Trauma-informed training should be part of basic health professions training.
2. Providers must understand the role of masculinity in health beliefs and develop systems that take into consideration how it affects male help-seeking behavior.
3. Co-location of physical and mental health services is critical to addressing the needs of men (and boys) of color.
4. Health outreach/navigator support is essential to help men move through systems of care. Because victims of violence are especially vulnerable to recurrent violence and retaliation, services should focus on interrupting the cycle of violence. Emergency department and hospital-based interventions have potential to accomplish this.
5. Coordination between systems including health care, schools, and community resources is necessary.

## Conclusion

Trauma exposure is common among African American men and health systems need to be sensitive to the unique needs of this population. Understanding neighborhood effects and various forms of racism are key to informing culturally sensitive trauma-informed systems of care. Interventions to implement and sustain trauma-informed care should be multimodal. At the level of the individual patient and provider, providers should allow time to develop bonds of trust with the patient, so that patients can, and will, be willing to persist in treatment (as was the case with Mr. J.). Considerable effort should be made to build trust and openness with one another over time. Providers should also consider the effects of cultural and historical incidents that can affect receipt of health care. At the clinic level, effort should be made to ensure patient safety, fairness, and respect at all levels from the front desk to the provider. Healthcare systems should consider models of care that promote active case management and primary care co-location with behavioral health and provide linkages to the community. Local and state governments can assist by funding programs that empower community organizations and lay workers in community-level partnerships, adjust health systems to accommodate patient needs, and support continued research to refine and test models of care.

## References

1. Black MC, Basile KC, Breiding MJ, Smith SG, Walters ML, Merrick MT, Chen J, Stevens MR. The National Intimate Partner and Sexual Violence Survey (NISVS): 2010 Summary Report. Atlanta, GA: National Center for Injury Prevention and Control, Centers for Disease Control and Prevention; 2011. Accessed 29 April 2018. Available at https://www.cdc.gov/ViolencePrevention/pdf/NISVS_Report2010-a.pdf.
2. Centers for Disease Control and Prevention. WISQARS™ (Web-based Injury Statistics Query and Reporting System) Atlanta, GA updated 2017. Accessed 3 May 2018. Available from: https://www.cdc.gov/injury/wisqars/index.html.
3. Centers for Disease Control and Prevention. Web based Injury Statistics Query and Reporting System (WISQARS)[online]. National Center for Injury Prevention and Control, Centers for Disease Control and prevention. Accessed 2018 May 10. Available from: https://www.cdc.gov/injury/wisqars.
4. Wiseman T, Foster K, Curtis K. Mental health following traumatic physical injury: an integrative literature review. Injury. 2013;44(11):1383–90.
5. Smith RN, Seamon MJ, Kumar V, Robinson A, Shults J, Reilly PM, et al. Lasting impression of violence: retained bullets and depressive symptoms. Injury. 2018;49(1):135–40.
6. Felitti VJ, Anda RF, Nordenberg D, Williamson DF, Spitz AM, Edwards V, et al. Relationship of childhood abuse and household dysfunction to many of the leading causes of death in adults. The Adverse Childhood Experiences (ACE) Study. Am J Prev Med. 1998;14(4):245–58.
7. Frayne SM, Chiu VY, Iqbal S, Berg EA, Laungani KJ, Cronkite RC, et al. Medical care needs of returning veterans with PTSD: their other burden. J Gen Intern Med. 2011;26(1):33–9.
8. Tudiver F, Talbot Y. Why don't men seek help? Family physicians' perspectives on help-seeking behavior in men. J Fam Pract. 1999;48(1):47–52.
9. Smith JA, Braunack-Mayer A, Wittert G. What do we know about men's help-seeking and health service use? Med J Aust. 2006;184(2):81–3.
10. Lindsey MA, Marcell AV. "We're going through a lot of struggles that people don't even know about": the need to understand African American males' help-seeking for mental health on multiple levels. Am J Mens Health. 2012;6(5):354–64.
11. Addis ME, Mahalik JR. Men, masculinity, and the contexts of help seeking. Am Psychol. 2003;58(1):5–14.
12. Powell W, Adams LB, Cole-Lewis Y, Agyemang A, Upton RD. Masculinity and race-related factors as barriers to health help-seeking among African American men. Behav Med. 2016;42(3):150–63.
13. Ashman JJ, Hing E, Talwalkar A. Variation in physician office visit rates by patient characteristics and state. NCHS Data Brief. 2012;2015(212):1–8.
14. Kessler RC, Sonnega A, Bromet E, Hughes M, Nelson CB. Posttraumatic stress disorder in the National Comorbidity Survey. Arch Gen Psychiatry. 1995;52(12):1048–60.
15. Casas JM. Male victims of domestic violence and the disparity in treatment trainings [dissertation]: California School of Forensic Studies Alliant International University Fresno; 2016.
16. Sorsoli L, Kia-Keating M, Grossman FK. "I keep that hush-hush": male survivors of sexual abuse and the challenges of disclosure. J Couns Psychol. 2008;55(3):333–45.
17. Parks SE, Johnson LL, McDaniel DD, Gladden M. Surveillance for violent deaths - National Violent Death Reporting System, 16 states, 2010. MMWR Surveill Summ. 2014;63(1):1–33.
18. Rich JA, Sullivan LM. Correlates of violent assault among young male primary care patients. J Health Care Poor Underserved. 2001;12(1):103–12.
19. Beard JH, Morrison CN, Jacoby SF, Dong B, Smith R, Sims CA, et al. Quantifying disparities in urban firearm violence by race and place in Philadelphia, Pennsylvania: a cartographic study. Am J Public Health. 2017;107(3):371–3.

20. Riddell CA, Harper S, Cerda M, Kaufman JS. Comparison of rates of firearm and nonfirearm homicide and suicide in black and white non-hispanic men, by U.S. state. Ann Intern Med. 2018;168(10):712–20.
21. Corbin TJ, Purtle J, Rich LJ, Rich JA, Adams EJ, Yee G, et al. The prevalence of trauma and childhood adversity in an urban, hospital-based violence intervention program. J Health Care Poor Underserved. 2013;24(3):1021–30.
22. Graves RE, Freedy JR, Aigbogun NU, Lawson WB, Mellman TA, Alim TN. PTSD treatment of African American adults in primary care: the gap between current practice and evidence-based treatment guidelines. J Natl Med Assoc. 2011;103(7):585–93.
23. Purtle J, Rich LJ, Rich JA, Cooper J, Harris EJ, Corbin TJ. The youth nonfatal violent injury review panel: an innovative model to inform policy and systems change. Public Health Rep. 2015;130(6):610–5.
24. Williams DR. Race and health: basic questions, emerging directions. Ann Epidemiol. 1997;7(5):322–33.
25. Jones CP. Invited commentary: "race," racism, and the practice of epidemiology. Am J Epidemiol. 2001;154(4):299–304. discussion 5–6
26. Macintosh T, Desai MM, Lewis TT, Jones BA, Nunez-Smith M. Socially-assigned race, healthcare discrimination and preventive healthcare services. PLoS One. 2013;8(5):e64522.
27. Williams DR, Lavizzo-Mourey R, Warren RC. The concept of race and health status in America. Public Health Rep. 1994;109(1):26–41.
28. Jones CP. Levels of racism: a theoretic framework and a gardener's tale. Am J Public Health. 2000;90(8):1212–5.
29. Chin MH, Walters AE, Cook SC, Huang ES. Interventions to reduce racial and ethnic disparities in health care. Med Care Res Rev. 2007;64(5 Suppl):7S–28S.
30. Yoo S. Racial threat to Salem Hospital Manager prompts a broader look at community. Statesman Journal [online] 2013 March 9. Accessed 17 June 2018. Available from: statesmanjournal.newspapers.com.
31. Hall WJ, Chapman MV, Lee KM, Merino YM, Thomas TW, Payne BK, et al. Implicit racial/ethnic Bias among health care professionals and its influence on health care outcomes: a systematic review. Am J Public Health. 2015;105(12):e60–76.
32. FitzGerald C, Hurst S. Implicit bias in healthcare professionals: a systematic review. BMC Med Ethics. 2017;18(1):19.
33. Phelan JC, Link BG, Tehranifar P. Social conditions as fundamental causes of health inequalities: theory, evidence, and policy implications. J Health Soc Behav. 2010;51(Suppl):S28–40.
34. Link BG, Phelan JC. Social conditions as fundamental causes of disease. J Health Soc Behav. 1995;35(Extra Issue):80–94.
35. Kramer T, Evans N, Garralda ME. Ethnic diversity among child and adolescent psychiatric clinic attenders. Child Psychol Psychiatry Rev. 2000;5(4):169–75.
36. Van Voorhees BW, Fogel J, Houston TK, Cooper LA, Wang NY, Ford DE. Attitudes and illness factors associated with low perceived need for depression treatment among young adults. Soc Psychiatry Psychiatr Epidemiol. 2006;41(9):746–54.
37. Zhang AY, Snowden LR. Ethnic characteristics of mental disorders in five U.S. communities. Cultur Divers Ethnic Minor Psychol. 1999;5(2):134–46.
38. Cooper LA, Gonzales JJ, Gallo JJ, Rost KM, Meredith LS, Rubenstein LV, et al. The acceptability of treatment for depression among African-American, Hispanic, and white primary care patients. Med Care. 2003;41(4):479–89.
39. Spoont M, Nelson D, van Ryn M, Alegria M. Racial and ethnic variation in perceptions of VA mental health providers are associated with treatment retention among veterans with PTSD. Med Care. 2017;55(Suppl 9 Suppl 2):S33–42.
40. The Belmont Report: Ethical Principles and Guidelines for the Protection of Human Subjects of Research. National Commission for the Protection of Human Subjects of Biomedical and Behavioral Research, US Department of Health and Human Services.1979. Accessed 2 March 2019. Available from: https://www.hhs.gov/ohrp/regulations-and-policy/belmont-report/read-the-belmont-report/index.html.

41. Powell W. How masculinity can hurt mental health [Internet]. Washington, DC: American Psychological Association (APA); 2016. Accessed 31 March 2019. Available from: https://www.apa.org/research/action/speaking-of-psychology/men-boys-health-disparities.
42. Hudson DL, Neighbors HW, Geronimus AT, Jackson JS. Racial discrimination, John Henryism, and depression among African Americans. J Black Psychol. 2016;42(3):221–43.
43. Williams DR, Collins C. Racial residential segregation: a fundamental cause of racial disparities in health. Public Health Rep. 2001;116(5):404–16.
44. Diez Roux AV, Merkin SS, Arnett D, Chambless L, Massing M, Nieto FJ, et al. Neighborhood of residence and incidence of coronary heart disease. N Engl J Med. 2001;345(2):99–106.
45. Fox GL, Benson ML. Household and neighborhood contexts of intimate partner violence. Public Health Rep. 2006;121(4):419–27.
46. Chae DH, Powell WA, Nuru-Jeter AM, Smith-Bynum MA, Seaton EK, Forman TA, et al. The role of racial identity and implicit racial bias in self-reported racial discrimination: implications for depression among African American men. J Black Psychol. 2017;43(8):789–812.
47. Powell WA, Taggart T, Richmond J, Adams LB, Brown A. They can't breathe: why neighborhoods matter for the health of African American men and boys. In: Burton LM, Burton D, McHale SM, King V, VanHook J, editors. Boys and men in African American families. National Symposium on Family Issues 7. 2016. p. 227–42.
48. Brown CA. Therapy utilization levels in African Americna men. [dissertation]. Ann Arbor, MI: Alliant International University; 203, 112 p.
49. Van Voorhees BW, Walters AE, Prochaska M, Quinn MT. Reducing health disparities in depressive disorders outcomes between non-Hispanic Whites and ethnic minorities: a call for pragmatic strategies over the life course. Med Care Res Rev. 2007;64(5 Suppl):157S–94S.
50. Victor RG, Ravenell JE, Freeman A, Leonard D, Bhat DG, Shafiq M, et al. Effectiveness of a barber-based intervention for improving hypertension control in black men: the BARBER-1 study: a cluster randomized trial. Arch Intern Med. 2011;171(4):342–50.
51. Kohn LP, Oden T, Muñoz RF, Robinson A, Leavitt D. Adapted cognitive behavioral group therapy for depressed low-income African American women. Community Ment Health J. 2002;38(6):497–504.
52. Purtle J, Dicker R, Cooper C, Corbin T, Greene MB, Marks A, et al. Hospital-based violence intervention programs save lives and money. J Trauma Acute Care Surg. 2013;75(2):331–3.
53. Wilson A, Rich J, Rich L, Bloom S, Evans S, Corbin T. Healing the hurt: trauma-informed approaches to the health of boys and young men of color. Philadelphia, PA: Center for Nonviolence and Social Justice and Department of Medicine, Drexel University; 2009, October 1.
54. Arean PA, Ayalon L, Hunkeler E, Lin EH, Tang L, Harpole L, et al. Improving depression care for older, minority patients in primary care. Med Care. 2005;43(4):381–90.

# Chapter 5
# Trauma-Informed Care of Sexual and Gender Minority Patients

**Tyler R. McKinnish, Claire Burgess, and Colleen A. Sloan**

## Interpersonal Trauma and the SGM Patient

Sexual and gender minority (SGM) individuals and communities have experienced and continue to suffer from marginalization, stress, and trauma. Relatedly, significant disparities in health and healthcare exist for this population, with significant variation across the many unique subgroups of this community. A large body of research has reliably documented increased risk of violence and victimization for SGM people compared to non-SGM people [1]. Appreciation and understanding of this context, particularly as it relates to clinical presentation, is necessary to provide affirming, competent, and effective care. As such, a trauma-informed approach to care when working with SGM patients is imperative. This chapter will aim to (1) provide a brief overview of important terminology relevant to the SGM community, (2) discuss SGM health disparities and their theoretical frameworks, (3) discuss SGM experiences of trauma and associated outcomes, (4) discuss the application of trauma-informed care when providing care to SGM patients, and (5) provide recommendations for healthcare providers and environments of care.

---

The original version of this chapter was revised. The correction to this chapter can be found at https://doi.org/10.1007/978-3-030-04342-1_12

T. R. McKinnish
Department of Obstetrics and Gynecology,
Washington University/Barnes-Jewish Hospital, St. Louis, MO, USA

C. Burgess
Instructor in Psychiatry, Harvard Medical School, Clinical Psychologist,
VA Boston Healthcare System, Boston, MA, USA

C. A. Sloan (✉)
Assistant Professor, Department of Psychiatry, Boston University School of Medicine,
Clinical Psychologist, VA Boston Healthcare System, Boston, MA, USA
e-mail: Colleen.Sloan2@va.gov

© Springer Nature Switzerland AG 2019
M. R. Gerber (ed.), *Trauma-Informed Healthcare Approaches*,
https://doi.org/10.1007/978-3-030-04342-1_5

## *Terminology*

Terminology relevant to the SGM community has a long history and is always evolving and varies considerably by community, geographic area, and individual. Language is incredibly important, as it reflects the user's understanding of self and others, validates culturally unique and diverse identities and experiences, and promotes effective communication between people. Related to this last point, knowledge of terminology is important for healthcare providers in order to engage and treat SGM patients competently. Below is a brief list of key terms [2]:

Cisgender (adj.): The term used to describe a person's identity or experience when their gender identity and sex assigned at birth correspond (i.e., not transgender).

Gender (noun): The behavioral, cultural, or psychological traits that a society associates with male or female sex.

Gender identity (noun): A person's inner sense of being a boy/man/male, girl/woman/female, another gender, or no gender.

Gender minority (adj): An umbrella term that describes identities that are not cisgender.

Gender expression (noun): The ways in which a person communicates their gender (e.g., maleness or masculinity, femaleness or femininity) to the world through their clothing, speech, behavior, etc. Gender expression is often fluid and is separate from assigned sex at birth or gender identity.

Genderqueer (adj.): The term that describes a person's self-identified gender identity that falls outside of the traditional gender binary structure. Other terms for people whose gender identity falls outside the traditional gender binary include gender nonconforming, gender expansive, etc. Sometimes written as two words (gender queer).

Heteronormativity (noun): The assumption that everyone is heterosexual and that heterosexuality is superior to all other sexualities.

Intersectionality (noun): The idea that identities are influenced and shaped by race, class, ethnicity, sexuality/sexual orientation, gender/gender identity, physical disability, national origin, etc., as well as by the interconnection of all of those characteristics.

Intersex (noun): A group of conditions in which the reproductive organs and genitals do not develop as expected. Some authors and patients prefer the term "disorders (or differences) of sex development." Intersex is also used as an identity term by some community members and advocacy groups.

Sex (noun): The classification of individuals as female or male on the basis of their reproductive organs. Many authors and patients prefer "sex assigned at birth."

Sexual minority (adj): An umbrella term that describes identities that are not heterosexual.

Sexual orientation (noun): A term that refers to how a person characterizes their emotional and sexual attraction to others. Terms like "gay," "lesbian," "bisexual," "straight," "asexual," "pansexual," and others are examples of sexual orientations.

Transgender (adj.): Used to describe a person's identity or experience when gender identity and assigned sex at birth do not correspond. Also used as an umbrella term to include gender identities outside of male and female. Sometimes abbreviated as trans.

Queer (adj.): An umbrella term used by some to describe people who think of their sexual orientation and/or gender identity as outside of societal norms. Some people view the term "queer" as more fluid and inclusive than traditional categories for sexual orientation and gender identity. Due to its history as a derogatory term, the term "queer" is not embraced or used by all members of the SGM community.

## Health Disparities in SGM Populations

Sexual and gender minority individuals experience a startling number of health disparities, from access and insurance to various mental health diagnoses and even physical conditions like cardiovascular disease and sexually transmitted infections (STIs). These disparities are distributed unevenly across the many identities and lived experiences that are condensed into acronyms like "SGM" or "LGBTQ." Many sources have indicated that the most acute disparities are found in gender minority populations, which have been given particular consideration in this chapter.

In an effort to understand gender minority disparities, the National Transgender Discrimination Survey (NTDS) was conducted in 2008–2009 [3]. This survey was the first of its kind to comprehensively examine health, healthcare, and other experiences (e.g., employment, housing) of the gender minority population within the USA. In 2015, the US Transgender Survey (USTS) added to the data of the NTDS and was the largest survey of gender minority people in the USA, including more than 27,000 individuals in all 50 states and US territories. Comparisons of results from both surveys evidenced improvements in disparities for some areas, while demonstrating no changes or worsening disparities in other areas. Nevertheless, results of the USTS 2015 survey showed alarmingly high rates of inequality, discrimination, and harassment in all areas of life: housing, employment, education, personal/family life, health and healthcare, encounters with the criminal justice system, and others.

The USTS 2015 survey revealed high rates of violence and victimization perpetrated against gender minority people by their families, employers and coworkers, law enforcement officials, and even their healthcare providers. Elevated rates of unemployment and homelessness, as well as low rates of health insurance coverage, were exacerbated by an absence of legal protections for gender minority people within many of these settings. Research has begun to examine the interrelationships among these variables and has suggested that the presence of one places an individual at greater risk for another. For example, homelessness increases the risk of victimization, such as physical and sexual assault. These data point to an all-too-common experience of trauma by gender minority people. One of the most remarkable results in the USTS was a strikingly high rate of suicide by gender minority people, nearly half having attempted suicide in their lifetime and 7% in the past year. This tragic reality is indelibly linked to the experiences of marginalization, stress, and traumatization.

While a comprehensive survey and collection of health data, such as the USTS, has not been conducted with sexual minority people in the USA, research has consistently documented disparities for this group as well. For example, Corliss et al. [4] reported that sexual minority youth are more likely to be homeless than their heterosexual counterparts and that this disparity increases sexual minority youth's risk of violence, substance use, and mental health problems [4]. Balsam et al. found that sexual minority people are not only at greater risk of victimization in childhood but across the entire life span [1]. Additionally, Roberts and colleagues found that sexual minority people are at greater risk of posttraumatic stress disorder (PTSD) than heterosexual people and that elevated rates of childhood abuse for sexual minority individuals account for much of this burden [5]. Lastly, a recent study by Hart and colleagues showed that both childhood trauma and stressors for sexual minority men were associated with adult psychological distress [6]. Taken as a whole, these results highlight both the increased prevalence and risk of victimization for sexual minority people, as well as the specific impact such experiences have on mental health.

This impact is far reaching, even into the realms of physical illness. Sexual minority men account for the majority of new HIV diagnoses in the USA, particularly young gay and bisexual men of color [7]. For transgender women, the prevalence of HIV is even more staggering: a 2012 meta-analysis by Baral et al. suggested it may be as high as 22% [8]. Herbst et al. demonstrated, also in a meta-analysis, the inequality of affliction, with 56% of black transwomen testing positive for HIV [9]. Substance abuse diagnoses, along with depression and anxiety disorders, are also slightly more common in the SGM community than the general population [10]. Even heart disease, stroke, asthma, cancer, chronic pain, and other physical conditions are more common in sexual minorities, though certainly not uniformly across different identities or the entire life span [11, 12]. Taken together, these data point to a constellation of unhealthy coping mechanisms, limited public health outreach, inadequate access to consistent healthcare, and a physiological stress response that predisposes sexual and gender minorities to certain health problems.

Formal theoretical models have been proposed to explain these disparities, which also provide a conceptual framework for the etiology and treatment of the same. Meyer's Minority Stress Model [13, 14] and its extension, the Gender Minority Stress Model [15], posit that SGM individuals experience chronic stress as a result of having a marginalized identity (or identities) that exists within a larger context that imposes stigma and discrimination against that identity. As a result, SGM people are simply more vulnerable and at greater risk for mental and medical health issues. Regarding gender minority identities in particular, Sloan, Berke, and Shipherd extended these models and proposed that the larger social context actively invalidates gender minority identities and experiences in various ways, including ignoring and failing to acknowledge these identities and even actively punishing them (e.g., discrimination) [16]. This chronic and pervasive invalidation negatively impacts the marginalized individual, who in turn may reasonably develop unhealthy coping mechanisms and more complex forms of distress (e.g., chronic suicidal behavior). This increased distress and associated expression likely elicits further invalidation (e.g., negative responses) from the environment, often marked by further stigmatization of the identities and/or blaming of the identity for the manifestations of distress [17]. Arguably, this model could also be applied to sexual minority people as well, given the ongoing stigmatization and invalidation of these identities, with one the most extreme forms of invalidation being interpersonal violence and victimization.

These theoretical models highlight the importance of the larger socio-cultural-political context and its impact on the physical and mental health of SGM people. Chap. 1 of this volume defines trauma (e.g., sexual assault), which is differentiated from general stress (e.g., getting fired), both of which may be experienced by SGM people within the aforementioned context. Additionally, SGM people may also experience unique stressors and trauma based on identity. For example, a gender minority person may be misgendered (i.e., addressed with the incorrect pronoun or name), which we can consider to be a "stressor"; a sexual minority person may suffer a physical assault due to their identity, which we might consider to be a "trauma." Regardless of the experience type, marginalization, stigma, discrimination, and trauma all contribute to increased rates of mental and physical health problems [14, 15, 17].

Perhaps king among the direct mental health consequences of trauma is PTSD. Not all victims of trauma will develop PTSD or struggle with recovery [18]; in fact, it has even been suggested that 92% of people who meet criteria at some point for PTSD will ultimately remit [19]. However, evidence has also indicated that remission is less likely when symptoms stem from childhood trauma and/or interpersonal violence, both of which are elevated in the SGM community [1, 20]. Furthermore, it has been suggested that complex childhood sexual trauma predicts PTSD, substance use, and risky sexual behavior in sexual minority men, providing a direct link between past trauma and physical illness in adulthood [17]. Additionally, a SGM-unique and specific risk factor for PTSD symptoms has also been noted, which is concealment of identity, a stressor specific to the SGM community and one that has been shown to relate to interpersonal problems [21] and increased mental health symptoms [22, 23].

As mentioned above, SGM people are at greater risk of experiencing violence and victimization compared to their cisgender and heterosexual counterparts. This violence may be perpetrated by an intimate partner, which is more common in many sexual minority groups than in their heterosexual counterparts [24]. It also may be perpetrated specifically because of a perceived identity (e.g., a hate crime), which is common and has been shown to contribute to complex and more severe symptomatology [25]. In fact, when controlling for discrimination, mental health disparities between sexual minority and heterosexual individuals diminish, which highlights the apparent effect of such stigma and its manifestation on the health of sexual minority people [26]. Collectively, these findings suggest that SGM people who are able and willing to seek healthcare services may be more likely to present with histories of trauma and significant stressors, possibly with unhealthy coping mechanisms, symptoms consistent with PTSD [27], or difficulties with behavioral and emotional regulation [16].

## Healthcare as a Stressor

SGM patients experience high rates of stressors across the life span outside of the healthcare setting [28–30]. Unfortunately, many healthcare settings may actually exacerbate stress, unknowingly prompting SGM persons to avoid care or risk distress [30–32]. Given this community's documented risk for marginalization, healthcare organizations must examine the current and historical practices that result in stress to patients.

Historically, SGM individuals have been condemned by the medical community, which labeled their identities as pathology. Homosexuality was listed as a mental disorder in the first three series of the Diagnostic and Statistical Manual of Mental Disorders, and medical doctors were charged with "fixing" LGBT individuals through treatment. In 1973, homosexuality was removed from the DSM with much debate and contention. Even though homosexuality has been declassified as a mental disorder, some mental health professionals and religious leaders continue to affirm that homosexual "tendencies" or "behaviors" can be removed and replaced with heterosexual ones. The Williams Institute estimates that nearly 700,000 adults in the USA have received some form of "reparative" or "conversion" therapy, many during psychologically vulnerable periods of childhood and adolescence [33]. The American Psychological Association [34], the American Medical Association (reaffirmed 2017) [35], and the National Association of Social Workers [36] have publicly denounced these practices as unethical, unscientific, and harmful to patients. Still, awareness of these practices may cause patients to anticipate negative experiences in healthcare or fear receiving invalidating treatment.

SGM patients may have had personal experiences or heard about stressors perpetrated by medical professionals through their peers. In a landmark report, Lambda Legal documented the frequency with which SGM patients are victimized by providers [31]. Seven percent of LGB participants and 26% of transgender and gender nonconforming (TGNC) persons reported being denied care outright. Eleven percent of sexual minorities reported that medical professionals either refused to touch them or used precautions in touching them that were excessive. Seven percent of TGNC respondents reported experiencing physically rough or abusive treatment from a healthcare professional. These findings were echoed in the USTS, in which 23% of the 27,000 respondents reported postponing medical care due to fear of mistreatment [3]. Of respondents who had seen a provider in the past year, one-third had experienced at least one negative interaction.

Medical providers have also been placed in the role of gatekeeping for TGNC individuals. Past editions of the World Professional Association for Transgender Health (WPATH) Standards of Care [37] and the Endocrine Treatment of Transsexual Persons [38] have discouraged providers from offering hormone therapy until patients have documented lengthy "real-life experiences" as their desired gender, have received letters of approval or attestation from mental health professionals, and many other long and costly barriers. Though recent guidelines have liberalized these requirements, some providers still practice under a more traditional, conservative model. This form of "gatekeeping" may discourage or preclude TGNC patients from accessing care—turning them instead to illicit sources for hormones or consigning them to remain in a gender incongruent body—and contribute to a mistrust of healthcare providers.

Effective patient-provider relationships require trust, the foundation of which is effective, humble, and empathetic communication. In order to be vulnerable with providers about their identities, patients must be confident in the provider's capacity for ethical care: including competence in modern care practices that are validating of their identity. Healthcare's long history of prejudice and outmoded systems of diagnosis may undermine open patient-provider communication and leave many sexual and gender minorities apprehensive about disclosing important facts about themselves in a healthcare setting.

## Current Status of Medical Competencies in SGM Care

A patient's presentation to care as their authentic self is only as effective as their caregiver's knowledge about SGM health. Many providers may lack education and comfort with issues related to a patient's SGM identity. Medical schools, leaders in healthcare training, have the opportunity to be beacons of knowledge and innovation in SGM health. Yet in one large survey, Obedin-Maliver found that most medical schools offer students few hours of SGM health training, some with no SGM-specific training at all [39]. Additional studies have found fewer training hours in pharmacy [40] and dental schools [41], as well as public health [42] and physician assistant programs [43].

When affirmative care practices are taught in medical settings, the effect is overwhelmingly positive. Exposure to SGM individuals increases medical students' self-reported positive attitudes about working with SGM [44]. Sanchez et al. [44] noted that exposure to SGM patients improves comfort with taking sexual histories and genitourinary exams, as well as increases the frequency with which medical students collect a sexual history. Sanchez and colleagues' finding has been replicated in a large study of first-year medical students in the USA [45]. White et al. [46] reported that education about SGM people in medical school makes students feel more prepared to care for these patients. Limited available data suggest that physician residency programs lack education hours dedicated to SGM health [47], leaving many physicians without any formal education in the care of SGM patients [48].

## *Documentation*

Many healthcare organizations continue to use outdated forms and assessments with gender-specific language with limited selections on questions concerning gender identity, sex, and sexual orientation. Sections that involve obstetric, gynecologic, or cancer histories may be designated as for "females only" or "males only," discouraging patients from reporting important information if their current gender identity or disorder of sexual development does not align with a binary category. Electronic health records (EHR) may additionally perpetuate the misgendering of patients, as gender markers are often difficult to find or change in the EHR. Patients' names and self-labels may be displayed incorrectly, and the health record may further lack prompts for appropriate health maintenance tasks (e.g., breast exams for transwomen, appropriate STI testing intervals for gay and bisexual men) and lab values.

## *Identity Disclosure and Privacy*

Patients made uncomfortable or uncertain by the healthcare environment may allow providers to assume that they are not a SGM person. Research indicates that nearly 30% of gay and bisexual men are not out to their primary care physicians, choosing instead to allow their provider to believe they are heterosexual [49, 50]. The avoidance of disclosure may preclude important medical conversations, preventing proper screening and counseling. Unfortunately, minority, low-income, and rural gay and bisexual men seem to be particularly susceptible to assumed heterosexuality, a problem that may be compounding health disparities in these communities [50].

Providers may also believe that the experiences of one SGM patient are overly generalizable to other SGM patients. Providers may confuse terms or questions about sexual health between sexual orientation and gender identity and apply them inappropriately to particular patients. When providers learn that their patients are SGM, they may overpathologize findings. Of particular concern, they may even blame the patient for their illness. Lambda Legal (2010) found that more than 12% of LGB respondents, 20% of TGNC respondents, and 26% of people with HIV reported being blamed for their own health conditions [31].

Additionally, providers may consider sexual orientation and gender as static identities, neglecting the fluidity of these constructs that may change with age, relationship status, and developmental stage. Ignorance of the fluidity of patients' identities may invalidate those for whom fluidity is a central feature (e.g., pansexual, gender fluid) or are in the process of transitioning between two identities [51]. Research by Rusow et al. [52] also reveals that sexual minority youth who adopt a nontraditional label or who changed labels over time were more likely to endorse histories of suicidal ideation and anxiety than youth who identified with a stable sexual minority label. These findings indicate a need for providers to share curiosity and explore labels with patients, rather than assume a patient's self-labels as they relate to identity. Empowering dialogues with patients about their understanding of their gender and sexuality can promote acceptance and self-confidence.

Patients may have privacy concerns over disclosure of stigmatizing information such as their sexual and gender identity. Therefore, how providers communicate with patients and families are both major concerns for patients. Disclosing one's identity may be part of the journey for SGM in safe contexts. In psychotherapy, in fact, disclosure may be the focus of treatment before someone moves forward with gender affirmation surgery. However, it can be distressing for someone's gender identity to be disclosed to their family without their consent. Young people, in particular, who disclose their identity in unsupportive environments, may be at risk of neglect, violence, and homelessness [53].

## Best Practices for Providers and Healthcare Systems

### Best Practices for SGM Patients

We have clearly shown that sexual and gender minority individuals are disproportionately burdened by the experience of stress, trauma, and many forms of violence and may be reticent to seek care and disclose personal information to their provider [3, 24, 54]. It is our recommendation that healthcare agencies be cognizant of the myriad ways that trauma influences the experience of and recovery from illness and utilize trauma-informed care principles to engage patients and enhance clinical efficacy. These agencies must seek to build trauma-informed care principles into everyday clinical processes for the benefit of all patients, while working to create intentionally welcoming spaces that facilitate disclosure of SGM identities and the provision of needed services.

## Screening for Trauma

Healthcare providers should consider routine screening for intimate partner violence for all sexual and gender minority patients. Additional research is needed to validate specific screening strategies and interventions, but standardized tools like the "HITS," a four-item questionnaire designed to determine if patients have been hurt, insulted, threatened with harm, or had a partner scream at them, can be easily administered and is appropriately neutral of assumptions about relationship type [55–57]. There are no data to support routine screening for other forms of trauma or violence in adults, including bias crime or police violence, but these may be discussed with patients when such forms of trauma are suspected by a clinician.

## Clinical Environment

A welcoming clinical environment is a critical component of encouraging SGM patients to seek care, disclose their identities and other relevant health information, and remain effectively engaged in care [58, 59]. Waiting rooms should prominently display representative imagery of SGM patients, with attention to intersectional identities of race, disability, age, gender, and religious symbolism. Small visual cues like rainbow or transgender pride flags or badge pins, signs that indicate a "safe space" or encourage patients to offer their pronouns, or a prominently displayed nondiscrimination policy, are simple and powerful invitations.

For gender minority patients, restroom location may be a source of significant anxiety, fearing being reprimanded or accused of wrongdoing by staff or other patients when using a bathroom consistent with their gender identity; in some states, this may even mean violating laws that restrict bathroom use not by gender identity but by sex assigned at birth [3]. Medical facilities should strongly consider designating a set of accessible bathrooms as gender neutral; in facilities where this capacity is limited by state or municipal regulations, clinics should display signage encouraging patients to use the restrooms most consistent with their gender identity [60]. Providers can serve as important resources, particularly when they are able to direct gender minority patients to gender-neutral bathrooms or provide maps of bathroom locations, both of which may help patients feel welcome in an unfamiliar space and less anxious about using restrooms.

## Personnel

Clinical personnel are uniquely situated to create a welcoming—or alienating—environment for SGM patients. Affirming providers will consistently use the patient's self-identified name and pronouns. Front desk and nursing staff, who may be calling patients from waiting areas, should be aware that names on insurance documents and in the EHR may not accurately reflect the patient's identified name. It is recommended that when the patient is in a public waiting area, they be addressed as indicated by the last name in the patient's chart. Once in a private space with the provider, the provider may ask the patient for name and pronouns and whether they are comfortable being addressed by these on the phone or in public spaces. These should be solicited at initial contact and documented in a visible location for subsequent points of contact between the patient and healthcare system. Open discussions between providers and SGM patients regarding these important components of care are strongly recommended.

Affirming providers can also use gender-neutral language in the collection of a clinical history. For example, when assessing relationship status, in lieu of using gendered terms like "wife" or "boyfriend," providers (and assessment forms) can use terms like "partner." Providers should work to respect differences of sexuality and gender identity or expression and, if unsure of terminology, may ask the patient to clarify, without judging or imposing personal beliefs on the patient. Providers should not assume that a patient is heterosexual and cisgender. Patients may use unique language to describe their identities and bodies including genital organs, which should be mirrored by the provider. However, providers may wish to consider further assessment if patients use pejorative or denigrating terms to describe themselves.

Patients who identify as transgender or any other identity consistent with a gender minority identity (e.g., genderqueer) should additionally be encouraged to complete an organ inventory in order to guide cancer screening and STI testing but only if it is anticipated to be relevant to the current visit. Providers should neither perseverate about the patient's genital organs nor conduct invasive components of the physical exam unless specifically clinically indicated. Transgender patients may not wish to be subjected to inspection of dysphoria-inducing organs and may be biologically predisposed to difficult exams (e.g., transmen taking testosterone frequently experience vaginal atrophy, making speculum insertion very uncomfortable) [61]. Additionally, nearly one-half of all transgender people are survivors of sexual violence, so the benefit to clinical decision-making must be carefully balanced against the risk of re-traumatization [3].

If sensitive exams are indicated, greet the patient when they are clothed and explain the rationale for each component of the exam. For example, a physician conducting a pelvic exam for a pap smear might describe the process step by step, highlighting the way each step might feel, and why each step is necessary (e.g., "the speculum is to help me find and visually inspect the cervix," "this swab will collect cells that we can examine for the features of early cancer"). Providers should offer the option to have a chaperone, friend, or family member accompany the patient or the use of headphones or other distraction techniques (e.g., a mobile device, magazine, or book). Alternatively, some patients may prefer to observe or participate in the exam. Reassure patients that they are in control of the exam and that they may stop or change the plan at any time. These practices can be implemented in both outpatient and inpatient settings, and many can be used for patients with limited decision-making capacity (e.g., when caring for involuntarily committed or incarcerated persons). When invasive tests are indicated (e.g., swabs for gonorrhoeae and chlamydia), patients should be offered the option to self-collect specimens, which are equivalent in validity to provider-collected specimens and acceptable to most patients [62]. Providers must be familiar with evidence-based recommendations for mental and physical health screening and counseling, as well as local SGM-competent resources for referral if necessary.

## Healthcare System

All healthcare systems should offer comprehensive cultural competency training to clinical and nonclinical staff, providers, and trainees, specifically relevant to SGM health and care. This might be delivered in-person or online via a learning management system but is recommended to be mandatory for new hires (or existing employees at initial implementation) and repeated every few years, as education and terminology are always evolving. Clinical departments should supplement this with additional opportunities where it pertains to their patient population and clinical services and as necessary following complaints. Examples of trainings are available to view with a free account at lgbthealtheducation.org.

Healthcare systems should take a nuanced approach to gendered services like trauma survivor support groups or "men's health" or "women's health" events. These should include patients based on current gender identity and the need being met; for example, the experience of violence in a transgender woman might be congruent with cisgender female peers and the patient best supported in a women's survivor group.

Healthcare systems with sufficient resources should additionally seek to expand the repertoire of clinical services available to SGM patients. Gender-diverse adults and adolescents may be candidates for gender-affirming hormone therapy, which can be prescribed by a variety of adequately trained providers [37]. Mental health organizations may facilitate gender-affirming therapies by hiring or training mental health professionals with specific interest in evaluating and supporting these patients.

Surgical interventions for gender affirmation are complex, and only some patients choose to pursue them [3]. They are ideally accomplished by an interdisciplinary team with specialized training in the panoply of considerations for these interventions. If appropriately trained specialists are unavailable within one healthcare system, organizations should seek to develop a referral network for patients desiring these therapies.

## Documentation and the Electronic Health Record

Intake documents should be updated to reflect modern, gender-neutral language [63]. This includes collecting sexual orientation and gender identity (SO/GI) data in three steps, which allows patients to identify (1) sexual orientation separately from (2) gender identity and (3) sex assigned at birth. This method has been studied and found to be a robust means of data collection and acceptable to patients [64–66]. Questions should be formatted (e.g., write-in fields for multiple choice or forgoing multiple choice options for blank spaces) to allow patients to identify with any of the multitude of terms used to describe gender and sexuality, a practice which affirms diverse identities.

The EHR should possess the capacity to display chosen name and pronouns prominently; we recommend that clinical staff be trained to collect and document this information in a consistent and visible location in the EHR. The necessary training, including example language for encounters and forms, can be provided to personnel along with a comprehensive cultural competency training.

Automated reminders for providers to conduct specific health screenings (e.g., HIV screening, mammography, and colon cancer screening) should be adapted to reflect differences in recommendations for SGM patients, particularly regarding periodicity. Automated reminders for gender minority patients should account for sex assigned at birth, gender identity, organs present, and duration of gender-affirming hormone therapies (if relevant). For instance, the EHR might offer an alert for breast cancer screening for a 60-year-old transgender woman with a lengthy history of estrogen usage, but not for a 60-year-old transgender man who has undergone mastectomy.

Organizations that provide care to children and adolescents should be aware of state regulations governing the privacy of medical records, so as not to unintentionally "out" patients to their legal guardians. They should also be cognizant that parents may see notes and "private" communications to patients via patient portals and be aware of what is provided to parents who request paper copies of records.

## Outreach and Visibility

Sexual and gender minorities are conspicuously absent from the marketing and outreach campaigns of many healthcare organizations. SGM patients seeking affirming care will notice inclusive language and imagery visible in online policies and statements and other literature. Many healthcare organizations provide a list of providers who identify as sexual or gender minorities and/or those with particular expertise in SGM health [67, 68]. This allows patients to see their community reflected in the healthcare system and seek care from clinicians who may better understand their lived experiences. Providers with specific knowledge about SGM health may additionally choose to identify themselves with the Gay and Lesbian Medical Association (http://www.glma.org/) or a similar entity.

Limited evidence suggests that SGM people are at least as likely as their heterosexual counterparts to interact with the healthcare system using health information technology [69, 70]. This includes scheduling appointments, filling prescriptions, and accessing health information. A lack of representation of minority groups may discourage patients from seeking care in a healthcare system [71]. It may also lead SGM patients to assume that no providers in the system will be able to meet their specific needs. Systems should capitalize on digital patient interactions by improving the representation of SGM patients in outreach material; highlighting SGM patients in pictures and bios on websites; using same-sex or queer couples in brochures, posters, and ads; announcing LGBT holidays; and using symbols like rainbow and trans-pride flags.

Other forms of outreach can also encourage SGM individuals to seek care within a particular system. For instance, sponsorship and participation in community events (e.g., pride celebrations, SGM sports leagues, health fairs) allows direct contact with potential patients and signals a commitment to equitable healthcare. Similarly, brochures, print advertisements, and television and radio spots are all opportunities to market both the services available and that the clinical environment is welcoming to SGM patients.

Systems should strive to hire and support SGM employees, with inclusion of SGM language in statements of equal employment opportunity. Hospitals and clinics should explicitly include "sexual orientation, gender identity, and gender expression" in nondiscrimination policies, harassment prevention, and reporting protocols.

## Exemplary Systems

A limited, but growing, number of healthcare systems have worked to enhance outreach and improve the clinical care provided to sexual and gender minority patients. Three of these systems are highlighted below. They vary in scale from a few providers to a few hundred facilities, embody different approaches and strengths, and illustrate the many ways in which an agent of healthcare—nurse, CEO, or entire hospital—can address the stress and trauma experienced by SGM individuals.

### *Veterans Health Administration*

The Veterans Health Administration (VHA) was the largest participant in the Human Rights Campaign's Healthcare Equality Index (HEI) 2017, a stringent evaluation of nearly 600 healthcare facilities in the USA with SGM-inclusive policies. With 101 participating facilities, the VHA handily outpaces its nearest rival, Kaiser Permanente, with only 38 participating facilities. The HEI evaluates each of these in four domains: nondiscrimination and staff training, patient services and support, employee benefits and policies, and patient and community engagement [72]. Of these 101, 85 were considered to be either a "Top Performer" or "Leader in LGBTQ Healthcare Equality," largely under VHA Directives 1340 and 2013-003, which ensure "clinically appropriate, comprehensive, Veteran-centered care with respect and dignity" to sexual minority and gender minority patients, respectively [73, 74]. These Directives include nondiscriminatory definitions of "family" and extend equal visitation rights to SGM patients at VHA hospitals. They also ensure a safe and confidential environment for disclosure and documentation of SGM identities, as well as the availability of appropriate clinical services (by referral if necessary). Patients are offered extensive guidance about specific healthcare needs and disparities in a series of "Get the Facts…" fact sheets [75]. Notably, LGBT Programs, which consist of a LGBT Veteran Care Coordinator and a number of SGM-specific resources, are available at 51 VHA facilities in 29 states [76].

The VHA also espouses a comprehensive Equal Employment Opportunity (EEO) policy (Directive 5975) and offers helpful guidance to particular groups, like transgender employees undergoing transition [77]. The VHA is unable to provide any gender-affirming surgeries ("sex reassignment surgery") as of the time of this writing, an indication that even exemplars have room to grow.

## *Fenway Health*

Fenway Health is a small system, just three clinics in Boston, MA, that was founded to serve a diverse mix of low-income residents, SGM people, students, and seniors. As a leader in HIV care and research since the earliest days of the pandemic, Fenway also pioneered the integration of holistic health practices into their care for a community ravaged by infection. Over time, the system has evolved to offer an incredibly robust array of clinical services, with a particular focus on SGM patients. Their offerings include the full spectrum of gender-affirming therapies, mental health, and specialty services like dermatology, podiatry, dentistry, gynecology, and optometry in addition to primary care.

Of particular note is the Violence Recovery Program, a bilingual support, counseling, and advocacy program for sexual and gender minority trauma survivors [78]. The program's mission encompasses survivors of intimate partner violence, bias crimes, and police misconduct and strives to offer trainings and consultation with other service providers in addition to direct patient care. Fenway Health collaborates with a number of other Boston-area agencies (the Hispanic Black Gay Coalition, The Network/La Red, and Renewal House of the Unitarian Universalist Urban Ministry) in a program called TOD@S, a prevention and intervention project for Black and Latinx community members affected by partner abuse [79]. Free services include English as a second language classes, social events, counseling, emergency housing, case management, and a 24-hour hotline. The program also conducts community education and offers technical assistance to other service providers.

Fenway's reach also extends far beyond its original mission as a community health clinic. The Fenway Institute is the system's education, research, and advocacy branch, which hosts the National LGBT Health Education Center [80]. This library of training videos, modules, and documents is an up-to-date and evidence-based SGM health resource that is accessible for free by any healthcare provider or trainee. The Institute also houses the LGBT Aging Project and an annual Transgender Health Conference and has a long publication record on scientific topics ranging from aging with HIV [81] to the relationship of sexual orientation to asthma [82] and the acceptability by patients of SO/GI data collection [66].

## *Duke Child and Adolescent Gender Care Clinic*

This Duke Health specialty clinic has been treating children and adolescents who experience gender dysphoria, identify as transgender or gender fluid, or have difference of sex development since the clinic opened in 2015 [83]. The clinic is one of only a handful like it in the southeast and has rapidly become a popular referral center with an impressively large patient population—new patients can expect to spend a few months on a waitlist before being seen [72]. However, the wait is a small price to pay for the clinic's impressive array of evidence-based, family-centered services.

Each patient receives a thorough evaluation from a multidisciplinary team comprising a pediatric endocrinologist, pediatric urologist, pediatric psychologist, adolescent medicine specialist, and social worker. This team can then prescribe medications that suppress puberty (giving the patient more time to explore their gender) or gender-affirming hormones. Though Duke Health doesn't perform gender-affirming surgeries, the clinic can facilitate surgical consultation elsewhere. The clinic leadership espouses a dedication to holistic care as well; they coordinate with aestheticians to facilitate the "look" of a patient's identified gender, community voice specialists to provide vocal coaching, and even specialized gender coaches to instruct patients in the social nuances of gendered behaviors. The clinic capitalizes on the expertise of the Duke School of Law to assist patients with changing the gender markers on birth certificate and passports.

In addition to clinical offerings, the faculty seek to enroll patients in research studies that could benefit the community at large. The clinic also utilizes a family advisory panel to engage with their patients' communities and crowdsource ideas for how to best support families [84]. Clinic leadership also advocates for the community they serve; Dr. Deanna Adkins, the clinic's founding pediatric endocrinologist, was a vocal opponent of North Carolina's oppressive House Bill 2, which restricted bathroom access for transgender people across the state [85].

## Conclusion

In this chapter, we have shown that for sexual and gender minority people, there are many reasons to use trauma-informed care principles in clinical settings. For these patients, trauma, victimization, violence, and the experience of stress may take immense tolls on emotional and physical well-being. We have highlighted the risks of marginalization and judgment that sexual and gender minorities take when presenting to the healthcare system and also offered solutions for fostering a welcoming environment. Professionals across the healthcare system can make a difference for sexual and gender minorities by seeking out education, implementing solutions pioneered by other healthcare systems, and advocating for SGM health in their organizations.

# References

1. Balsam KF, Rothblum ED, Beauchaine TP. Victimization over the life span: a comparison of lesbian, gay, bisexual, and heterosexual siblings. J Consult Clin Psychol. 2005;73(3):477.
2. Glossary of LGBT Terms for Health Care Teams. National LGBT Health Education Center. Last updated July 2017. Accessed 8 June 2018. Available from: https://www.lgbthealtheducation.org/wp-content/uploads/2018/03/Glossary-2018-English-update-1.pdf.
3. James SE, Herman JL, Rankin S, Keisling M, Mottet L, Anafi M. The report of the 2015 US transgender survey. National Center for Transgender Equality 2016. Accessed 30 May 2018. Available from: https://transequality.org/sites/default/files/docs/usts/USTS-Full-Report-Dec17.pdf.
4. Corliss HL, Goodenow CS, Nichols L, Austin SB. High burden of homelessness among sexual-minority adolescents: findings from a representative Massachusetts high school sample. Am J Public Health. 2011;101(9):1683–9.
5. Roberts AL, Rosario M, Corliss HL, Koenen KC, Austin SB. Elevated risk of posttraumatic stress in sexual minority youths: mediation by childhood abuse and gender nonconformity. Am J Public Health. 2012;102(8):1587–93.
6. Hart TA, Noor SW, Vernon JR, Kidwai A, Roberts K, Myers T, et al. Childhood maltreatment, bullying victimization, and psychological distress among gay and bisexual men. J Sex Res. 2018;55(4–5):604–16.
7. HIV in the United States: at a glance. Centers for Disease Control and Prevention. Updated November 2017. Accessed 8 June 2018. Available from: https://www.cdc.gov/hiv/statistics/overview/ataglance.html.
8. Baral SD, Poteat T, Stromdahl S, Wirts AL, Guadamuz TE, Beyrer C. Worldwide burden of HIV in transgender women: a systematic review and meta-analysis. Lancet Infect Dis. 2013;13(3):214–22.
9. Herbst JH, Jacobs ED, Finlayson TJ, McKleroy VS, Neumann MS, Crepaz N. Estimating HIV prevalence and risk behaviors of transgender persons in the United States: a systematic review. AIDS Behav. 2008;12(1):1–17.
10. King M, Semlyen J, Tai SS, Killapsy H, Osborn D, Popelyuk D, Nazarareth I. A systematic review of mental disorder, suicide, and deliberate self-harm in lesbian, gay and bisexual people. BMC Psychiatry. 2008;8(70)
11. Fredriksen-Goldsen KI, Kim H-J, Shui C, Bryan AEB. Chronic health conditions and key health indicators among lesbian, gay, and bisexual older US adults, 2013–2014. Am J Public Health. 2017;107(8):1332–8. https://doi.org/10.2105/AJPH.2017.303922.
12. Conron KJ, Mimiaga MJ, Landers SJ. A population-based study of sexual orientation identity and gender differences in adult health. Am J Public Health. 2010;100(10):1953–60. https://doi.org/10.2105/AJPH.2009.174169.
13. Meyer IH. Minority stress and mental health in gay men. J Health Soc Behav. 1995;1:38–56.
14. Meyer IH. Prejudice, social stress, and mental health in lesbian, gay, and bisexual populations: conceptual issues and research evidence. Psychol Bull. 2003;129(5):674–97.
15. Hendricks ML, Testa RJ. A conceptual framework for clinical work with transgender and gender nonconforming clients: an adaptation of the minority stress model. Prof Psychol Res Pract. 2012;43(5):460.
16. Sloan CA, Berke DS, Shipherd JC. Utilizing a dialectical framework to inform conceptualization and treatment of clinical distress in transgender individuals. Prof Psychol Res Pract. 2017;48(5):301.
17. Boroughs MS, Valentine SE, Ironson GH, Shipherd JC, Safren SA, Taylor SW, et al. Complexity of childhood sexual abuse: predictors of current post-traumatic stress disorder, mood disorders, substance use, and sexual risk behavior among adult men who have sex with men. Arch Sex Behav. 2015;44(7):1891–902.

18. Butler LD, Critelli FM, Rinfrette ES. Trauma-informed care and mental health. Dir Psychiatry. 2011;31(3):197–212.
19. Chapman C, Mills K, Slade T, McFarlane AC, Bryant RA, Creamer M, Silove D, Teesson M. Remission from post-traumatic stress disorder in the general population. Psychol Med. 2012;42(8):1695–703.
20. Roberts AL, Austin SB, Corliss HL, Vandermorris AK, Koenen KC. Pervasive trauma exposure among US sexual orientation minority adults and risk of posttraumatic stress disorder. Am J Public Health. 2010;100(12):2433–41.
21. Newheiser AK, Barreto M. Hidden costs of hiding stigma: ironic interpersonal consequences of concealing a stigmatized identity in social interactions. J Exp Soc Psychol. 2014;52:58–70.
22. Pachankis JE. The psychological implications of concealing a stigma: a cognitive-affective-behavioral model. Psychol Bull. 2007;133(2):328.
23. Cochran BN, Balsam K, Flentje A, Malte CA, Simpson T. Mental health characteristics of sexual minority veterans. J Homosex. 2013;60(2–3):419–35.
24. Walters ML, Chen J, Breiding MJ. The National Intimate Partner and Sexual Violence Survey (NISVS): 2010 findings on victimization by sexual orientation. National Center for Injury Prevention and Control, Centers for Disease Control and Prevention. 2013. Accessed 8 June 2018. Available from: https://www.cdc.gov/violenceprevention/pdf/nisvs_sofindings.pdf.
25. Herek GM, Gillis JR, Cogan JC. Psychological sequelae of hate-crime victimization among lesbian, gay, and bisexual adults. J Consult Clin Psychol. 1999;67(6):945.
26. Mays VM, Cochran SD. Mental health correlates of perceived discrimination among lesbian, gay, and bisexual adults in the United States. Am J Public Health. 2001;91(11):1869–76.
27. Mustanski B, Andrews R, Puckett JA. The effects of cumulative victimization on mental health among lesbian, gay, bisexual, and transgender adolescents and young adults. Am J Public Health. 2016;106(3):527–33.
28. Andersen JP, Blosnich J. Disparities in adverse childhood experiences among sexual minority and heterosexual adults: results from a multi-state probability-based sample. Chao L, ed. PLoS One. 2013;8(1):e54691. https://doi.org/10.1371/journal.pone.0054691.
29. Brotman S, Ryan B, Cormier R. The health and social service needs of gay and lesbian elders and their families in Canada. Gerontologist. 2003;43(2):192–202.
30. Ray CM, Tyler KA, Simons L. Risk factors for forced, incapacitated, and coercive sexual victimization among sexual minority and heterosexual male and female college students. J Interpers Violence. 2018. https://doi.org/10.1177/0886260518758332.
31. When health care isn't caring: Lambda legal's survey of discrimination against LGBT people and people with HIV. Lambda legal. 2010. Accessed 1 June 2018. Available from: www.lambdalegal.org/health-care-report.
32. Waters E. Lesbian, gay, bisexual, transgender, queer, and HIV-affected hate violence in 2016. National Coalition of Anti-Violence Programs (NCAVP). 2016. Accessed 1 June 2018. Available from: https://avp.org/wp-content/uploads/2017/06/NCAVP_2016HateViolence_REPORT.pdf.
33. Mallory C, Brown TNT, Conron KJ. Conversion therapy and LGBT youth. The Williams Institute. 2018. Accessed 1 June 2018. Available from: https://williamsinstitute.law.ucla.edu/wp-content/uploads/Conversion-Therapy-LGBT-Youth-Jan-2018.pdf.
34. Report of the American Psychological Association Task Force on Appropriate Therapeutic Responses to Sexual Orientation. American Psychological Association, Task Force on appropriate therapeutic responses to sexual orientation. 2009. Accessed 1 June 2018. Available from: http://www.apa.org/pi/lgbc/publications/therapeutic-resp.html.
35. Policies on Lesbian, Gay, Bisexual, Transgender & Queer (LGBTQ) Issues. American Medical Association. Accessed 1 June 2018. Available from: https://www.ama-assn.org/delivering-care/policies-lesbian-gay-bisexual-transgender-queer-lgbtq-issues.
36. Sexual Orientation Change Efforts (SOCE) and Conversion therapy with lesbians, gay men, bisexuals, and transgender persons. National Association of Social Workers, National Committee on Lesbian, Gay, Bisexual, and Transgender Issues. 2015. Accessed 1 June 2018.

Available from: https://www.socialworkers.org/LinkClick.aspx?fileticket=IQYALknHU6s%3D&portalid=0.
37. World Professional Association for Transgender Health. Standards of care for the health of transsexual, transgender, and gender nonconforming people. 7th Ed. 2011. Accessed 30 Apr 2018. Available from: https://www.wpath.org/publications/soc.
38. Hembree WC, Cohen-Kettenis P, Delemarre-van de Waal HA, Gooren LJ, Meyer WJ, Spack NP, et al. Endocrine treatment of transsexual persons: an Endocrine Society clinical practice guideline. J Clin Endocrinol Metab. 2009;94(9):3132–54. https://doi.org/10.1210/jc.2009-0345.
39. Obedin-Maliver J, Goldsmith ES, Stewart L, White W, Tran E, Brenman S, et al. Lesbian, gay, bisexual, and transgender–related content in undergraduate medical education. JAMA. 2011;306(9):971–7. https://doi.org/10.1001/jama.2011.1255.
40. Braun HM, Ramirez D, Zahner GJ, Gillis-Buck EM, Sheriff H, Ferrone M. An evaluation of lesbian, gay, bisexual, and transgender (LGBT) health education in pharmacy school curricula. Curr Pharm Teach Learn. 2014;6(6):752–8. https://doi.org/10.1016/j.cptl.2014.08.001.
41. Hillenburg KL, Murdoch-Kinch CA, Kinney JS, Temple H, Inglehart MR. LGBT coverage in U.S. dental schools and dental hygiene programs: results of a national survey. J Dent Educ. 2016;80(12):1440–9.
42. Corliss HL, Shankle MD, Moyer MB. Research, curricula, and resources related to lesbian, gay, bisexual, and transgender health in US schools of public health. Am J Public Health. 2007;97(6):1023–7.
43. Seaborne LA, Prince RJ, Kushner DM. Sexual health education in U.S. physician assistant programs. J Sex Med. 2015;12(5):1158–64. https://doi.org/10.1111/jsm.12879.
44. Sanchez NF. Medical students' ability to care for lesbian, gay, bisexual, and transgendered patients. Fam Med. 2006;38(1):21–7.
45. Burke SE, Dovidio JF, Hovland CI, Przedworski JM, Hardeman RR, Perry SP, et al. Do contact and empathy mitigate bias against gay and lesbian people among heterosexual medical students? A report from medical student CHANGES. Acad Med. 2015;90(5):645–51.
46. White W, Brenman S, Paradis E, Goldsmith ES, Lunn MR, Obedin-Maliver J. Lesbian, gay, bisexual, and transgender patient care: medical students' preparedness and comfort. Teach Learn Med. 2015;27(3):254–63. https://doi.org/10.1080/10401334.2015.1044656.
47. Moll J, Krieger P, Moreno-Walton L, Lee B, Slaven E, James T, et al. The prevalence of lesbian, gay, bisexual, and transgender health education and training in emergency medicine residency programs: what do we know? Acad Emerg Med. 2014;21(5):608–11.
48. Smith DM, Mathews WC. Physicians' attitudes toward homosexuality and HIV: survey of a California Medical Society- revisited (PATHH-II). J Homosex. 2007;52(3–4):1–9.
49. Petroll AE, Mosack KE. Physician awareness of sexual orientation and preventive health recommendations to men who have sex with men. Sex Transm Dis. 2011;38(1):63–7. https://doi.org/10.1097/OLQ.0b013e3181ebd50f.
50. Coleman TA, Bauer GR, Pugh D, Aykroyd G, Powell L, Newman R. Sexual orientation disclosure in primary care settings by gay, bisexual, and other men who have sex with men in a Canadian City. LGBT Health. 2017;4(1):42–54. https://doi.org/10.1089/lgbt.2016.0004.
51. MacDonnell JA, Grigorovich A. Gender, work, and health for trans health providers: a focus on transmen. ISRN Nursing. 2012. https://doi.org/10.5402/2012/161097.
52. Rusow JA, Burgess C, Gibbs J, Goldbach J. The role of supportive adults on sexual minority mental health symptoms and isolating behaviors. Poster presented at the Society for Social Work and Research 20th annual conference, Washington, DC. 2016.
53. Durso LE, Gates GJ. Serving our youth: findings from a national survey of service providers working with lesbian, gay, bisexual, and transgender youth who are homeless or at risk of becoming homeless. The Williams Institute with true colors fund and the palette fund. 2012. Accessed 1 June 2018. Available from: https://williamsinstitute.law.ucla.edu/wp-content/uploads/Durso-Gates-LGBT-Homeless-Youth-Survey-July-2012.pdf.

54. Willis DG. Hate crimes against gay males: an overview. Issues Ment Health Nurs. 2009;25(2):115–32.
55. Feltner C, Wallace I, Berkman N, et al. Screening for intimate partner violence, elder abuse, and abuse of vulnerable adults: evidence report and systematic review for the US preventive services task force. JAMA. 2018;320(16):1688–701. https://doi.org/10.1001/jama.2018.13212.
56. Sherin KM, Sinacore JM, Li XQ, Zitter RE, Shakil A. HITS: a short domestic violence screening tool for use in a family practice setting. Fam Med. 1998;30(7):508–12.
57. Shakil A, Donald S, Sinacore JM, Krepcho M. Validation of the HITS domestic violence screening tool with males. Fam Med. 2005;37(3):193–8.
58. National LGBT Health Education Center. 10 things: creating inclusive health care environments for LGBT People. The Fenway Institute. 2015. Accessed 30 Apr 2018. Available from: https://www.lgbthealtheducation.org/wp-content/uploads/Ten-Things-Brief-Final-WEB.pdf.
59. The Joint Commission. Advancing effective communication, cultural competence, and patient- and family centered care for the lesbian, gay, bisexual, and transgender (LGBT) community: a field guide. 2011. Accessed 30 Apr 2018. Available from: https://www.jointcommission.org/assets/1/18/LGBTFieldGuide_WEB_LINKED_VER.pdf.
60. American Medical Association. Access to basic human services for transgender individuals H-65.964. Last modified 2017. Accessed 30 Apr 2018. Available from: https://policysearch.ama-assn.org/policyfinder/detail/Access%20to%20Basic%20Human%20Services%20for%20Transgender%20Individuals%20H-65.964?uri=%2FAMADoc%2FHOD.xml-H-65.964.xml.
61. Center of Excellence for Transgender Health, Department of Family and Community Medicine, University of California San Francisco. Guidelines for the primary and gender-affirming care of transgender and gender nonbinary people. 2nd ed. Deutsch MB, ed; 2016. Accessed 30 Apr 2018. Available from: www.transhealth.ucsf.edu/guidelines.
62. Workowski KA, Bolan GA. Sexually transmitted disease treatment guidelines, 2015. MMWR Recomm Rep. 2015;64(2):51–65.
63. National LGBT Health Education Center. Focus on forms and policy: creating an inclusive environment for LGBT patients. 2017. Accessed 30 Apr 2018. Available from: https://www.lgbthealtheducation.org/wp-content/uploads/2017/08/Forms-and-Policy-Brief.pdf.
64. The Gender Identity in U.S. Surveillance (GenIUSS) Group. Best practices for asking questions to identify transgender and other gender minority respondents on population-based Surveys. Herman JL, editor. The Williams Institute, Los Angeles, CA; 2014. Accessed 30 Apr 2018. Available from: https://williamsinstitute.law.ucla.edu/wp-content/uploads/geniuss-report-sep-2014.pdf.
65. Sexual Minority Assessment Research Team (SMART). Best practices for asking questions about sexual orientation on surveys. The Williams Institute; 2009. Accessed 30 Apr 2018. Available from: https://williamsinstitute.law.ucla.edu/wp-content/uploads/SMART-FINAL-Nov-2009.pdf.
66. Cahill S, Singal R, Grasso C, King D, Mayer K, Baker K, et al. Do ask, do tell: high levels of acceptability by patients of routine collection of sexual orientation and gender identity data in four diverse American community health centers. PLoS One. 2014;9(9):e107104.
67. LGBT OutList. Accessed 30 Apr 2018. Available from: http://www.feinberg.northwestern.edu/diversity/programs-groups/outlist.html.
68. Outlist. Accessed 30 Apr 2018. Available from: https://www.pennmedicine.org/for-patients-and-visitors/find-a-program-or-service/lgbt-health/outlist.
69. Dahlhamer JM, Galinsky AM, Joestl SS, Ward BW. Sexual orientation and health information technology use: a nationally representative study of US Adults. LGBT Health. 2017;4(2):121–9.
70. GLSEN, CiPHR, & CCRC. Out online: the experiences of lesbian, gay, bisexual and transgender youth on the Internet. GLSEN. 2013. Accessed 30 Apr 2018. Available from: https://www.glsen.org/sites/default/files/Out%20Online%20FINAL.pdf.
71. Whitehead J, Shaver J, Stephenson R. Outness, stigma, and primary health care utilization among rural LGBT populations. Newman PA, ed. PLoS One. 2016;11(1):e0146139.

72. Human Rights Campaign. Healthcare equality index 2017. 2017. Accessed 21 Dec 2018. Available online at: https://assets2.hrc.org/files/assets/resources/HEI-2017.pdf?_ga=2.148874162.468495970.1518802432-366372500.1518802432.
73. Veterans Health Administration. VHA directive 1340 transmittal sheet. Department of Veterans Affairs. July 6, 2017. Accessed 30 Apr 2018. Available from: https://www.patientcare.va.gov/lgbt/va_lgbt_policies.asp.
74. Veterans Health Administration. VHA directive 2013-003. Revised Department of Veterans Affairs. January 19, 2017. Accessed 30 Apr 2018. Available from: https://www.patientcare.va.gov/lgbt/va_lgbt_policies.asp.
75. Veterans Health Administration. VA LGBT outreach. Accessed 30 Apr 2018. Available from: https://www.patientcare.va.gov/LGBT/VA_LGBT_Outreach.asp.
76. Veterans Health Administration. VA facilities with LGBT program websites. Accessed 30 Apr 2018. Available from: https://www.patientcare.va.gov/LGBT/VAFacilities.asp.
77. Veterans Health Administration. Office of Diversity and Inclusion (ODI) directive and handbooks. Accessed 30 Apr 2018. Available from: https://www.diversity.va.gov/policy/diversity.aspx.
78. Violence Recovery Program Fenway Health. Accessed 30 Apr 2018. Available from: http://fenwayhealth.org/care/behavioral-health/violence-recovery/.
79. Transforming Ourselves Through Dialogue, Organizing and Services (TOD@S). Mission. Accessed 30 Apr 2018. Available from: http://todosinaction.org/mission/.
80. The National LGBT Health Education Center. Fenway Health. Accessed 30 Apr 2018. Available from: http://fenwayhealth.org/the-fenway-institute/education/the-national-lgbt-health-education-center/.
81. Cahill S, Valadéz R. Growing older with HIV/AIDS: new public health challenges. Am J Public Health. 2013;103(3):e7–e15.
82. Landers SJ, Mimiaga MJ, Conron KJ. Sexual orientation differences in asthma correlates in a population-based sample of adults. Am J Public Health. 2011;101(12):2238–41.
83. Gender Care for Children and Adolescents. Duke Health. Accessed 30 Apr 2018. Available from: https://www.dukehealth.org/pediatric-treatments/adolescent-transgender-program.
84. Gillis B. Clinic for transgender children and teens and children with differences in sex development. Duke Health Blog. October 25, 2016. Accessed 30 Apr 2018. Available from: https://www.dukehealth.org/blog/clinic-transgender-children-and-teens-and-children-differences-sex-development.
85. Phillips A. The tumultuous history of North Carolina's bathroom bill, which is on its way to repeal. The Washington Post. 2017, March 30. Accessed 2 March 2019. Available from: https://www.washington-post.com/news/the-fix/wp/2016/12/19/the-tumultuous-recent-history-of-north-carolinas-bath-room-bill-which-could-be-repealed/?utm_term=.cf04f08a57ee.

# Chapter 6
# Trauma-Informed Care of Veterans

Megan R. Gerber

## Introduction

While trauma-informed care (TIC) is relevant for all clinicians who work with Veterans, this chapter is designed to assist those who work in community settings and may encounter Veterans routinely or may not be aware of the Veteran status of those they work with.

On July 1,1973, the US military became an all-volunteer force. Currently it is estimated that less than 0.5% of the US population has served in the military [1]. This marked a decrease from World War II when approximately 12% of the US population served [1]. The result of this is that the experiences of Veterans in combat and in military service in support of combat operations are seldom shared, or understood, by the majority of society. Therefore, it is critical to include an assessment of military service status as part of all initial intakes and visits. Occasionally, an individual will not self-identify as a Veteran, this is particularly common among women who have served in the US military [2]. In order to provide TIC to Veterans, working knowledge of the unique aspects of each era of service is needed, as is some sense of military culture which many Americans have never been personally exposed to.

The roots of the current Veterans Administration (VA) date back to the seventeenth century [3]. However the modern VA, as we know it, came into being when President Abraham Lincoln signed a law to establish a national soldiers and sailors asylum. Renamed as the National Home for Disabled Volunteer Soldiers in 1873, it was the first-ever government institution created specifically for honorably discharged volunteer soldiers. The first national home opened on November 1, 1866, near Augusta, Maine. The national homes were often called "soldiers' homes" or

---

M. R. Gerber (✉)
Section of General Internal Medicine, Boston University School of Medicine, Veterans Affairs (VA) Boston Healthcare System, Boston, MA, USA
e-mail: meggerber@post.harvard.edu

© Springer Nature Switzerland AG 2019
M. R. Gerber (ed.), *Trauma-Informed Healthcare Approaches*,
https://doi.org/10.1007/978-3-030-04342-1_6

"military homes," and only soldiers who fought for the Union Army (including African American soldiers) were eligible for admission [4]. These institutions became the foundation for subsequent generations of federal Veterans' hospitals. Consolidation of federal Veterans programs took place in 1921 when Congress created the Veterans Bureau, and a hospital construction program for World War I Veterans began [4, 5]. Today, the VA is the second-largest government agency [6] and the largest integrated healthcare system in the United States, providing care at 172 VA Medical Centers and 1062 outpatient sites of care [7]. Over nine million Veterans are enrolled in the VA healthcare program, [5] which provides specialized care often not found in community healthcare settings.

## Healthcare Usage of Veterans

A number of population-based surveys, including the Centers for Disease Control and Prevention (CDC) Behavioral Risk Factor Survey (BRFSS) conducted annually and the US Census, query Veteran status. The BRFSS has enabled population-based comparisons between Veteran and non-Veteran health indicators. Typically, Veterans who use VA have poorer overall health than those who do not access VA care [8–10]. VA users are more likely than non-VA users to be elderly, non-Hispanic black, and of lower income [10].

According to the 2017 Survey of Veteran Enrollees' Health and Use of Health Care [11], 51% of Veterans enrolled in VA also had Medicare benefits, 28% had private insurance, 19.8% had Tricare, 6.6% had Medicaid, and 20% were uninsured. Sizable portions of the Veteran community do not access VA health care [10, 12]; the reasons for this are complex and multifactorial [9, 13, 14]. For this reason, community clinicians and systems of care must be cognizant of the presence of Veterans on their patient panels and in their catchment areas. Attrition from VA care has also been examined; for example, women Veterans who leave VA care tend to be healthier than those who remain [14].

Concomitant use of VA and non-VA care is known as "dual care" use; estimates of this vary based on the data source and payor. Approximately 80% of Veterans dually eligible for VA and Medicare services use both [15], and distance from VA services is a big driver of dual care utilization [16]. After passage of the Veterans Choice Act in 2014, dual care use has become increasingly common and creates challenges for coordinating care [17, 18].

## Combat Trauma and Era-Specific Injury

Veterans of all eras are a highly trauma-exposed population [19]. Although Veterans who have experienced trauma—and may be diagnosed with posttraumatic stress disorder (PTSD) or other mental health diagnoses—may share challenges and presentations similar to those of other clinical populations, serving in the military carries cultural values/beliefs that impact Veterans' systems of meaning [20]. Providers and organizations can better provide TIC to Veterans by understanding military culture and the unique aspects of each era of service. Warfare has changed over the years, as have combat medicine and protective gear. The unique context of each war, and society's view of it, impacts current Veteran health and well-being.

## World War II

Currently, the oldest living Veterans are those of World War II (WWII), who are now in their 80s and 90s [21]. While during World War I, most soldiers were wounded by enemy bullets and chemical agents such as mustard gas, in WWII, artillery and bombs inflicted the most injuries—more severe than previous conflicts. Head wounds and traumatic amputations were common [22]. The Veterans who fought in WWII are known as "the greatest generation" [23] and despite gruesome exposures and injuries, there is an enduring sense of historical pride and appreciation of WWII and those who fought in it. As discussed above, a considerable percentage of the population served in WWII, and the population at home was also mobilized into the war effort as "Home Front workers" [24]. It was impossible to ignore the war, and it became part of everyone's daily life and experience.

## The Korean War

Five years after WWII, the Korean conflict began when North Korea invaded South Korea in June 1950; it was essentially an expansion of a war between the Koreas that began with Japan's defeat in 1950 [25]. It lasted 37 months, ending in what has been described as "a truce," it is often known as the "Forgotten War" [26]. Relatively less is understood about this conflict, which began while the United States was still in recovery from WWII and the "baby boom" had begun. James Wright wrote in *The Atlantic*, *"There were no celebrations in Times Square–or anywhere else. The Washington Post noted, 'Washington greeted news of the Korean truce yesterday with a matter-of-fact attitude–quietly, without evident jubilation....' It was peace without a clear victory"* [26].

Nearly 1.8 million Americans served in Korea from 1950 to 1953, and 36,574 died there. Combat was often brutal and injuries from extreme cold and radiation were common [4]. What was termed a "police action" by President Truman was not congressionally recognized as a "war" until 1998 [26]. The conflict in Korea ushered in an era in which wars were fought by increasingly less representative sectors of the American society; this further enabled many Americans to pay little attention to the details of these military encounters [26].

By the end of the war in 1953, US armed forces remained much larger than they had been in 1950 and were ensured a steady supply of manpower through the retention of conscription. The military shifted its focus away from preparing for a WWII-type mobilization to maintaining forces ready for immediate use. Our military might was widely dispersed around the world, including in Indochina, where American advisers assisted the new Republic of Vietnam [25].

## Vietnam

Much of our modern understanding of trauma and treatment of PTSD comes from the Vietnam War era [27, 28]. 2.7 million Americans served in Vietnam [29], which was the first ever televised war [4]. Vietnam was also the first true US guerilla war [30], and the witness and/or use of "abusive violence" was conceptualized as an additional stressor [30]. Unlike WWII and Korea where the enemy had a defined uniform and battle lines were clear, Vietnam had unclear conflict zones and boundaries which created unprecedented challenges for soldiers [4]. In addition, many Vietnam era soldiers also reported often not feeling any sense of gratitude from the South Vietnamese they were supposed to be aiding [4]. In essence, Vietnam Veterans fought an unpopular war for a country that often confused the soldier with the policymakers [28].

Keane et al [28] in an early study of PTSD in Vietnam Veterans noted that war combatants experienced multiple stressors or traumatic events during a combat tour. The typical Vietnam combat Veteran, deployed for a 12–13-month tour, saw high levels of combat, unprecedented at the time due to capabilities in mechanization and mobilization [28]. The constant hypervigilance of guerilla warfare led to a high prevalence of PTSD [4]. Vietnam also brought about the understanding that killing in combat is one of the most traumatic psychological experiences for military personnel; it is a well-established precursor to both PTSD and suicide [31, 32] and often results in "moral injury" [33].

The military environment typically does not encourage expressions of emotion subsequent to traumatic combat events [28]. For many Vietnam Veterans, a parallel experience occurred when they returned to the United States. Upon return, they were discouraged from sharing their combat exposures and narratives; thus, many Vietnam Veterans never fully disclosed their experiences [28]. Furthermore, improvements in medical and surgical trauma therapy meant that more severely wounded soldiers had higher survival rates and were living with severe and disabling injuries that made reintegration even more difficult [4]. Substance use disorder (SUD) is common with PTSD (this is true for all eras of conflict); Vietnam Veterans' longitudinal experiences with both conditions have provided better understanding of this comorbidity, and in comparative studies, those who served in Vietnam exhibit the highest rate of this [34]. Ideally PTSD and SUD should be treated concurrently [35, 36], which may be challenging in non-VA care settings.

## Gulf Wars

### *The Persian Gulf War (Gulf War I)*

The invasion of Kuwait by Iraq in 1990 led to mobilization of a coalition of forces led by the United States that liberated Kuwait rapidly, allowing our ground troops to leave the following year. Veterans of this brief conflict experienced multiple environmental toxins, burning petrochemicals and other substances, as well as radiation exposure to depleted uranium [4]. Many Veterans returned with diffuse pain, fibromyalgia, memory loss, and other multisystem symptoms, now known as "Gulf War Syndrome" [37]. Respiratory problems and amyotrophic lateral sclerosis (ALS) are also recognized as being linked to exposures during this conflict [38].

### *Operations Enduring Freedom, Iraqi Freedom, and New Dawn*

The war on terror began on September 11, 2001 [39], after simultaneous attacks on the World Trade Center, the Pentagon, and a foiled airliner attack and crash in Pennsylvania. Beginning in October 2001, approximately 1.64 million US troops were deployed in Operation Enduring Freedom (Afghanistan 2001–2014), Operation Iraqi Freedom (Iraq 2003–2011), and Operation New Dawn (2010–2011). Significant numbers of US service members have remained in Iraq, Afghanistan, and Syria since the end dates of these conflicts, and at the time of this writing, the precise number of deployed personnel is unknown [40].

Due to the overall length of these conflicts, and the volunteer nature of the armed forces, many have served multiple tours and deployments, which is unprecedented in the history of US warfare. Overall about 40% of current military service members have been deployed more than once [41]. Pressure on troops needed for deployment resulted in some combat units serving longer tours and spending shorter periods at home between tours (referred to as dwell time) [41]. This resulted in prolonged and repeated exposure to combat-related stress not seen in prior conflicts.

In this most recent war era, service members survived blasts that would have been lethal previously, and rates of traumatic brain injury (TBI) are unprecedented [42]. The Defense and Veterans Brain Injury Center estimated that 22% of all OEF/OIF combat wounds were brain injuries [42]. This was compared to TBI in 12% of Vietnam-era combat wounds [43]. In addition, it is estimated that 23% of these newer Veterans meet criteria for probable PTSD [44], and this may be an underestimate. War-related trauma has resulted in an increasing number of suicides and self-injury among Veterans [19].

## Women Veterans

Women have served in the US military throughout history; however, since September 11, the population of women joining the military is at an all-time high. Women now comprise 15% of Active Duty personnel [45] and 19% of the National Guard/Reserves [46]. They are the fastest-growing segment of the Veteran population [47]. In the most recent conflicts, women reported experiencing combat exposures and combat-related stressors [48, 49], even before the combat exclusion policy (which dated to 1948) was lifted in 2013 [50]. While their numbers are growing, they remain a distinct minority in all military branches.

Services for women in VA have expanded dramatically over the last two decades [46]. Women do not always self-identify as Veterans; for this reason, VA recommends that providers ask patients: "Have you served in the military?" [2] This is particularly important for women Veterans who are at higher risk for interpersonal trauma than males and who also lacked the same degree of social support while serving. Women Veterans, in particular, are a commonly trauma-exposed population and often enter the military with significant histories of child abuse, sexual assault, and intimate partner violence (IPV) [51, 52]. These exposures may be compounded by combat exposure and military sexual trauma (MST), which is discussed in detail below.

## Veterans and Interpersonal Violence Exposure

When compared to non-Veterans, Veterans consistently report higher levels of adverse childhood experiences (ACEs) across studies. Using data from CDC, two recent studies have examined the burden of ACEs in the military Veteran population and found elevated levels of adverse childhood events [53, 54]. In the current all-volunteer era, it is not uncommon for individuals to join the military to escape difficult family situations and adversity, Veterans from the draft era report lower overall ACE scores [53]. Veterans were more than twice as likely to endorse four or more ACEs than were non-Veterans [53]. ACEs in Veterans were associated with smoking, drinking, and obesity [54], as well as greater risk of PTSD in adulthood [55], even after controlling for combat exposure [55]. Additional research showed that some ACEs were correlated with greater homelessness risk and mental and physical health conditions [56].

In population-based studies, Veterans have demonstrated higher rates of exposure to IPV, parental separation or divorce, household member incarceration, drug and alcohol misuse, mental illness, as well as emotional, physical, and sexual abuse during childhood and adolescence compared to non-Veterans [20, 53, 54]. In recent years, VA has developed a national IPV Assistance Program (https://www.socialwork.va.gov/IPV/Index.asp) and embarked on novel programming, informed by research with Veterans, to address both experience [57] and use [58] of IPV.

While a detailed discussion of the multiple evidence-based trauma-focused treatments for Veterans is beyond the scope of this chapter, clinicians and health systems should be aware of the existence of these [59], including a unique self-care smartphone app called "PTSD Coach" which is free and available to anyone [60]. To date, "PTSD Coach" has been downloaded over 100,000 times in 74 different countries and can be used by all trauma-exposed persons, not just Veterans [61].

## *Military Sexual Trauma*

The Department of Veterans Affairs (VA) uses the term military sexual trauma (MST) to refer to experiences, defined in 38 US Code Sec. 1720D as *physical assault of a sexual nature, battery of a sexual nature, or sexual harassment which occurred while the Veteran was serving on active duty or active duty for training.* Sexual harassment and assault are conceptualized as experiences along a continuum of sexual trauma for the purposes of addressing Veterans' healthcare needs [62]. MST is considered a duty-related hazard [62], and an electronic health record prompt for screening occurs once for each Veteran. MST has been experienced by male and female service members and occurred throughout all eras of service [63–65]. VA data estimate that 1 in 4 women and 1 in 100 men screen positive for MST during medical visits, this may be an underestimate [66]. Women are disproportionately impacted, and their ranks are growing rapidly [63].

Like all forms of trauma, MST has been linked to poorer mental and physical health [67, 68]. MST, like other interpersonal traumas, is underreported in part due to military culture in which toughness and unit cohesion are emphasized [69, 70]. It is difficult for service members to disclose MST, and sometimes they are met with disbelief or dismissal or—at worst—reprisal; men may face even greater social pressures not to mention MST [65, 69]. Male Veterans are less likely than women to receive MST care even though the overall number of men reporting MST is similar to that for women because the Veteran population is mostly male [62, 69].

It is also common for those who have experienced MST to already have prior interpersonal trauma histories [62, 71]; prior traumatic experiences also predispose to MST [71, 72]. MST has been linked to adverse mental and physical health [71]; the odds of developing PTSD after MST are higher than the odds of PTSD after combat exposure for both genders [73]. In addition, MST and combat trauma interact to increase the risk of developing PTSD; in one study of women Veterans who served in Afghanistan and Iraq under conditions of high combat exposure, those with MST had significantly higher PTSD symptomatology when compared to female Veterans without MST. While the Department of Defense (DoD) does not use the term MST, it does conduct its own surveillance of current Active Duty service members [62].

MST prevalence data derived from self-report measures and interviews appear to yield higher estimates than rates derived from the VA medical record [74]. For example, a 2018 meta-analysis of MST prevalence indicated that 15.7% of military personnel and Veterans report any MST (3.9% of men, 38.4% of women), when the measure includes both harassment and assault. Assault-only rates reveal that 13.9%

report MST (1.9% of men, 23.6% of women). Finally, when the measure assesses harassment only, 31.2% report MST (8.9% of men, 52.5% of women) [74].

A recent study of MST was derived from the population-based National Health Study for a New Generation of US Veterans (NewGen) which surveyed 60,000 OEF/OIF Veterans [62]. The study included VA users and non-users, and in this cohort, 41% of women reported MST and sexual harassment and 10% reported sexual assault; 4% of men reported MST and sexual harassment and 0.5% reported sexual assault [62]. Surveyed Veterans accessing VA health care had higher rates; 49% of women and 5% of men using VA reported MST [62]. The Marine Corps had the highest rates of MST for women (52%); the Air Force had the lowest. National Guard and Reserve Veterans were less likely to report MST than Active Duty service members. In this study, deployment itself did not increase risk of MST for men or women, but combat exposure did. Notably, men with combat exposure were three times more likely to report experiencing sexual assault than men without combat exposure. The authors of this study hypothesized that rates of disclosure on confidential surveys may be higher than rates obtained in screening at VA medical visits due to social stigma and trauma-related avoidance during medical visits [62]. The high rates of MST among Veterans not using VA care underscore that non-VA clinicians must remain aware of the possibility of MST among Veteran patients cared for in the community.

All VA medical centers are mandated to have an MST coordinator. All treatment for mental and physical health conditions related to MST is provided free of charge to Veterans. This includes outpatient, inpatient, residential, and pharmaceutical treatment. To receive this free MST-related care, Veterans do not need to be service connected; care is given independent of receipt of other VA benefits. Veterans may be able to receive free MST-related care even if they are not eligible for other VA care. These services are a permanent benefit by law [70], and there is no length of service or income requirement to receive MST-related care. Veterans do not need to have reported the incidents when they happened or have other documentation that they occurred [64].

All healthcare providers, including community providers, should be aware of the importance of MST as a potential contributor to poor health when caring for Veteran patients. Veterans seeking community mental health services, or homelessness services, are likely to be survivors of multiple forms of trauma [75]. From the standpoint of implementing TIC, the national MST program can provide an important paradigm for all systems of care that seek to provide programming that is sensitive to survivors' preferences and needs [76].

## *Homeless Veterans*

While Veterans make up approximately 7% of the US population, they represent more than 12% of the homeless adult population [77]. Veteran homelessness has been aggressively targeted in recent years by programs such as the Mayors' Challenge to End Veteran Homelessness. According to the US Interagency Council to End Homelessness (USICH), between 2011 and 2017, Veteran homelessness has dropped by 46%, and a 50% reduction in Veterans experiencing unsheltered homelessness has also occurred [78]. Rural Veterans, however, have actually experienced an increase in homelessness [78], in part due to a lack of service infrastructure in rural areas and the need for long-distance travel to access resources. Veterans in rural areas are likely to be homeless for longer periods of time [77] and are often invisible to the public which associates homelessness with urban environments. Thus, homelessness among Veterans remains a critical public health issue.

Trauma and PTSD are common in the homeless population, and both often precede housing loss [77]. Often the risk of trauma exposure increases when an individual becomes homeless [79]. For Veterans, PTSD and any mental health diagnosis are the strongest predictors of homelessness [77], and PTSD is associated with a risk of recurrent or chronic homelessness [80]. It is a common misconception that homelessness among Veterans is solely the result of combat exposure and post-war adjustment issues; this was demonstrated by higher rates of homelessness among post-Vietnam, pre-Gulf War era Veterans [77] who did not experience the exposure to combat seen in prior conflicts.

As more women enter military service, homelessness among women Veterans is growing. The number of homeless women Veterans more than doubled between 2006 and 2010 [81]. Many women Veterans are not aware of housing services, and an estimated 60% of government-funded Veteran housing programs do not house children [82]. Those that do impose restrictions on the number of children per Veteran and age limits [82]. Homeless women Veterans were three times as likely as their housed peers to have experienced MST [83]. In one study, the majority (75%) of homeless women Veterans also reported combat trauma [84]. Many women Veterans are single mothers; by 2010, 30,000 single mothers were deployed to Afghanistan and Iraq, and at least 40% of Active Duty women had children [81], suggesting that the magnitude of this issue could increase. Trauma is common among homeless mothers, and the combined experience of trauma and homelessness may be compounded by feelings of guilt and shame [77].

Common barriers to TIC among homeless Veterans include a lack of routine trauma screening in this population [77], along with the multiple layers of psychosocial need and competing health issues that can result in providers failing to recognize the association between trauma and homelessness [77]. Many homeless Veterans have also had past negative reporting experiences and a betrayal of trust in relationships [77]. Routinely asking all homeless persons about prior military service is recommended in order to connect them with Veteran-specific housing benefits and programs. Non-VA community providers may commonly see homeless Veterans in rural settings where the nearest VA is not readily geographically accessible.

## *VA Mental Health and Primary Care*

Returning service members may not be identified as having mental health conditions or adequately treated while on active duty and deployment [19]. Many Veterans avoid, or delay, seeking mental health care due to stigma or fear of negative career impact [85, 86]. Veterans are often more likely to present in primary care, or other medical settings, than in mental health practices [19]. Colocation of primary care and mental health services is ideal for this population; the VA Primary Care-Mental Health Integration (PC-MHI) program is designed to provide short-term collaborative care to Veterans in primary care settings [87]. Some Veterans decline specialized mental health treatment, such as trauma-focused care in a dedicated PTSD program [87]. Similar collaborative care models outside VA are becoming increasingly common.

Community providers should be aware of local Vet Centers [88], which are VA-affiliated, free-standing clinics that provide readjustment counseling to Veterans, service members (including members of the Reserves) who have served in combat zones, and their families [89]. Patients may self-refer. Records are kept separate from those of VA and DoD, and many Veterans prefer to be seen in Vet Centers which commonly resemble a typical outpatient clinical setting as opposed to a government hospital.

On a practical level (Table 6.1), TIC processes for Veterans should include providing privacy when asking a Veteran to complete sensitive forms related to trauma

**Table 6.1** Recommendations for Veteran-focused trauma-informed care [19, 20, 90]

| |
|---|
| *Trauma awareness:*<br>Be aware of Veteran status and potential trauma related to Veteran characteristics like gender, age, and era of service. Ask "Have you served in the military?" and not "Are you a Veteran?" Understand how various mental and physical symptoms may be adaptations to traumatic exposures. |
| *Safety:* An emphasis on safety can help Veterans build physical and emotional security<br>Not all Veterans access VA, in part because it can reproduce aspects of military service [91, 92]. Some may find community settings less triggering.<br>Avoid closing the door to an office without the Veteran's consent [20].<br>Do not ask Veterans to recount traumatic events multiple times for multiple staff for the purposes of completing paperwork [20] or staff convenience.<br>Relaxation techniques that include closed eyes should only be undertaken after ensuring feelings of emotional and physical safety [20].<br>Inquire about possible triggers the Veteran may already be aware of. |
| *Collaboration/rebuild control:*<br>Give the Veteran opportunities to rebuild control (trauma has resulted in past loss of control). Collaborative decision-making with the Veteran is critical; military medicine is often about readiness, and medical providers and nurses are officers.<br>For example, a Veteran should not be "ordered" to have an exam or vaccination. (*Discussions of providing TIC in clinical examination settings, and holistic, trauma-informed nursing care, are included in chapters 7 and 10 of this volume.*) |
| *Empowerment/use of a strengths-based approach:*<br>Be aware of stigmatization, employ recovery-oriented models, and identify the Veteran's strengths.<br>Remember that many, if not most, of the Veterans you see have volunteered to serve, acknowledge this, and thank her/him/them for their service. Military service, alone, requires strength and self-sacrifice.<br>Promote self-advocacy within the organizational structure [20]. In the Military Health System (MHS), Veterans do not have to negotiate care/treatment.<br>Providers should become familiar with and cultivate ties to governmental (municipal, state, federal) agencies and Veterans' service organizations [20]; a member of the extended care team can assist with this. |

and mental health issues, reducing "noise pollution" [20], including loud, startling sounds like slamming doors. Veterans should be allowed to decide where to sit in an exam or consultation room [20]; many Veterans prefer never to be seated with their back facing a door. Clinicians should avoid sudden, potentially startling movements during an exam, especially those that involve approaching a Veteran from behind.

A trauma-informed approach to Veteran care necessitates inquiring about military service and being aware of conditions unique to military Veterans. We recommend that providers routinely ask patients "have you served in the military?" Others recommend inquiring about a family member's military service: "Do you have a close family member who has served in the military?" Asking whether your patient/client has close family members who have served in the military can (1) lead to a deeper understanding of the individual's family context and (2) allow you to assess whether family functioning could benefit from connection with relevant resources [93]. Additional Veteran-centric TIC recommendations include [94] (1) posting a simple sign letting Veterans and service members know that you would like to know if they have served, (2) respecting a Veteran or service member's choice not to discuss their experiences, (3) conveying a willingness to listen to their experiences if the Veteran or service member wants to discuss them in the future, and (4) remembering that if a Veteran discloses sexual assault in the military (MST), that individual is eligible for treatment regardless of other eligibility/income/time served.

In summary, the increased dependence of the military on National Guard and Reserve forces [41] means that community providers and systems of care are often seeing these Veterans who return to their homes, communities and jobs after deployment. Many Veterans choose to access care outside VA, and developing an understanding of their unique needs is critical to delivering excellent care.

**Disclaimer** The views expressed in this chapter are those of the author and do not necessarily reflect the position or policy of the Department of Veterans Affairs or the US government.

# References

1. Eiekenberry KW, Kennedy DM. Americans and their military, drifting apart. The New York Times. 2013 May 23;Sect. Opinion. Accessed 13 May 2018. Available at https://www.nytimes.com/2013/05/27/opinion/americans-and-their-military-drifting-apart.html.
2. US Department of Veterans Affairs WVHC. Resources for non-VA providers, medical students. Washington, DC. 2017. Accessed 20 May 2018. Available from: https://www.womenshealth.va.gov/programoverview/providers.asp.
3. US Department of Veterans Affairs. History – Department of Veterans Affairs (VA). Washington, DC. 2018. Accessed 20 May 2018. Available from: https://www.va.gov/about_va/vahistory.asp.
4. Module 9: The Experience of Veterans from Different War Eras. In: Emanuel LL, Hauser JM, Bailey FA, Ferris FD, von Gunten CF, Von Ronn J, editors. EPEC For Veterans: Education in Palliative and End-of- life Care for Veterans Chicago, IL; Washington, DC. 2012.
5. Veterans Health Administration. Restoring trust in veterans healthcare fiscal year 2016 annual report 2017. Accessed 10 June 2018. Available from: https://www.va.gov/HEALTH/docs/VHA_AR16.pdf.

6. Office of Personnel Management (OPM). Workforce information. Accessed 19 May 2018. Available from: https://www.opm.gov/FAQs/QA.aspx?fid=56538f91-625a-4333-84ba-28b3574b7942&pid=013be2c9-8ae5-455d-889c-6e74063441ba.
7. Veterans Health Administration. About VHA: US Department of Veterans Affairs. 2018. Accessed 29 July 2018. Available from: https://www.va.gov/health/aboutvha.asp.
8. Phillips BR, Shahoumian TA, Backus LI. Surveyed enrollees in veterans affairs health care: how they differ from eligible veterans surveyed by BRFSS. Mil Med. 2015;180(11):1161–9.
9. Washington DL, Farmer MM, Mor SS, Canning M, Yano EM. Assessment of the healthcare needs and barriers to VA use experienced by women veterans: findings from the National Survey of women veterans. Med Care. 2015;53:S23–31.
10. Machlin SR, Muhuri P. Characteristics and Health Care Expenditures of VA Health System Users versus Other Veterans, 2014–2015 (Combined). Statistical Brief (Medical Expenditure Panel Survey (US)). Rockville (MD): Agency for Healthcare Research and Quality (US); 2018.
11. Huang G, Muz B, Kim SGJ. 2017 survey of veteran enrollees' health and use of health care. Data findings report. Rockville; 2018. Accessed 10 June 2018. Available from: https://www.va.gov/HEALTHPOLICYPLANNING/SoE2017/VA_Enrollees_Report_Data_Findings_Report2.pdf.
12. Nelson KM, Starkebaum GA, Reiber GE. Veterans using and uninsured veterans not using Veterans Affairs (VA) health care. Public Health Rep. 2007;122(1):93–100.
13. Elnitsky CA, Andresen EM, Clark ME, McGarity S, Hall CG, Kerns RD. Access to the US Department of Veterans Affairs health system: self-reported barriers to care among returnees of operations enduring freedom and Iraqi freedom. BMC Health Serv Res. 2013;13:498.
14. Hamilton AB, Frayne SM, Cordasco KM, Washington DL. Factors related to attrition from VA healthcare use: findings from the National Survey of women veterans. J Gen Intern Med. 2013;28(Suppl 2):S510–6.
15. Petersen LA, Byrne MM, Daw CN, Hasche J, Reis B, Pietz K. Relationship between clinical conditions and use of Veterans Affairs health care among medicare-enrolled veterans. Health Serv Res. 2010;45(3):762–91.
16. Gaglioti A, Cozad A, Wittrock S, Stewart K, Lampman M, Ono S, et al. Non-VA primary care providers' perspectives on comanagement for rural veterans. Mil Med. 2014;179(11):1236–43.
17. Gellad WF. The Veterans Choice Act and dual health system use. J Gen Intern Med. 2016;31(2):153–4.
18. Gellad WF, Thorpe JM, Zhao X, Thorpe CT, Sileanu FE, Cashy JP, et al. Impact of dual use of Department of Veterans Affairs and Medicare Part D drug benefits on potentially unsafe opioid use. Am J Public Health. 2018;108(2):248–55.
19. Kelly U, Boyd MA, Valente SM, Czekanski E. Trauma-informed care: keeping mental health settings safe for veterans. Issues Ment Health Nurs. 2014;35(6):413–9.
20. Currier JM, Stefurak T, Carroll TD, Shatto EH. Applying trauma-informed care to community-based mental health services for military veterans. Best Pract Ment Health. 2017;13(1):47–65.
21. National Center for Veterans Analysis and Statistics. Veteran population. Washington, DC: US Department of Veterans Affairs; 2016. Accessed 22 May 2018. Available from: https://www.va.gov/vetdata/veteran_population.asp.
22. Manring MM, Hawk A, Calhoun JH, Andersen RC. Treatment of war wounds: a historical review. Clin Orthop Relat Res. 2009;467(8):2168–91.
23. Brokaw T. The greatest generation. New York: Random House; 1998.
24. National Park Service. The WWII home front. Washington, DC. Accessed 13 May 2018. Available from: https://www.nps.gov/articles/the-wwiihome-front.htm.
25. Stewart RW. The United States Army in a global era, 1917–2008. 2nd ed. Center of Military History United States Army: Washington, DC; 2010.
26. Wright J. What we learned from the Korean war. The Atlantic. 2013. Accessed 16 Dec 2018. Available from: https://www.theatlantic.com/international/archive/2013/07/what-we-learned-from-the-korean-war/278016/.
27. Herman J. Trauma and recovery. New York: Basic Books; 2015.
28. Keane TM, Zimering RT, Caddell JM. A behavioral formulation of posttraumatic stress disorder in Vietnam veterans. Behav Ther. 1985;8(1):9–12.

29. Vietnam Veterans [Internet]. 2015 Apr 30. Accessed 19 May 2018. Available from: https://www.benefits.va.gov/persona/veteran-vietnam.asp.
30. Laufer RS, Gallops MS, Frey-Wouters E. War stress and trauma: the Vietnam veteran experience. J Health Soc Behav. 1984;25(1):65–85.
31. Maguen S, Metzler TJ, Litz BT, Seal KH, Knight SJ, Marmar CR. The impact of killing in war on mental health symptoms and related functioning. J Trauma Stress. 2009;22(5):435–43.
32. Maguen S, Burkman K, Madden E, Dinh J, Bosch J, Keyser J, et al. Impact of killing in war: a randomized, controlled pilot trial. J Clin Psychol. 2017;73(9):997–1012.
33. Litz BT, Stein N, Delaney E, Lebowitz L, Nash WP, Silva C, et al. Moral injury and moral repair in war veterans: a preliminary model and intervention strategy. Clin Psychol Rev. 2009;29(8):695–706.
34. Petrakis IL, Rosenheck R, Desai R. Substance use comorbidity among veterans with posttraumatic stress disorder and other psychiatric illness. Am J Addict. 2011;20(3):185–9.
35. Manhapra A, Stefanovics E, Rosenheck R. Treatment outcomes for veterans with PTSD and substance use: impact of specific substances and achievement of abstinence. Drug Alcohol Depend. 2015;156:70–7.
36. Ouimette PC, Brown PJ, Najavits LM. Course and treatment of patients with both substance use and posttraumatic stress disorders. Addict Behav. 1998;23(6):785–95.
37. Minshall D. Gulf war syndrome: a review of current knowledge and understanding. J R Nav Med Serv. 2014;100(3):252–8.
38. Institute of Medicine. Committee on Gulf War and Health. Gulf war health: update on health effects of serving in the Gulf war. Washington, DC: Institute of Medicine; 2009.
39. Stevenson RW. President makes it clear: phrase is 'war on terror'. The New York Times. 2005 Aug 4;Sect. Politics. Accessed 11 June 2018. Available from https://www.nytimes.com/2005/08/04/politics/president-makes-it-clear-phrase-is-war-on-terror.html.
40. Copp T. Your military: Pentagon strips Iraq, Afghanistan, Syria troop numbers from web. Military Times. 2018 Apr 9. Accessed 27 July 2018. Available from: https://www.militarytimes.com/news/your-military/2018/04/09/dod-strips-iraq-afghanistan-syria-troop-numbers-from-web/.
41. Institute of Medicine. Operation Enduring Freedom and Operation Iraqi Freedom: demographics and impact. Washington, DC: Returning Home from Iraq and Afghanistan: Preliminary Assessment of Readjustment Needs of Veterans, Service Members, and Their Families; 2010.
42. Defense and Veterans Brain Injury Center. Department of Defense (DoD) worldwide numbers for TBI 2018. Accessed 20 May 2018. Available from: http://dvbic.dcoe.mil/dod-worldwide-numbers-tbi.
43. National Center for PTSD. Traumatic brain injury and PTSD: focus on veterans. 2017 Nov 6. Accessed 20 May 2018. Available from: https://www.ptsd.va.gov/professional/co-occurring/traumatic-brain-injury-ptsd.asp.
44. Fulton JJ, Calhoun PS, Wagner HR, Schry AR, Hair LP, Feeling N, et al. The prevalence of posttraumatic stress disorder in Operation Enduring Freedom/Operation Iraqi Freedom (OEF/OIF) veterans: a meta-analysis. J Anxiety Disord. 2015;31:98–107.
45. Parker K, Cilluffo A, Stepler R. 6 facts about the U.S. military and its changing demographics. Washington, DC: Pew Research Center; 2017. Accessed 19 May 2018. Available from: http://www.pewresearch.org/fact-tank/2017/04/13/6-facts-about-the-u-s-military-and-its-changing-demographics/.
46. Women Veterans Report: The Past, Present, and Future of Women Veterans. Washington, DC: National Center for Veterans Analysis and Statistics, Department of Veterans Affairs; 2017 Feb. Accessed 19 May 2018. Available from: https://www.va.gov/vetdata/docs/SpecialReports/Women_Veterans_2015_Final.pdf.
47. Sourcebook: Women Veterans in the Veterans Health Administration. Volume 4: Longitudinal Trends in Sociodemographics, Utilization, Health Profile, and Geographic Distribution. [Internet]. Women's Health Services, Veterans Health Administration. 2018. Accessed 17 Mar 2019. Available from: https://www.womenshealth.va.gov/WOMENSHEALTH/docs/WHS_Sourcebook_Vol-IV_508c.pdf.
48. Street AE, Vogt D, Dutra L. A new generation of women veterans: stressors faced by women deployed to Iraq and Afghanistan. Clin Psychol Rev. 2009;29(8):685–94.

49. Vogt D, Vaughn R, Glickman ME, Schultz M, Drainoni ML, Elwy R, et al. Gender differences in combat-related stressors and their association with postdeployment mental health in a nationally representative sample of U.S. OEF/OIF veterans. J Abnorm Psychol. 2011;120(4):797–806.
50. Bumiller E, Shanker T. Pentagon is set to lift combat ban for women. The New York Times. 2013 Jan 23. Accessed 20 May 2018. Available from: https://www.nytimes.com/2013/01/24/us/pentagon-says-it-is-lifting-ban-on-women-in-combat.html.
51. Zinzow HM, Grubaugh AL, Monnier J, Suffoletta-Maierle S, Frueh BC. Trauma among female veterans: a critical review. Trauma Violence Abuse. 2007;8(4):384–400.
52. Gerber MR, Iverson KM, Dichter ME, Klap R, Latta RE. Women veterans and intimate partner violence: current state of knowledge and future directions. J Womens Health (Larchmt). 2014;23(4):302–9.
53. Blosnich JR, Dichter ME, Cerulli C, Batten SV, Bossarte RM. Disparities in adverse childhood experiences among individuals with a history of military service. JAMA Psychiat. 2014;71(9):1041–8.
54. Katon JG, Lehavot K, Simpson TL, Williams EC, Barnett SB, Grossbard JR, et al. Adverse childhood experiences, military service, and adult health. Am J Prev Med. 2015;49(4):573–82.
55. Van Voorhees EE, Dedert EA, Calhoun PS, Branco M, Runnels J, Beckham JC. Childhood trauma exposure in Iraq and Afghanistan war era veterans: implications for post traumatic stress disorder symptoms and adult functional social support. Child Abuse Negl. 2012;36:423–32.
56. Montgomery AE, Cutuli JJ, Evans-Chase M, Treglia D, Culhane DP. Relationship among adverse childhood experiences, history of active military service, and adult outcomes: homelessness, mental health, and physical health. Am J Public Health. 2013;103(Suppl 2):S262–8.
57. Iverson KM, Gregor K, Gerber MR. Recovering from intimate partner violence through strengths and empowerment (RISE). Unpublished 2019.
58. Creech SK, Benzer JK, Ebalu T, Murphy CM, Taft CT. National implementation of a trauma-informed intervention for intimate partner violence in the Department of Veterans Affairs: first year outcomes. BMC Health Serv Res. 2018;18(1):582.
59. National Center for PTSD. PTSD treatment, White River Junction, VT. 2017 Aug 18. Accessed 16 May 2018. Available from: https://www.ptsd.va.gov/public/treatment/therapy-med/treatment-ptsd.asp.
60. Miner A, Kuhn E, Hoffman JE, Owen JE, Ruzek JI, Taylor CB. Feasibility, acceptability, and potential efficacy of the PTSD coach app: a pilot randomized controlled trial with community trauma survivors. Psychol Trauma. 2016;8(3):384–92.
61. National Center for PTSD. Mobile app: PTSD coach: US Department of Veterans Affairs; 2018 Jan 31. Accessed 1 June 2018. Available from: https://www.ptsd.va.gov/public/materials/apps/ptsdcoach.asp.
62. Barth SK, Kimerling RE, Pavao J, McCutcheon SJ, Batten SV, Dursa E, et al. Military sexual trauma among recent veterans: correlates of sexual assault and sexual harassment. Am J Prev Med. 2016;50(1):77–86.
63. Gibson CJ, Gray KE, Katon JG, Simpson TL, Lehavot K. Sexual assault, sexual harassment, and physical victimization during military service across age cohorts of women veterans. Womens Health Issues. 2016;26(2):225–31.
64. Department of Veterans Affairs. Military Sexual Trauma. Washington, DC. 2018 Apr 18. Accessed 20 May 2018. Available from: https://www.mentalhealth.va.gov/msthome.asp.
65. Morris EE, Smith JC, Farooqui SY, Suris AM. Unseen battles: the recognition, assessment, and treatment issues of men with military sexual trauma (MST). Trauma Violence Abuse. 2014;15(2):94–101.
66. US Department of Veterans Affairs. Military sexual trauma. 2015. Accessed 22 May 2018. Available from: https://www.mentalhealth.va.gov/docs/mst_general_factsheet.pdf.
67. Suris A, Lind L. Military sexual trauma: a review of prevalence and associated health consequences in veterans. Trauma Violence Abuse. 2008;9(4):250–69.
68. Frayne SM, Skinner KM, Sullivan LM, Tripp TJ, Hankin CS, Kressin NR, et al. Medical profile of women veterans administration outpatients who report a history of sexual assault occurring while in the military. J Womens Health Gend Based Med. 1999;8(6):835–45.

69. Turchik JA, McLean C, Rafie S, Hoyt T, Rosen CS, Kimerling R. Perceived barriers to care and provider gender preferences among veteran men who have experienced military sexual trauma: a qualitative analysis. Psychol Serv. 2013;10(2):213–22.
70. Kimerling R, Gima K, Smith MW, Street A, Frayne S. The Veterans Health Administration and military sexual trauma. Am J Public Health. 2007;97(12):2160–6.
71. Kelly UA, Skelton K, Patel M, Bradley B. More than military sexual trauma: interpersonal violence, PTSD, and mental health in women veterans. Res Nurs Health. 2011;34(6):457–67.
72. Surís A, Lind L, Kashner TM, Borman PD, Petty F. Sexual assault in women veterans: an examination of PTSD risk, health care utilization, and cost of care. Psychosom Med. 2004;66(5):749–56.
73. Kang H, Dalager N, Mahan C, Ishii E. The role of sexual assault on the risk of PTSD among gulf war veterans. Ann Epidemiol. 2005;15(3):191–5.
74. Wilson LC. The prevalence of military sexual trauma: a meta-analysis. Trauma Violence Abuse. 2018;19(5):584–97. 1524838016683459.
75. Tsai J, Rosenheck RA. Risk factors for homelessness among US veterans. Epidemiol Rev. 2015;37:177–95.
76. Ming Foynes M, Makin-Byrd K, Skidmore WC, King MW, Bell ME, Karpenko J. Developing systems that promote Veterans' recovery from military sexual trauma. Recommendations from the Veterans Health Administration national program implementation. Mil Psychol. 2018;30(3):270–81.
77. Dinnen S, Kane V, Cook JM. Trauma-informed care: a paradigm shift needed for services with homeless veterans. Prof Case Manag. 2014;19(4):161–70. quiz 71-2
78. United States Interagency Council on Ending Homelessness. Ending veteran homelessness. Updated 30 November 2018. Accessed 2 March 2019. Available from: https://www.usich.gov/goals/veterans.
79. Perron BE, Alexander-Eitzman B, Gillespie DF, Pollio D. Modeling the mental health effects of victimization among homeless persons. Soc Sci Med. 2008;67(9):1475–9.
80. O'Connell MJ, Kasprow W, Rosenheck RA. Rates and risk factors for homelessness after successful housing in a sample of formerly homeless veterans. Psychiatr Serv. 2008;59(3):268–75.
81. National Coalition for Homeless Veterans (NCHV). Homeless Female Veterans. Washington, DC. Available from: http://www.nchv.org/images/uploads/HFVpaper.pdf.
82. US Government Accountability Office (GAO). Homeless Women Veterans: Actions needed to ensure safe and appropriate housing Washington, DC. 2012, January 23. Available from: https://www.gao.gov/products/GAO-12-182.
83. Washington DL, Yano EM, McGuire J, Hines V, Lee M, Gelberg L. Risk factors for homelessness among women veterans. J Health Care Poor Underserved. 2010;21(1):82–91.
84. Tsai J, Pietrzak RH, Rosenheck RA. Homeless veterans who served in Iraq and Afghanistan: gender differences, combat exposure, and comparisons with previous cohorts of homeless veterans. Admin Pol Ment Health. 2013;40(5):400–5.
85. Kim PY, Thomas JL, Wilk JE, Castro CA, Hoge CW. Stigma, barriers to care, and use of mental health services among active duty and National Guard soldiers after combat. Psychiatr Serv. 2010;61(6):582–8.
86. Coleman SJ, Stevelink SAM, Hatch SL, Denny JA, Greenberg N. Stigma-related barriers and facilitators to help seeking for mental health issues in the armed forces: a systematic review and thematic synthesis of qualitative literature. Psychol Med. 2017;47(11):1880–92.
87. Post EP, Metzger M, Dumas P, Lehmann L. Integrating mental health into primary care within the Veterans Health Administration. Fam Syst Health. 2010;28(2):83–90.
88. US Department of Veterans Affairs. Vet Center Program. Washington, DC. 2018 May 28. Accessed 11 June 2018. Available from: https://www.vetcenter.va.gov/.
89. Vet Centers. Final rule. Fed Regist. 2016;81(41):10764–5.
90. Substance Abuse and Mental Health Services Administration (SAMHSA). SAMHSA's concept of trauma and guidance for a trauma-informed approach. 2014. Accessed 2 June 2018. Available from: https://store.samhsa.gov/shin/content/SMA14-4884/SMA14-4884.pdf.

91. Gilmore AK, Davis MT, Grubaugh A, Resnick H, Birks A, Denier C, et al. "Do you expect me to receive PTSD care in a setting where most of the other patients remind me of the perpetrator?": Home-based telemedicine to address barriers to care unique to military sexual trauma and Veterans Affairs hospitals. Contemp Clin Trials. 2016;48:59–64.
92. Kehle-Forbes SM, Harwood EM, Spoont MR, Sayer NA, Gerould H, Murdoch M. Experiences with VHA care: a qualitative study of U.S. women veterans with self-reported trauma histories. BMC Womens Health. 2017;17(1):38.
93. Veterans Health Administration Mental Health Services. Understanding your client's military background. Military Screening Questions. 2018. Accessed 10 June 2018. Available from: https://www.mentalhealth.va.gov/communityproviders/docs/Military_Service_Screening.pdf.
94. Veterans Health Administration. Why Screen for Military Service? Understanding your client's military background. Military Screening Questions. 2018. Accessed 2 March 2019. Available from: https://www.mentalhealth.va.gov/communityproviders/screening.asp.

# Part III
# Clinical Strategies

# Chapter 7
# Trauma-Informed Adult Primary Care

Megan R. Gerber

## Introduction: The Challenge of Trauma-Informed Care in Adult Primary Care

This chapter will focus on the provision of primary care services to adults. In the United States (US), primary care is delivered by allopathic and osteopathic physicians trained in internal medicine and family practice and by advanced practice nurses and physician assistants all of whom will be referred to here collectively as primary care providers (PCPs). Obstetrician-gynecologists provide aspects of primary health care to women, and this discussion is relevant to their outpatient office practices as well. Many of the principles outlined in this chapter are also derived from, and are relevant to, pediatric and adolescent medical settings.

Aspects of the US primary care delivery system—short visits, large patient panels, shortages of PCPs [1], and challenges to access in some communities [2],— make primary care settings potentially difficult environments for the trauma-exposed adult. Some argue that primary care is more complex than other specialties due to the sheer breadth of patient presentations and the number of inputs and outputs managed during each visit [3]. PCPs must manage each patient's comorbidities, disease severity, medication tolerance, beliefs, desires, and socioeconomic factors [4], typically in 20 minutes or less for the average visit [5]. Burnout among physicians alone has become rampant and is most common in the specialties of family practice and internal medicine [6]. Yet, if underlying trauma results in chronic disease and drives utilization of care, the primary care delivery system cannot ignore it. One potential solution lies in fully integrating a trauma-informed care (TIC) approach into primary

---

M. R. Gerber (✉)
Section of General Internal Medicine, Boston University School of Medicine, Veterans Affairs (VA) Boston Healthcare System, Boston, MA, USA
e-mail: meggerber@post.harvard.edu

© Springer Nature Switzerland AG 2019
M. R. Gerber (ed.), *Trauma-Informed Healthcare Approaches*,
https://doi.org/10.1007/978-3-030-04342-1_7

care workflow, "baking it in," so to speak, which will benefit both patients and clinicians. In one study, PCPs perceptions of a clinic's ability to address patients' social needs were associated with lower burnout scores [7]. While much of the current literature on TIC focuses on mental health and pediatric settings, adult primary care is an ideal setting for thoughtful and innovative approaches to implementation of TIC.

The landmark Adverse Childhood Experiences (ACEs) study, which first shed light on the linkage between childhood adversity and adult disease, was conducted in a cohort of adults drawn from primary care patient panels at Kaiser Permanente, a large group model health maintenance organization in California [8]. These patients were mostly White, employed, middle- and upper-income persons who one might have assumed had more stable childhood environments [9]. The study found that a higher number of ACEs increased poor health behaviors including smoking, severe obesity, physical inactivity, alcohol, and illicit drug use. Odds of ischemic heart disease, any cancer, stroke, chronic bronchitis/emphysema, sexually transmitted disease, and diabetes were elevated most notably when four or more ACEs were endorsed by patients [8]. Adults with six or more ACEs had on average a life expectancy of 20 years less than those with a lower score [10]. Addressing adverse health behaviors and managing chronic disease are at the heart of adult primary care practice, and we are in daily contact with survivors of trauma.

Multiple studies have demonstrated high rates of multiple forms of interpersonal trauma and posttraumatic stress disorder (PTSD) among primary care patients [11–14]. It also appears that many primary care patients with trauma exposure and psychiatric conditions are not receiving mental health care, for example, in one urban setting, 65% of African American primary care patients had experienced trauma, and 51% had PTSD, yet only 21% of these patients were receiving treatment [14]. Trauma-exposed patients are often not well served by traditional healthcare delivery systems. Patients with trauma histories and PTSD also report more negative perceptions of, and interactions with, clinicians [15, 16]. In the US, access to mental and behavioral health is commonly lacking [17, 18], and primary care has often been dubbed "the de facto US mental health system" [19].

## How Trauma "Looks" in Primary Care

In addition to an increased burden of disease including cardiovascular conditions, diabetes, and cancer [8], primary care patients with trauma histories often exhibit a high burden of somatic symptoms [20], some of which remain medically unexplained [21]. These patients are often high utilizers who revisit practices frequently [22–24]. However, repeat medical visits and diagnostic tests are not ultimately therapeutic for them. Others avoid medical care entirely or minimize physical symptoms that might require an intrusive exam [25]. Patients with trauma histories may appear uncooperative, anxious, or jumpy during seemingly benign interactions. They often exhibit strong emotional reactions such as crying, showing signs of panic, irritability, or becoming tearful during an exam without obvious cause [25]. An overwhelmed trauma survivor might dysregulate, appear angry, or shut down emotionally [26].

It is important that PCPs and their teams remain vigilant for signs and symptoms of dissociation which is defined in the *Diagnostic and Statistical Manual of Mental Disorders, Fifth Edition (DSM-5)*, as a "disruption of and/or discontinuity in the normal, subjective integration of one or more aspects of psychological functioning, including – but not limited to – memory, identity, consciousness, perception, and motor control" [27]. Dissociative phenomena occur across a clinical spectrum [28]; the mildest (and most common) form is "spacing out" in which the patient would report experiencing this as a memory gap or time that cannot be accounted for [28, 29]. Other presenting signs of dissociation include a glazed look, appearing "frozen," or physically withdrawn [25]. Patients can become suddenly quiet/uncommunicative during an episode of dissociation and can seem disoriented and distractible [25]; they are often unable to make or sustain eye contact. Other presentations include blinking, eye rolling, changes in body posture, and trance-like behavior [29]. Episodes of pseudoseizure have been linked to dissociation [30]. A dissociative patient may have difficulty concentrating and can seem disconnected from the present.

Many PCPs have not been trained to recognize and manage dissociative episodes [29]. Management recommendations include stopping an invasive exam or procedure and helping the patient with "grounding" (returning control to the patient and refocusing on the present). This can be done through words or physical sensations such as offering the patient a glass of water and providing a tactile object such as a stuffed animal, squishy ball, or even a coarse medical washcloth. Another grounding technique is to focus on concrete, simple tasks that are free of abstract connotations and can return a sense of control back to the patient [29]. Examples include counting aloud with the patient, discussing the color of the room, or suggesting that the patient focus on their breathing [29]. Well-meaning clinicians and staff may have the impulse to touch the patient to reassure and provide comfort. This is not recommended as it can be a sensory reminder of previous trauma and can be misinterpreted by the patient [29]. Trauma-informed practice, through its emphasis on identifying patient experience and ascertaining what may help an individual feel more comfortable in the medical environment, can help deter or prevent dissociation.

Other common stigmata of trauma exposure in primary care include non-participation in treatment plans, for example, patients with PTSD can fail to adhere to medication regimens [31] or miss appointments. Patients' chronic conditions can seem stubbornly refractory to treatment because we are not addressing the underlying trauma and PTSD that perpetuate them [32].

## History of Interpersonal Trauma, Chronic Pain and Substance Use

Adult primary care settings bear much of the burden of treating patients with chronic pain, and severe pain is common among primary care patients with substance use disorder (SUD) [33]. Chronic pain in trauma-exposed patients is common [34–36], and these patients can also present with an increased prevalence of somatic symptoms [36, 37]. The opioid epidemic has provided additional challenges in healthcare delivery

[38], and PCPs are on the "front lines" [39]. Chronic pain patients report high rates of trauma exposure throughout the lifespan [40]. Past abuse, especially in childhood, can predispose toward addiction and may complicate treatment of pain [41]. The widely employed Opioid Risk Tool weights history of preadolescent sexual abuse as equivalent to alcohol misuse in predicting risk of future aberrant medication taking behavior [41]. Adding to the challenges faced in primary care, trauma-exposed patients prescribed controlled substances have reported that repeated negotiations of prescription refills are a source of anxiety and distress [24]; this may result in what can appear to be difficult behaviors or "drug seeking" presentations.

Interpersonal trauma exposure is linked to subsequent development of SUD across the population [42, 43]. Women with SUD, in particular, have high rates of past sexual or physical abuse [44]; these rates may exceed those found among other medical populations using the same measures [45]. While many healthcare systems offer addiction services, availability of treatment in the US is poor overall, and many who need care for SUD cannot access it [46]. This results in PCPs and their care teams taking the lead in caring for patients with comorbid trauma histories and substance misuse [47, 48].

## Inquiry: Patients Want to Be Asked

Trauma-exposed patients support inquiry in primary care settings; this has been demonstrated for a number of forms of interpersonal violence including child abuse [24, 49], intimate partner violence (IPV) [50], and sexual assault [51]. However, many PCPs feel ill-prepared to address trauma directly with their patients [52]. Patients without significant trauma histories also support screening [49]. Inquiry about traumatic experiences has been shown to increase patient satisfaction with care [53].

## TIC in Primary Care: Better Care

Data supporting improved patient outcomes after implementation of TIC in primary care settings is currently sparse [54]. In a randomized study of a trauma-informed medical care training for PCPs, family medicine physician participants demonstrated a significant increase in patient centeredness after the training [55]. Their patients subsequently rated the trained PCPs higher on a post-training partnership scale [56].

We do know that good communication in primary care is critical and does influence patient satisfaction and adherence [57]. TIC is truly a variant of patient-centered care which has been shown to improve outcomes in some domains, notably patient satisfaction and self-management [58, 59]. Increasing patient engagement and activation leads to improved health outcomes [60]. There remains a general consensus that equipping PCPs and their care teams to engage high-utilizing, "high-needs" patients in primary care is necessary [61] and that a strong patient–clinician relationship does improve some health outcomes [62, 63]. Often understanding the connection between traumatic experiences and health can be transformative and healing, enabling patients to understand that childhood and adult trauma underlie many illnesses and unhealthy behaviors for which many may blame themselves [32].

Raja et al. have proposed an approach to TIC in medical settings [64] that begins with small changes in practice that can be used with all patients, "universal trauma precautions." Knowledge of a patient's detailed trauma history is not necessary and these strategies may enable trust and rapport with survivors [64]. Trauma-specific strategies, typically interdisciplinary in nature, are deployed once the provider is aware that a given patient has a trauma history [64]. Purkey notes that clinicians and staff can "bear witness" to the patient's experience of trauma, not "in all its terrible detail, but in general outlines." Doing this, and identifying how the abuse may have led to maladaptive coping strategies, can be life changing and ensures that patients do not feel responsible for the trauma they have experienced [65].

## Screening for Traumatic Exposures in Primary Care

Trauma-informed care typically includes routine and deliberate identification of traumatic experiences with referral to appropriate services and care [66]. Others point out that not all systems have the capacity to carry out universal trauma screening but can and should employ basic TIC or "universal trauma precautions" [32, 64]. The Institute of Medicine [67] has also called for identification and a response to trauma in primary care settings. Currently, the US Preventive Services Task Force (USPSTF) [68] and a number of professional organizations, including the American Medical Association (AMA) [69], the American Academy of Family Physicians (AAFP) [70], and the American College of Obstetricians and Gynecologists (ACOG) [71], among others, recommend routine screening for IPV. The USPSTF evaluated a number of screens and found six brief tools [68] that showed the highest sensitivity and specificity and can be self-administered or used in a clinician interview format; these include the brief Hurt, Insult, Threaten, Scream (HITS) [72] and Humiliation, Afraid, Rape, Kick (HARK) [73] measures. Multiple other validated IPV screens exist, and the CDC has published a guide entitled "Intimate Partner Violence and Sexual Violence Victimization Assessment Instruments for Use in Healthcare Settings" [74]. There are currently no evidence-based population-level recommendations for routinely screening adults for a history of childhood abuse or sexual assault; ACOG recommends inquiry for both [48, 75], and many favor routine inquiry despite a lack of formal guidelines [76]. A sensitive and specific screen for detecting a history of childhood abuse in adults is the Modified Childhood Trauma Questionnaire–Short Form (CTQ-SF) [77]. Some have used versions of the

ACE questionnaire in primary care and found it feasible and worthy of additional study [78], although this remains controversial.

Another trauma-informed strategy that has been proposed is "task-centered disclosure" [76]. Task-centered disclosure is a form of screening relevant to the examination to be performed. When using this form of screening, sensitive questions are asked when the patient is fully dressed and sitting, using a question such as *"Is there anything about your past experiences that makes this exam particularly difficult for you?"* Then a follow-up question is asked, for example, *"What can I do to make it easier for you?"* [79].

Some authors recommend screening all adults for PTSD [80], making the argument that (1) some providers may find it easier to screen for PTSD than to ask behaviorally based questions about specific traumas; (2) PTSD is an important mediator of many of the long-term health effects of trauma; (3) a number of time-limited, evidence-based treatments exist for PTSD; and (4) a large proportion of cases of PTSD remit over time [25, 28] (Table 7.1). Identification of other treatable conditions that commonly result from past trauma, such as anxiety, depression, chronic pain and SUD, is another feasible approach [81].

A number of screening tools have been developed for primary care; one of the most widely used is the PC-PTSD-5 [82] (Table 7.2). Detailed, but brief, screening questions are only asked if a patient endorses a traumatic event in the initial stem question.

Prior to any routine screening, it is essential that resources be in place and identified, either within the healthcare organization itself or in the broader community or both. A listing of these resources and appropriate contacts should be readily available and can be developed by the organization for use across all departments. Primary care teams should not be scrambling to identify resources during an already busy patient care visit. Ideally, social work and mental health colleagues are available in the practice or onsite for a warm handoff and collaborative care. Lastly, any patient disclosure should be met with support and validation. Consider the process of asking, listening, and accepting as an intervention in and of itself [54].

**Table 7.1** Trauma-specific screening versus PTSD screening [25]

| Trauma-specific screening | Screening for PTSD |
| --- | --- |
| Connectivity to safety planning, advocacy in medical/community setting | Potentially easier for some PCPs (talking about traumatic experiences and violence is difficult for many) |
| The mental health effects of trauma are heterogeneous (differing treatment may be needed based on the exposure or multiple exposures) | Diagnosis of PTSD is strongly linked to health effects after trauma |
| Can capture temporality (recent and current risk of trauma) | Better fits biomedical model of screening (PTSD is a treatable condition with defined interventions) |
| May provide validation of difficult/shameful experience(s) | PTSD remits in the majority of patients |

**Table 7.2** PC-PTSD-5 questions and scoring [82]

| |
|---|
| Patients answer one stem question first, "Sometimes things happen to people that are unusually or especially frightening, horrible, or traumatic" |
| *For example:*<br>  A serious accident or fire<br>  A physical or sexual assault or abuse<br>  An earthquake or flood<br>  A war<br>  Seeing someone be killed or seriously injured<br>  Having a loved one die through homicide or suicide |
| Have you ever experienced this kind of event?<br>If the answer is no, no further items need to be completed |
| If yes, continue with screening |
| In the past month, have you...<br>1. had nightmares about the event(s) or thought about the event(s) when you did not want to? YES/NO<br>2. tried hard not to think about the event(s) or went out of your way to avoid situations that reminded you of the event(s)? YES/NO<br>3. been constantly on guard, watchful, or easily startled? YES/NO<br>4. felt numb or detached from people, activities, or your surroundings? YES/NO<br>5. felt guilty or unable to stop blaming yourself or others for the events(s) or any problems the event(s) may have caused? YES/NO |
| Scoring: Each YES response is one point. Three points is a positive screen |

## Guidance for TIC in Primary Care

The Substance Abuse and Mental Health Services Administration (SAMHSA) has been a leader in the field of TIC. According to SAMHSA principles, trauma-informed care settings [66]:

- *Realize the widespread impact of trauma and understand potential paths for recovery.* In trauma-informed primary care, there is understanding of the impact of trauma on patients, and the practice seeks to understand the origins of trauma faced by the communities that practice serves [83]. Resources such as community and healthcare-based programs are known to all staff, and staff are made aware of cultural issues and needs of the patient community.
- *Recognize the signs and symptoms of trauma in clients, families, staff, and others involved with the system.* All primary care staff are trained to recognize signs and symptoms of trauma in patients, including some of the more subtle or indirect manifestations.
- *Respond by fully integrating knowledge about trauma into policies, procedures, and practices.* Primary care practices incorporate TIC processes into their everyday workflow. A more detailed discussion follows.
- *Seek to actively resist re-traumatization.* All members of primary care teams are aware that the healthcare environment has the capacity to cause distress and contains many potential triggers. Through training and routine processes, they are familiar with common examples of frequently distressing and triggering situations.

Finally, to accomplish this, and help patients heal from trauma and become healthy, there must also be an ongoing focus on staff wellness [32, 83]. Machtinger aptly summarized this, *"For both patients and providers moving toward trauma-informed primary care has the potential to transform the experience and efficacy of primary care from treatment to genuine healing"* [32]. In adult primary care, the challenge is to not allow the pressures of high visit volumes, short appointment times, and large numbers of health indicators and screenings to result in care that is not trauma-informed. This can best be accomplished by creating trauma-informed clinical processes and anticipating, when possible, the needs of trauma survivors ahead of time.

## Before the Visit: A Welcoming and Trauma-Sensitive Environment

The clinical environment should be as quiet as possible (this may be very difficult in ambulatory settings within hospitals), mechanisms should be installed on older doors to keep them from slamming shut, sound proofing measures and mechanical sound screens/white noise machines can also be employed. While many safety net settings that serve trauma-exposed populations may be located in older buildings (and subject to budgetary constraints), when possible soothing colors and artwork should be used; some research suggests that lighting and views of nature may be more important than color [84].

When patients with trauma histories enter healthcare facilities, they may feel very anxious. Clear and linguistically appropriate signage is very important to help maintain a sense of control. Patients with trauma histories may not feel comfortable sitting close to others [24]. Waiting rooms should be set up, whenever possible, to reduce crowding and to allow patients some choice of where to sit. The check-in area and process should allow for confidentiality.

All staff, including clerical/administrative and phone center personnel, should undergo training on the prevalence of traumatic exposures in the population they serve and understand that some behaviors (e.g., irritability or rapidity to anger) may be related to anxiety or even a sense of fear or dread. When possible, patients who appear distressed or "triggered" in waiting room settings should be brought to an exam room or a more private waiting area as soon as possible.

Primary care practices should be aware of the resources available in the larger healthcare system or in the surrounding community. Pamphlets, palm cards, and posters should be available and visible in waiting and other public areas. Patients who may not directly disclose trauma often benefit from the information itself and may infer that the practice is open to discussing and addressing these issues. TIC also includes being sensitive to cultural, historical, and gender issues; all information should be inclusive and welcoming, written in the languages commonly spoken in the community, and accessible to those with low vision. Patients should always be informed ahead of time of clinician gender and offered alternative appointments if gender is a concern. Both women and men who have experienced trauma often have strong preferences around visit provider gender. While not always possible, continuity of care creates safety and fosters trust. In one study of women with trauma histories, participants reported feeling a connection to staff and providers who had known them for a long time and expressed more forgiveness if physicians appeared rushed or inattentive on a given day [24]. Fostering continuity and trust in primary care is a challenge as modern health care is often fragmented by use of urgent care clinics, multiple specialty referrals, and trainees in the system. The medical home model is an ideal platform on which to build TIC [83, 85].

A number of professional organizations recommend preplanning [86] for scheduled medical visits as a means of enhancing patient centeredness and efficiency; during chart review, the presence of trauma-related documentation can be helpful in preparing for the patient encounter [87], especially if the scheduled appointment may include an invasive exam. As patients with trauma histories may present with more somatic complaints, or need a longer visit for other reasons, preplanning enables the primary care team to potentially offload some routine care (lab orders, preventive care prompts/reminders, chronic disease management) from the visit itself, maximizing the time the patient and clinician have to talk.

## The Appointment

In many primary care practices, there is an initial clinical intake with a member of the healthcare team (often a medical assistant or nurse). During this intake, clinical care prompts/reminders, aspects of medication reconciliation, and even vaccinations may be performed along with vital signs. At this point, support staff can be trained to be vigilant for signs of distress and unease and can then communicate with the PCP. Practices will vary in the nature and amount of information they collect from patients on the visit day, prior to the encounter, but being trauma aware is important even when sensitive questions are not being asked. Anxious feelings about an office visit may be amplified for a trauma survivor [26]. When a patient expresses a concern or fear, all staff must be equipped to identify and, acknowledge it as understandable (or even as a normal reaction); this kind of validation is very important for trauma survivors [26].

## PCP Encounter and Examination

Medical visits may often be perceived as invasive by patients. In primary care, encounters often involve being asked potentially sensitive questions, undressing, examination of intimate body parts, vulnerable physical positions, and sometimes receipt of uncomfortable—even painful—treatments; even an injection/vaccination can be difficult for some. Patients, even those who have not experienced significant trauma, can feel a lack of control over the situation or be intimidated by the power dynamics of the clinician-patient relationship. So, it is critical that PCPs and teams be aware of the possibility of a trauma history and take steps to ensure all actions are as trauma-informed as possible. Patients may also have experienced serious illness or negative experiences in the medical setting or may have witnessed difficult healthcare interactions for a loved one. One brief question that may help tailor the visit is *"Is there anything in your history that makes seeing a practitioner or having a physical examination difficult?"* [88]. This creates an opportunity for patients to advocate for themselves by explaining their past medical experiences, potential anxiety, and what has been helpful and harmful previously. This simple question also enables patients to feel that they have some control over what will happen during the encounter and fosters trust. Detailed TIC actions and strategies for the primary care encounter (Table 7.3), examination (Table 7.4), and invasive examinations/procedures (Table 7.5) are summarized below.

**Table 7.3** Recommendations for TIC during the PCP-patient encounter [24, 64, 87]

| |
|---|
| Allow your patient to choose where she/he/they sit in the exam room. |
| Patients should always be asked for permission before another person (i.e., staff, trainee) is brought into the exam room. |
| Always take the time to sit down and be sure you are at eye level with a patient. |
| It is strongly recommended that you meet patients when they are fully clothed. Detailed discussions and decision-making should occur when the patient is fully clothed as well. |
| If you will be using a computer and typing during the visit, explain briefly why, and make eye contact as much as possible. |
| Always stop typing if a patient discloses something sensitive or becomes distraught. |
| Ask patients about their priorities for the visit. |
| If an interpreter is being used, ask if there is a gender or cultural preference for this service. |
| Obtain the patient's consent before the exam. Comments like "it's time for your exam" *or* "please get undressed" can be very distressing for some patients. |
| Explain beforehand what the exam today will consist of and what parts of the body will be examined preferably while the patient is fully clothed. |
| When possible, ask patients to remove clothing to their level of comfort. If feasible, offer the patient the option of shifting an item of clothing out of the way rather than putting on a gown. |
| Always provide an after-visit summary or written instructions/referral information in case the patient is not able to attend to details, feels overwhelmed, or dissociates. |
| Some recommend allowing the door to be left slightly open; in some settings it may not be possible to safeguard the privacy of the patient and others if this is done. |

**Table 7.4** TIC recommendations for the examination [24, 64, 87]

| |
|---|
| Obtain the patient's consent/permission to begin the exam. |
| Ask the patient before starting if she/he/they have concerns about the exam. |
| Give the patient as much control and choice as possible. |
| Survivors have reported difficulty with dark/confined exam rooms. Be attentive to lighting; if it is necessary to darken the room for an examination, warn the patient, and explain why this is needed. Raise the level of light as soon as possible. |
| Patients who are anxious in a fully supine position may feel more comfortable propped up with a pillow; this also allows them to see you and staff. |
| Avoid unexpected physical contact. |
| Ask the patient for permission as you go through the examination, describe what you are doing ("in order to examine your thyroid gland, I will need to place my fingers on the front of your neck"), and avoid sudden, abrupt movements. |
| Talk to the patient throughout and explain what you are doing and why. |

**Table 7.5** TIC strategies for pelvic and other invasive exams/procedures [64, 87, 89]

| |
|---|
| Give the patient the choice of whether to have the exam, and ask the patient what can help them feel more comfortable during the exam. Defer the exam as needed. |
| Bates et al. recommend that when a patient describes a prior negative experience, gently elicit specific details and strategize together to minimize discomfort [89]. |
| Ask the patient if having another person in the room for support would be helpful. There are no universal guidelines on chaperone use; experts recommend routine use of chaperones by male clinicians. Female clinicians may offer a chaperone to accommodate individual patients' preferences [89]. |
| Remind patients they are the expert on their bodies! |
| Be sure you or an assistant is monitoring the patient's facial expressions and body language during the exam. Drape the patient so you can see them during the exam. |
| Use the smallest speculum possible. |
| For pelvic exams, offer self-insertion of swabs when cultures are needed. |
| Offer guided self-insertion of speculum. |
| Use neutral terms and language like "foot holders" and "drape." |
| If a patient needs a smaller (or differently shaped) speculum, put a note in the chart for future reference. |
| At the beginning of the exam, remind the patient that s/he is in charge of the exam, and it will stop any time s/he asks. Describe what you will be doing, and ask permission/obtain consent for each component of the exam. |
| Warn of possible sounds and sensations: "the speculum will click when I open it," "you may have some light spotting after the pap smear." |
| Patients can be offered the opportunity to listen to music during the exam (either with a personal device/headphones or a staff smartphone) or to choose the topic of conversation. |
| Do not give orders (e.g., telling the patient, "relax"); employ suggestions like "some find it helpful to take a deep breath during this part of the exam." |

## Caring for Primary Care Staff

An essential part of TIC is maintaining the physical and emotional health and well being of staff; it is critical that the healthcare environment also support its clinicians and teams [32]. Techniques and approaches to self-care and wellness are covered in detail later in Chapter 11. As discussed above, primary care teams manage complex patients with multiple morbidities and psychosocial challenges. The potential emotional impact of caring for patients with trauma histories, and listening to their stories can add to the already demanding and overwhelming nature of primary care practice [90]. Clinicians in under-resourced settings may have few referral sources and tools to aid in the care of such patients. Trauma-exposed patients bring chronic health issues, distress, relationship, authority issues and somatization to encounters with PCPs [91]. It is important that staff understand their own histories and reactions to patients' experiences. Given the prevalence of interpersonal trauma, it is likely that many staff have had their own adverse life experiences [32, 64, 90]. When combined with the pressures of primary care practice, these issues may lead to vicarious, or secondary, traumatization and exacerbate burnout and compassion fatigue.

Burnout is a syndrome characterized by a loss of enthusiasm for work (emotional exhaustion), feelings of cynicism (depersonalization), and a low sense of personal accomplishment. It can result in feelings of physical, emotional, and mental exhaustion along with feelings of being overwhelmed [6]. As mentioned above, it is common among PCPs [6] and may result in low job satisfaction and powerlessness and can adversely influence quality of care, increase the risk for medical errors, and promote early retirement. Compassion fatigue refers to diminished capacity of a health professional when he/she experiences repeated distress at knowing about or witnessing the suffering of patients; it is often the result of helping and knowing about trauma [90, 92].

Burnout and compassion fatigue are common among healthcare personnel and are not unique to those who work with survivors of trauma. Conversely, vicarious traumatization is unique to those who work with trauma-exposed patients and occurs when a clinician experiences negative transformative processes [92], a change in their inner experience, or a system of meaning, as a result of engagement with survivors; at times, it can be as debilitating as the primary trauma [90]. Vicarious traumatization can afflict the entire care team, including administrative staff [90]. Higher risk of vicarious traumatization is conferred by personal trauma history, chronicity of trauma work, combining service provision and research, younger age of the clinician, and the individual's capacity for empathy [90, 92]. Most of the literature on vicarious traumatization focuses on mental health providers, social workers, first responders, and humanitarian workers, although work on primary care providers and health professions trainees is emerging [92, 96].

While not specifically studied among PCPs and their teams, it is likely that risk of vicarious traumatization would be greater when working with communities that have a high prevalence of trauma, including sexual assault survivors, trafficked persons, and areas with high rates of community violence and historical trauma. Lastly, secondary traumatic stress is similar to vicarious traumatization but differs in that it is identified based on clinical symptoms and more closely parallels PTSD. Providers can experience intrusive symptoms, hyperarousal, numbing and nightmares. The prevalence of secondary traumatic stress among PCPs is unknown [92], but likely less common than compassion fatigue, burnout and vicarious traumatization [90]. Nimmo has reviewed validated scales that can be used to measure all four of these constructs [92].

The impact of caring for trauma survivors underscores the need not only for practices but for entire organizations to adopt a TIC approach; safeguarding the health of providers and teams underlies good care. While a detailed discussion of wellness and self-care is out of the scope of this chapter, it is important for individuals working with trauma-exposed persons to be aware of the potential for burnout, compassion fatigue, and vicarious traumatization and to seek assistance. Good self-care practices (covered in Chapter 11) must be combined with organizational support and teamwork [7]. Mental health has a much more developed practice and culture of providing support and supervision to those who work with trauma survivors [90]; building on those models, interdisciplinary teams can be built in primary care in close collaboration with other services. Finally, trauma-sensitive health professions training beginning early on—and continuing throughout careers—may also mitigate some of the responses described above [55, 90, 93, 94, 97]. Patients with trauma histories also favor enhanced training on trauma and can perceive a lack of skill in some encounters [24].

## Resilience

One of the critiques of the TIC model is that it focuses too much on negative experiences [9] and does not place adequate focus on protective, resilience-oriented approaches. Even the most vulnerable have strengths, dreams for the future, and have endured numerous challenges and have "bounced back" [9]. Recognizing the "phenomenal resilience" [24] of so many can be tremendously rewarding in primary care practice. A clearly stated goal of TIC is to promote resilience and healing [66], so one of the challenges in primary care will be to emphasize strengths and promote patient self-efficacy. Incorporating strengths-based interviewing, or using a whole health approach and asking the patient *"what really matters to you, what do you need to be healthy for?"* [95], can begin to incorporate and promote patient activation and self efficacy into the, albeit too brief, primary care discourse. This approach similarly aids healthcare teams and some have described the concept of "compassion satisfaction" which emphasizes the gratifying and rewarding aspects of care [92].

## Conclusion

Primary care clinicians and care teams work longitudinally with adults, many of whom are aging, medically complex and commonly experiencing the cumulative effect of a lifetime of trauma and psychosocial stressors. We are in a unique position to make a difference for our patients, primary care has the power to prevent, identify, and address trauma-related problems [83]. By offering longitudinal connection with patients, primary care offers a consistent and compassionate relationship that can aid in promoting healing and recovery [96]. While primary care in the US has been challenged and often under-resourced, it remains the setting in which a patient's entire well-being is addressed; primary care teams address health behavior change and chronic illness, both of which are impacted by trauma exposure. Research demonstrates that patients with trauma histories favor inquiry and that connecting traumatic pasts to present-day health can be highly effective. Applying principles of TIC to primary care settings, even slowly and incrementally, enhances patient experience, augments existing efforts at making care patient-centered and has the promise to improve patient health outcomes. Primary care practices are busy and often strained by multiple competing demands, high volumes, performance metrics, and productivity requirements and cannot accomplish implementation of TIC on their own. Practice-managers, healthcare organizations, and even insurance companies, must support rollout and sustainment of trauma-informed, patient-centered primary care. We have the opportunity and the responsibility to actively prevent retraumatization in our practices, develop resources to support survivors [96], and to partner with our patients and their communities to move toward healing and better health.

# References

1. Dall T, West T, Chakrabarti R, Reynolds R, Iacobucci W. The complexities of physician supply and demand: projections from 2016 to 2030. 2018 Update. American Association of Medical Colleges, Washington, DC; 2018. Accessed 16 June 2018. Available from: https://aamc-black.global.ssl.fastly.net/production/media/filer_public/85/d7/85d7b689-f417-4ef0-97fb-ecc129836829/aamc_2018_workforce_projections_update_april_11_2018.pdf.
2. Altschuler J, Margolius D, Bodenheimer T, Grumbach K. Estimating a reasonable patient panel size for primary care physicians with team-based task delegation. Ann Fam Med. 2012;10(5):396–400.
3. Katerndahl DA, Wood R, Jaén CR. A method for estimating relative complexity of ambulatory care. Ann Fam Med. 2010;8(4):341–7.
4. Young RA, Roberts RG, Holden RJ. The challenges of measuring, improving, and reporting quality in primary care. Ann Fam Med. 2017;15(2):175–82.
5. Shaw MK, Davis SA, Fleischer AB, Feldman SR. The duration of office visits in the United States, 1993 to 2010. Am J Manag Care. 2014;20(10):820–6.
6. Shanafelt TD, Boone S, Tan L, Dyrbye LN, Sotile W, Satele D, et al. Burnout and satisfaction with work-life balance among US physicians relative to the general US population. Arch Intern Med. 2012;172(18):1377–85.
7. Olayiwola JN, Willard-Grace R, Dube K, Hessler D, Shunk R, Grumbach K, et al. Higher perceived clinic capacity to address Patients' social needs associated with lower burnout in primary care providers. J Health Care Poor Underserved. 2018;29(1):415–29.
8. Felitti VJ, Anda RF, Nordenberg D, Williamson DF, Spitz AM, Edwards V, et al. Relationship of childhood abuse and household dysfunction to many of the leading causes of death in adults. The Adverse Childhood Experiences (ACE) Study. Am J Prev Med. 1998;14(4):245–58.
9. Leitch L. Action steps using ACEs and trauma-informed care: a resilience model. Health Justice. 2017;5(1):5.

10. Brown DW, Anda RF, Tiemeier H, Felitti VJ, Edwards VJ, Croft JB, et al. Adverse childhood experiences and the risk of premature mortality. Am J Prev Med. 2009;37(5):389–96.
11. Liebschutz J, Saitz R, Brower V, Keane TM, Lloyd-Travaglini C, Averbuch T, et al. PTSD in urban primary care: high prevalence and low physician recognition. J Gen Intern Med. 2007;22(6):719–26.
12. Stein MB, McQuaid JR, Pedrelli P, Lenox R, McCahill ME. Posttraumatic stress disorder in the primary care medical setting. Gen Hosp Psychiatry. 2000;22(4):261–9.
13. Spottswood M, Davydow DS, Huang H. The prevalence of posttraumatic stress disorder in primary care: a systematic review. Harv Rev Psychiatry. 2017;25(4):159–69.
14. Alim TN, Graves E, Mellman TA, Aigbogun N, Gray E, Lawson W, et al. Trauma exposure, posttraumatic stress disorder and depression in an African-American primary care population. J Natl Med Assoc. 2006;98(10):1630–6.
15. Bassuk EL, Dawson R, Perloff J, Weinreb L. Post-traumatic stress disorder in extremely poor women: implications for health care clinicians. J Am Med Womens Assoc (1972). 2001;56(2):79–85.
16. Green BL, Kaltman SI, Chung JY, Holt MP, Jackson S, Dozier M. Attachment and health care relationships in low-income women with trauma histories: a qualitative study. J Trauma Dissociation. 2012;13(2):190–208.
17. Cunningham P, McKenzie K, Taylor EF. The struggle to provide community-based care to low-income people with serious mental illnesses. Health Aff (Millwood). 2006;25(3):694–705.
18. Gillespie L. Even with coverage expansion, access to mental health services poses challenges. Kaiser Health News [Internet]. 2014, Dec 18. Accessed 22 June 2018. Available from: https://khn.org/news/even-with-coverage-expansion-access-to-mental-health-services-poses-challenges/.
19. Kessler R, Stafford D. Primary care is the De facto mental health system. In: Kessler R, Stafford D, editors. Collaborative medicine case studies: evidence in practice. New York: Springer New York; 2008. p. 9–21.
20. Stein MB, Lang AJ, Laffaye C, Satz LE, Lenox RJ, Dresselhaus TR. Relationship of sexual assault history to somatic symptoms and health anxiety in women. Gen Hosp Psychiatry. 2004;26(3):178–83.
21. Katon W, Sullivan M, Walker E. Medical symptoms without identified pathology: relationship to psychiatric disorders, childhood and adult trauma, and personality traits. Ann Intern Med. 2001;134(9 Pt 2):917–25.
22. Rosenberg HJ, Rosenberg SD, Wolford GL, Manganiello PD, Brunette MF, Boynton RA. The relationship between trauma, PTSD, and medical utilization in three high risk medical populations. Int J Psychiatry Med. 2000;30(3):247–59.
23. Kartha A, Brower V, Saitz R, Samet JH, Keane TM, Liebschutz J. The impact of trauma exposure and post-traumatic stress disorder on healthcare utilization among primary care patients. Med Care. 2008;46(4):388–93.
24. Purkey E, Patel R, Beckett T, Mathieu F. Primary care experiences of women with a history of childhood trauma and chronic disease: trauma-informed care approach. Can Fam Physician. 2018;64(3):204–11.
25. Street AE, Gerber MR. Using lessons from VA to improve care for women with mental health and trauma histories, Part II. Washington, DC; 2014, Oct 1. Accessed 2 July 2018. Available from: https://www.hsrd.research.va.gov/for_researchers/cyber_seminars/archives/video_archive.cfm?SessionID=900.
26. Substance Abuse and Mental Health Services Administration (SAMHSA). Trauma-informed practice series: trauma survivors in medical and dental settings. Accessed 17 June 2018. Available from: https://www.integration.samhsa.gov/clinicalpractice/Trauma_Survivors_in_Medical_and_Dental_Settings.pdf.
27. Spiegel D, Loewenstein RJ, Lewis-Fernandez R, Sar V, Simeon D, Vermetten E, et al. Dissociative disorders in DSM-5. Depress Anxiety. 2011;28(12):E17–45.
28. Morgan CA, Hazlett G, Wang S, Richardson EG, Schnurr P, Southwick SM. Symptoms of dissociation in humans experiencing acute, uncontrollable stress: a prospective investigation. Am J Psychiatry. 2001;158(8):1239–47.

29. Bradley A. Dissociation. In: Liebschutz JM, Frayne SM, Saxe GN, editors. Violence against women: a physician's guide to identification and management. Philadelphia: Am Coll Phys; 2003. p. 262–7.
30. Harden CL. Pseudoseizures and dissociative disorders: a common mechanism involving traumatic experiences. Seizure. 1997;6(2):151–5.
31. Kronish IM, Lin JJ, Cohen BE, Voils CI, Edmondson D. Posttraumatic stress disorder and medication nonadherence in patients with uncontrolled hypertension. JAMA Intern Med. 2014;174(3):468–70.
32. Machtinger EL, Cuca YP, Khanna N, Rose CD, Kimberg LS. From treatment to healing: the promise of trauma-informed primary care. Womens Health Issues. 2015;25(3):193–7.
33. Alford DP, German JS, Samet JH, Cheng DM, Lloyd-Travaglini CA, Saitz R. Primary care patients with drug use report chronic pain and self-medicate with alcohol and other drugs. J Gen Intern Med. 2016;31(5):486–91.
34. Fishbain DA, Pulikal A, Lewis JE, Gao J. Chronic pain types differ in their reported prevalence of post-traumatic stress disorder (PTSD) and there is consistent evidence that chronic pain is associated with PTSD: an evidence-based structured systematic review. Pain medicine. 2017;18(4):711–35.
35. Sprang G, Bush HM, Coker AL, Brancato CJ. Types of trauma and self-reported pain that limits functioning in different-aged cohorts. J Interpers Violence. 2017: 886260517723144.
36. McCall-Hosenfeld JS, Winter M, Heeren T, Liebschutz JM. The association of interpersonal trauma with somatic symptom severity in a primary care population with chronic pain: exploring the role of gender and the mental health sequelae of trauma. J Psychosom Res. 2014;77(3):196–204.
37. Eberhard-Gran M, Schei B, Eskild A. Somatic symptoms and diseases are more common in women exposed to violence. J Gen Intern Med. 2007;22(12):1668–73.
38. Seal K, Becker W, Tighe J, Li Y, Rife T. Managing chronic pain in primary care: it really does take a village. J Gen Intern Med. 2017;32(8):931–4.
39. Bachhuber MA, Weiner J, Mitchell J, Samet JH. Primary care: on the front lines of the opioid crisis. Philadelphia: Penn Leonard Davis Institute of Health Economics, University of Pennsylvania; 2016.
40. Driscoll MA, Higgins DM, Seng EK, Buta E, Goulet JL, Heapy AA, et al. Trauma, social support, family conflict, and chronic pain in recent service veterans: does gender matter? Pain Med. 2015;16(6):1101–11.
41. Webster LR, Webster RM. Predicting aberrant behaviors in opioid-treated patients: preliminary validation of the opioid risk tool. Pain Med. 2005;6(6):432–42.
42. Hughes T, McCabe SE, Wilsnack SC, West BT, Boyd CJ. Victimization and substance use disorders in a national sample of heterosexual and sexual minority women and men. Addiction (Abingdon, England). 2010;105(12):2130–40.
43. Ullman SE, Relyea M, Peter-Hagene L, Vasquez AL. Trauma histories, substance use coping, PTSD, and problem substance use among sexual assault victims. Addict Behav. 2013;38(6):2219–23.
44. Covington SS. Women and addiction: a trauma-informed approach. J Psychoactive Drugs. 2008;Suppl 5:377–85.
45. McCloskey LA, Lichter E, Ganz ML, Williams CM, Gerber MR, Sege R, et al. Intimate partner violence and patient screening across medical specialties. Acad Emerg Med. 2005;12(8):712–22.
46. Hoge MA, Stuart GW, Morris J, Flaherty MT, Paris M Jr, Goplerud E. Mental health and addiction workforce development: federal leadership is needed to address the growing crisis. Health Aff (Millwood). 2013;32(11):2005–12.
47. Saitz R, Daaleman TP. Now is the time to address substance use disorders in primary care. Ann Fam Med. 2017;15(4):306–8.
48. American College of Obstetricians and Gynecologists (ACOG). Sexual assault. Committee opinion no. 592. Obstet Gynecol. 2014;123:905–9.

49. Goldstein E, Athale N, Sciolla AF, Catz SL. Patient preferences for discussing childhood trauma in primary care. Perm J. 2017;21:16–055.
50. Iverson KM, Huang K, Wells SY, Wright JD, Gerber MR, Wiltsey-Stirman S. Women veterans' preferences for intimate partner violence screening and response procedures within the Veterans Health Administration. Res Nurs Health. 2014;37(4):302–11.
51. Friedman LS, Samet JH, Roberts MS, Hudlin M, Hans P. Inquiry about victimization experiences. A survey of patient preferences and physician practices. Arch Intern Med. 1992;152(6):1186–90.
52. Green BL, Kaltman S, Frank L, Glennie M, Subramanian A, Fritts-Wilson M, et al. Primary care providers' experiences with trauma patients: a qualitative study. Psychol Trauma Theory Res Pract Policy. 2011;3(1):37–41.
53. Jackson JL, Kroenke K. The effect of unmet expectations among adults presenting with physical symptoms. Ann Intern Med. 2001;134(9 Pt 2):889–97.
54. Felitti VJ, Anda RF. The lifelong effects of adverse childhood experiences. In: Chadwick DL, Giardino AP, Alexander R, Thackeray JD, Esernio-Jenssen D, editors. Chadwick's child maltreatment: sexual abuse and psychological maltreatment. 4th ed. Florissant: STM Learning, Inc; 2014. p. 203–15.
55. Green BL, Saunders PA, Power E, Dass-Brailsford P, Schelbert KB, Giller E, et al. Trauma-informed medical care: CME communication training for primary care providers. Fam Med. 2015;47(1):7–14.
56. Green BL, Saunders PA, Power E, Dass-Brailsford P, Schelbert KB, Giller E, et al. Trauma-informed medical care: patient response to a primary care provider communication training. J Loss Trauma. 2016;21(2):147–59.
57. Haskard KB, Williams SL, DiMatteo MR, Rosenthal R, White MK, Goldstein MG. Physician and patient communication training in primary care: effects on participation and satisfaction. Health Psychol. 2008;27(5):513–22.
58. Rathert C, Wyrwich MD, Boren SA. Patient-centered care and outcomes:a systematic review of the literature. Med Care Res Rev. 2013;70(4):351–79.
59. Zolnierek KB, Dimatteo MR. Physician communication and patient adherence to treatment: a meta-analysis. Med Care. 2009;47(8):826–34.
60. Hibbard JH, Greene J. What the evidence shows about patient activation: better health outcomes and care experiences; fewer data on costs. Health Aff (Millwood). 2013;32(2):207–14.
61. Yedidia MJ. Competencies for engaging high-needs patients in primary care. Healthc (Amst). 2018;6(2):122–7.
62. Kelley JM, Kraft-Todd G, Schapira L, Kossowsky J, Riess H. The influence of the patient-clinician relationship on healthcare outcomes: a systematic review and meta-analysis of randomized controlled trials. PLoS One. 2014;9(4):e94207.
63. Kerse N, Buetow S, Mainous AG, Young G, Coster G, Arroll B. Physician-patient relationship and medication compliance: a primary care investigation. Ann Fam Med. 2004;2(5):455–61.
64. Raja S, Hasnain M, Hoersch M, Gove-Yin S, Rajagopalan C. Trauma informed care in medicine: current knowledge and future research directions. Fam Community Health. 2015;38(3):216–26.
65. Purkey E, Patel R, Phillips SP. Trauma-informed care: better care for everyone. Can Fam Physician. 2018;64(3):170–2.
66. Substance Abuse and Mental Health Services Administration (SAMHSA). SAMHSA's concept of trauma and guidance for a trauma-informed approach. 2014, October. Accessed 15 December 2018. Available from: https://store.samhsa.gov/product/SAMHSA-s-Concept-of-Trauma-and-Guidance-for-a-Trauma-Informed-Approach/SMA14-4884.htm
67. Institute of Medicine. Clinical preventive services for women: closing the gaps. Washington, DC; 2011. Accessed 15 Dec 2018. Available from: http://nationalacademies.org/hmd/~/media/Files/Report%20Files/2011/Clinical-Preventive-Services-for-Women-Closing-the-Gaps/preventiveservicesforwomenreportbrief_updated2.pdf.

68. Curry SJ, Krist AH, Owens DK, Barry MJ, Caughey AB, Davidson KW, et al. Screening for intimate partner violence, elder abuse, and abuse of vulnerable adults: US preventive services task force final recommendation statement. JAMA. 2018;320(16):1678–87.
69. Council on Ethical and Judicial Affairs (CEJA)/American Medical Association. Amendment to opinion E-2.02, "Physicians' obligations in preventing, identifying, and treating violence and abuse". Chicago; 2007.
70. American Academy of Family Practice. Intimate partner violence, vol. 2014. Leawood: COD; 2002.
71. American College of Obstetricians and Gynecologists (ACOG). Intimate partner violence: committee opinion No. 518. Washington, DC, 2012, February. Contract No.: 518.
72. Sherin KM, Sinacore JM, Li XQ, Zitter RE, Shakil A. HITS: a short domestic violence screening tool for use in a family practice setting. Fam Med. 1998;30(7):508–12.
73. Sohal H, Eldridge S, Feder G. The sensitivity and specificity of four questions (HARK) to identify intimate partner violence: a diagnostic accuracy study in general practice. BMC Fam Pract. 2007;8:49.
74. Basile KC, Hertz MF, Back SE. Intimate partner violence and sexual violence victimization assessment instruments for use in healthcare settings: Version 1. Atlanta, GA: Centers for Disease Control and Prevention, National Center for Injury Prevention and Control; 2007. Accessed 12 June 2018. Available from: https://www.cdc.gov/violenceprevention/pdf/ipv/ipvandsvscreening.pdf.
75. American College of Obstetricians and Gynecologists (ACOG). Adult manifestations of childhood sexual abuse. Committee opinion no. 498. Obstet Gynecol. 2011;118:392–5.
76. Tudiver S, McClure L, Heinonen T, Scurfield C, Kreklewetz C. Women survivors of childhood sexual abuse: knowledge and preparation of health care providers to meet client needs. Final Report. 2000, April.
77. Bernstein DP, Stein JA, Newcomb MD, Walker E, Pogge D, Ahluvalia T, et al. Development and validation of a brief screening version of the childhood trauma questionnaire. Child Abuse Negl. 2003;27(2):169–90.
78. Glowa PT, Olson AL, Johnson DJ. Screening for adverse childhood experiences in a family medicine setting: a feasibility study. J Am Board Fam Med. 2016;29(3):303–7.
79. Seng JS, Petersen BA. Incorporating routine screening for history of childhood sexual abuse into well-woman and maternity care. J Nurse Midwifery. 1995;40(1):26–30.
80. Ursano RJ, Benedek DM, Engel CC. Trauma-informed care for primary care: the lessons of war. Ann Intern Med. 2012;157(12):905–6.
81. Machtinger EL, Davis KB, Kimberg LS, Khanna N, Cuca YP, Dawson-Rose C, et al. From treatment to healing: inquiry and response to recent and past trauma in adult health care. Womens Health Issues. 2018.
82. Prins A, Bovin MJ, Smolenski DJ, Marx BP, Kimerling R, Jenkins-Guarnieri MA, et al. The primary care PTSD screen for DSM-5 (PC-PTSD-5): development and evaluation within a veteran primary care sample. J Gen Intern Med. 2016;31(10):1206–11.
83. Earls MF. Trauma-informed primary care: prevention, recognition, and promoting resilience. N C Med J. 2018;79(2):108–12.
84. Salonen H, Lahtinen M, Lappalainen S, Nevala N, Knibbs LD, Morawska L, et al. Physical characteristics of the indoor environment that affect health and wellbeing in healthcare facilities: a review. Intell Buildings Int. 2013;5(1):3–25.
85. Bair-Merritt MH, Mandal M, Garg A, Cheng TL. Addressing psychosocial adversity within the patient-centered medical home: expert-created measurable standards. J Prim Prev. 2015;36(4):213–25.
86. Sinsky C. Pre-visit planning: American Medical Association; 2014, October. Accessed 17 June 2018. Available from: https://www.stepsforward.org/Static/images/modules/3/downloadable/PreVisit_Planning.pdf.
87. Ravi A, Little V. Providing trauma-informed care. Am Fam Physician. 2017;95(10):655–7.

88. Tello M. Trauma-informed care: what it is, and why it's important. Harvard Health Blog [Internet]. October 16, 2018. Accessed 14 December 2018. Available from: https://www.health.harvard.edu/blog/trauma-informed-care-what-it-is-and-why-its-important-2018040413562.
89. Bates CK, Carroll N, Potter J. The challenging pelvic examination. J Gen Intern Med. 2011;26(6):651–7.
90. Coles J, Dartnall E, Astbury J. "Preventing the pain" when working with family and sexual violence in primary care. Int J Family Med. 2013;2013:198578.
91. McKegney CP. Surviving survivors. Coping with caring for patients who have been victimized. Prim Care. 1993;20(2):481–94.
92. Nimmo A, Huggard P. A systematic review of the measurement of compassion fatigue, vicarious trauma, and secondary traumatic stress in physicians. Australasia J Disaster Trauma Stud. 2013;1:37–44.
93. Strait J, Bolman T. Consideration of personal adverse childhood experiences during implementation of trauma-informed care curriculum in graduate health programs. Perm J. 2017;21:16–061.
94. Goldstein E, Murray-García J, Sciolla AF, Topitzes J. Medical Students perspectives on trauma-informed care training. Perm J. 2018;22:17–050.
95. Krejci LP, Carter K, Gaudet T. Whole health: the vision and implementation of personalized, proactive, patient-driven health care for veterans. Med Care. 2014;52(12 Suppl 5):S5–8.
96. Rittenberg, E., Trauma-Informed Care - Reflections of a Primary Care Doctor in the Week of the Kavanaugh Hearing N Engl J Med. 2018;379(22):2094–5
97. Elisseou S, Puranam S, Nandi M. A Novel, Trauma-Informed Physical Examination Curriculum for First-Year Medical Students. MedEdPORTAL. 2019;15:10799.

# Chapter 8
# Trauma-Informed Maternity Care

Megan R. Gerber

## Introduction

### Trauma and Women's Reproductive Health

Exposure to interpersonal trauma is common worldwide and adversely impacts the reproductive health of women. This chapter will address trauma-informed care (TIC) specifically for pregnant women in maternity (obstetric) care, many of the principles and techniques reviewed in the previous chapter on primary care also apply to routine outpatient obstetrics and gynecology (OB-GYN) practice. Women have a higher risk of experiencing many forms of interpersonal trauma including childhood maltreatment [1], intimate partner violence (IPV), and sexual assault [2]. The practice of human trafficking, which is common worldwide, also more commonly exploits girls and women [3]. Contraceptive coercion (including birth control sabotage and coerced pregnancy) is a form of IPV that can result in unintended pregnancy [4]. Unfortunately, it is not unusual for women to experience multiple forms of violence and abuse across the lifespan [5]. While all women can experience interpersonal trauma, clinicians should be particularly aware of populations at very high risk for trauma; these include homeless and incarcerated women, those with substance use disorder, refugees, and members of groups with high historical trauma burden including African and Native Americans (see Chap. 1 of this volume) [6]. These populations are often cared for in low-resource settings sometimes under suboptimal conditions, for example, in the US, many incarcerated women are still shackled during labor; at the time of this writing, fewer than half of all states had legislation against this practice [7].

M. R. Gerber (✉)
Section of General Internal Medicine, Boston University School of Medicine,
Veterans Affairs (VA) Boston Healthcare System, Boston, MA, USA
e-mail: meggerber@post.harvard.edu

© Springer Nature Switzerland AG 2019
M. R. Gerber (ed.), *Trauma-Informed Healthcare Approaches*,
https://doi.org/10.1007/978-3-030-04342-1_8

The direct and indirect effects of lifetime traumatic exposure cumulatively impact women's health [8, 9], including their reproductive health and the health of their babies [10]. Current and past trauma exposure may impact reproductive choice, health, and birth outcomes; for example, women experiencing emotional and physical abuse are less likely to be using their preferred method of contraception [11]. Trauma-exposed women have higher rates of pelvic pain [12, 13], sexually transmitted infections [1, 14], infertility [15] and experience poorer perinatal and post-partum outcomes [10, 16]. Women with abuse histories, and those who have developed PTSD, are more likely to develop post-partum depression [17]. A prospective study of pregnancy outcomes demonstrated that women who reported verbal abuse had a significantly higher risk of low birth weight infants than the unabused group; physical abuse was strongly associated with increased risk of neonatal death [16]. Women with trauma histories may delay seeking prenatal care [18], in part because intimate contact during well-woman, perinatal, and peripartum care can trigger posttraumatic stress disorder (PTSD) symptoms such as flashbacks, dissociation, hyperarousal, and avoidance [6]. Finally, childbirth itself has the ability to induce traumatic stress and, less commonly, posttraumatic stress disorder (PTSD) [19]. The data on sexual abuse in childhood, alone, indicates that at least one in four expectant women will have a history of sexual abuse [20]. The Centers for Disease Control and Prevention (CDC) recently estimated that one in five adult women experience lifetime completed or attempted rape [21]. These data underscore that trauma-informed care (TIC) is especially important during pregnancy and childbirth [6], and in this chapter, we review the approach to TIC in maternity care settings.

## *Goals of Trauma-Informed Maternity Care*

Trauma-informed maternity care practice incorporates these main principles: (1) detection of new or ongoing abuse and/or violence enabling staff to offer support and referral, (2) prevention of new trauma (childbirth itself can be traumatic), (3) avoidance of re-traumatization of women who have histories of either interpersonal (or other) trauma or prior "birth trauma," and (4), when appropriate, referral of women with trauma histories to trauma-focused treatment. Trauma-focused treatment may not be a priority, or option, for those women who prefer to avoid focusing on triggers during pregnancy and birth, and routine application of TIC throughout maternity care is critical [6]. Clinical teams and staff may not always know who has a trauma history, and sometimes a "trauma reaction" is the first sign of a patient's history. Much the way preparation for birth includes prevention of "vertical transmission" of certain infections; trauma-informed maternity care has potential to reduce/prevent vertical (intergenerational) transmission of trauma [22].

## *Posttraumatic Stress Disorder in Maternity Settings*

Pregnancy is a life-changing event, and in the US, nearly half of all pregnancies are unintended [23]. Apart from routine disrobing and genital examinations, other features of the prenatal and peripartum care environments such as raised side rails, restraint or entrapment in bed by equipment (fetal monitors leads/belts, oxygen masks, intravenous lines), and delayed response for calls to assistance can also trigger memories of past abuse [24]. In the second stage of labor, the stretching and pressure of the baby moving through the vaginal canal can evoke powerful memories of past forced intercourse [25]. Not surprisingly, pregnancy and childbirth can evoke strong feelings and reactions, particularly for survivors of child and adult sexual abuse [26]. Estimates of posttraumatic stress disorder (PTSD) prevalence in pregnancy range from 3% to 14%; the highest rates are found in low-resource settings [6, 27]. Abuse in childhood is the biggest risk factor for PTSD during pregnancy [28], and PTSD has been linked to poorer perinatal health outcomes including low birth weight, short gestation, adverse maternal mental health, and impaired bonding [29, 30]. Pre-existing PTSD [27] is a risk factor for women perceiving and identifying a birth experience as traumatic and for experiencing PTSD symptoms in the postpartum period [29]. This can impact subsequent parenting and infant attachment [29] and may contribute to intergenerational impact of the original traumatic exposure.

As discussed, childbirth itself is a complex process and life event that can be associated with both positive and negative psychological responses [19]. A woman who was healthy before labor and delivery may develop acute stress disorder (an acute stress reaction that occurs in the initial month after exposure to a traumatic event and before the possibility of diagnosing PTSD) [31] after a difficult and traumatic birth. The majority of these cases do not progress to PTSD [6]. The term birth trauma has been used to refer to a birth experience that is not only characterized by actual or threatened injury or death to the mother or her baby but also by negative interactions with care providers resulting in women feeling unsupported, disconnected, helpless, and isolated during birth [32]. Negative interactions with care providers can result in even higher odds of PTSD than those seen with obstetric complications [33]. When giving birth is experienced as particularly traumatic, it this can have a negative impact on a woman's postnatal emotional well-being and health, health of the baby, and subsequent attachment [34–36].

While much of the experience of childbirth occurs at the individual patient-provider-care team level, health system factors can contribute strongly to perpetuating conditions in which the patient is not allowed to take an active role in decision-making. System-driven power dynamics can also predispose to traumatic birth experiences [32]. In obstetric medicine in particular, risk aversion and concerns over litigation often result in focusing efforts on mitigation of perceived risks to physical outcomes for mothers and babies, to the detriment of emphasizing patient-centered care and psychosocial outcomes [32]. Being supportive and flexible, *within the limits of safety,* is challenging but critical for providing maternity care to women with trauma histories [25]. Systems of care need to recognize these constraints and make a deliberate effort to support and extend patient-centered, trauma-informed models of care.

A recent qualitative study of pregnancy and childbirth after sexual trauma [63] demonstrated that survivors desired clear communication between prenatal care providers and the labor and delivery team, they expressed frustration when the team was not aware of a sexual trauma history disclosed prenatally. Some of the women developed birth plans and shared that this was a way of having some control during delivery. Participants felt that disclosing their history of sexual trauma would change their care. During delivery, women wanted control over who was present during cervical examinations, and the degree of exposure of their bodies during labor. They suggested clinicians avoid triggering language [63].

## *Implementing Trauma-Informed Maternity Care*

Trauma-informed health settings [37] design services based on an understanding of the vulnerabilities or triggers of trauma survivors so as to be more supportive and avoid re-traumatization [38]. Applying TIC principles to maternity care includes routine screening for history of trauma, including childhood sexual abuse and IPV, in order to tailor care and plan ahead for childbirth [39]. The American College of Obstetricians and Gynecologists (ACOG) advocates routine screening for child and adult sexual abuse [40], as well as IPV [41]. A recent study evaluated the feasibility of screening for adverse childhood experiences (ACEs), including sexual abuse, during routine prenatal visits [42]; the majority of patients reported that sharing ACEs with a healthcare provider was acceptable and comfortable and even helped their provider know them better. Clinicians felt that the screening worked well when incorporated into a standard workflow and paired with referral resources like social work and mental health [42].

The six key TIC principles [37, 38] which include 1) safety, 2) trustworthiness and transparency, 3) peer support, 4) collaboration and mutuality, 5) empowerment, voice and choice, and 6) awareness of cultural/historical and gender issues have important implications for prenatal and peripartum care (Table 8.1). Birth is not just a physical experience; it is a family event influenced by community, cultural context, and beliefs [43]. Even seemingly benign childbirth education classes can be difficult for survivors, for example, lying down in a group to practice breathing techniques may have the opposite effect for a woman who has experienced sexual abuse [25]. Having a positive pregnancy and birth is possible and can be a powerful healing experience [25] with the potential to offer a turning point in time for survivors to explore possibilities that can occur with this new beginning [44].

A number of authors have proposed pathways to more woman-centered maternity care and shared decision-making (SDM) [43], and these approaches can be conduits for implementing TIC (Table 8.1). SDM [43] is an approach that enables the patient and clinician to share information and best evidence when decisions need to be made. When SDM is employed, the care team supports the patient in considering options; during this collaborative process, opportunities for greater

**Table 8.1** Applying trauma-informed principles to maternity care [6, 22, 25, 26, 43, 47, 50, 51, 55, 60, 61]

| Trauma-informed principle | Action, intervention, or program example |
|---|---|
| Safety | Obtain consent for/explain even the most routine procedures ("May I check your cervix now?"). |
| | Minimize vaginal exams, and remove monitors when possible. |
| | Allow partners/support persons to accompany patient to appointments/be present during birth when requested by the patient. |
| | Develop a care plan for possible trauma triggers in advance. |
| | Provide a doula, especially for women who do not have support from a trusted birth partner. |
| | Place a sign on the door of the birthing or delivery room asking staff to knock and announce themselves before proceeding to attend to/examine the birthing woman. |
| | Keep the birthing woman covered in between exams, unless she asks otherwise. |
| | Be aware that statements/ commands such as "relax" and "let go" can be triggering and advice should be delivered in suggestion form. |
| Trustworthiness | Keep women informed and aware of all options available to them/engage in shared decision-making. |
| | Provide "holding" during care (Sanctuary principle). |
| | Minimize the number of personnel entering the room when possible. |
| Transparency | Obtain informed consent for even the most routine interventions. |
| | Antenatal education around unplanned emergencies. |
| Peer support | Prenatal shared medical appointments (e.g., Centering Pregnancy). |
| | Peer-to-peer support (e.g., Centering Pregnancy, B'more fit for babies). |
| | Designate a staff person on every shift who is knowledgeable about trauma/TIC. |
| Collaboration/ mutuality | Antenatal education. |
| | Shared decision-making. |
| | Birth planning. |
| | Use of co-constructed handheld written/electronic maternity records (pregnancy passports) |
| | Negotiate and use a variety of means to communicate with women, and remind them of appointments [24]. |
| | Provide more flexibility in scheduling appointments [24]. |
| | Even if in the room briefly, staff should endeavor to position themselves at eye level with the patient (do not stand above/over her). |
| Empowerment (voice and choice) | Waiting room pamphlets/literature on giving birth as a survivor. |
| | Individualized trauma-informed birth plan [44]. |
| | Shared decision-making. |
| | Provide doula support [55]. |
| | During labor respect the woman's physical space and change the environment as requested. |
| | In both very routine and emergent situations, take time to obtain consent |

(continued)

**Table 8.1** (continued)

| Trauma-informed principle | Action, intervention, or program example |
|---|---|
| Awareness of cultural, historical, and gender issues | Social support (may address racial disparities in outcomes like preterm birth), e.g., B'more fit for babies [58] and Centering and Racial Disparities (CRADLE) Study [47]/Centering Pregnancy [46]. |
| | Use of professional interpreters. |
| | Combined interpreter/doula program [62]. |
| | Address potential biases on the part of staff. |
| | Be aware of relevant racial disparities in maternal-fetal outcomes within your institution. |

mutual understanding emerge and trust is built. With SDM [43], there is an interactive exchange of professional information, personal information, and deliberation by both patient and clinician; lastly a consensus-based decision is arrived at. SDM in maternity care begins with prenatal care and ends after birth; it has potential to improve birth experiences and satisfaction with care [43]. The challenges of applying SDM in the perinatal period include the very nature of labor and birth – dynamic processes in which time to make decisions can be limited by emergent developments, and pain of contractions can interfere with interaction and deliberation [43]. Advance planning through creation of a "birth plan" is especially important for trauma survivors. Birth planning enables an expectant woman to be an agent in her own birth through education, empowerment, and trauma-informed planning preferably in advance [44]. For example, one survivor wrote [45]:

> These adjustments can appear minor, but have a lasting impact on survivors. I experienced this myself: In the midst of the chaos of my first birth, the surgeon took 15 seconds to stop, look me in the eye, and explain what was happening. She let me give consent – real consent – to the C-section. Those 15 seconds stuck with me as a single moment of empowerment in an otherwise powerless situation.

Additional interventions have been identified that are consonant with TIC principles; one of these is "Centering Pregnancy," first developed in the late 1990s [46]. Centering Pregnancy is a shared medical appointment for pregnant women that can be tailored to the needs of communities and ethnic groups [47–49]. The use of co-constructed handheld paper [50] or electronic health records [51] has shown mixed, but promising, results and requires further study. Decision aids to support women in their choices during pregnancy and birth [52, 53] are important tools, but typically focus on the information component of SDM [43]. Some have found that mobile applications may reduce patient activation and thus require more study [54]. Finally, doula (birth companion) care has been demonstrated to improve birth outcomes, even among traditionally underserved women. The communication, encouragement, and advocacy provided by a doula can enhance women's self-efficacy during labor and delivery [55]. Many organizations that train and provide doulas to birthing women have developed trauma-informed guidance [44], and when possible having a doula attend a trauma survivor's birth may be a facilitator or pathway to ideal trauma-informed maternity care.

## *Programmatic Examples*

The two examples that follow provide two different approaches that can be adapted to a variety of maternity care settings. The first is a manualized psychoeducation program that any practice or health system can implement. The second provides an example of delivering culturally specific TIC in a community public health context. Sperlich et al. [6] review a number of other trauma-informed maternity care interventions which provide additional exemplars.

1. *The Survivor Mom's Companion* [56, 57] is a manualized 10-module self-study psychoeducational program in workbook form designed to help pregnant women with a history of childhood maltreatment break the cycles of abuse and psychiatric vulnerability in their lives and in the lives of their newborns. The program was developed to address the adverse impact prenatal PTSD can have on pregnancy and subsequent attachment and bonding of the newborn as discussed above. Survivor Mom's Companion was designed to address issues and concerns beyond PTSD symptoms themselves, and it can be useful even for women who do not meet full diagnostic criteria for PTSD. Women may self-refer and participate in self-study using each module to problem-solve through acompanying vignettes. Clinicians and care teams may also refer women to the program.

    The first four modules are fundamental and provide an overview of how trauma and PTSD can affect childbearing and early mothering. These modules teach *reaction skills* to manage PTSD in the aftermath of being triggered, *soothing skills* to improve affect regulation, and in*terpreting skills* to improve interpersonal reactivity [57]. A 30-min session with a trained tutor is then offered either in person or by phone. During the session, the woman shares her work on the module. Tutors can be perinatal nurses, social workers, or health educators who have undergone a standardized training program. The program also allows case finding for past and present trauma and can promote treatment engagement when referral is requested. Demonstrated outcomes of the program are improved interpersonal reactivity and reduction in PTSD symptoms among completers [56]. The program is available to individuals, healthcare organizations, and agencies (www.survivormoms.org).

2. *B'more Fit for Babies* [58]: B'more fit for babies is a project that targeted obesity among trauma-exposed post-partum women in Baltimore. While it does not specifically address prenatal care, it has a goal of improving women's health, reducing adverse pregnancy outcomes, and enhancing parenting skills through a TIC lens.

    Exposure to violence is widespread in Baltimore; a study of children ages 6–9 found that 87% had experienced multiple traumatic events and 28% met partial or full criteria for posttraumatic stress disorder [59]. Exposure to community violence is compounded by historic trauma and gendered racism in this population. A number of poor health outcomes were identified as prevalent in Baltimore; rates of obesity were high especially among African American women. As a major contributor toward infant mortality and poor maternal health, obesity was selected as the target of this initiative. At the outset, trauma-related issues were identified during focus groups, for example, the influence of traumatic experiences on food and exercise choices. The program was developed with the input of the women toward whom it was directed and utilized a trauma-informed policy framework. A peer-led model evolved, and programming was designed to be culturally sensitive. Participants developed strategies for weight loss, improved nutrition, and better parenting which also prepared them for their next possible pregnancy. The program then participated in spreading trauma-informed care across other city institutions. B'more Fit is a model that can inform trauma-informed community public health in other US urban centers and systems of care.

## Conclusion

Trauma is common among women and directly impacts reproductive health. Survivors of sexual trauma, and other forms of violence and abuse, face challenges during childbirth. Through trauma-informed care the birthing experience can be less frightening and re-traumatizing and more of a positive and empowering experience. Clinical practices, agencies, and healthcare institutions can draw on the suggestions and guidance outlined in this chapter to begin to create an environment that is more sensitive to the needs of survivors during this important phase in their lives.

## References

1. Felitti VJ, Anda RF, Nordenberg D, Williamson DF, Spitz AM, Edwards V, et al. Relationship of childhood abuse and household dysfunction to many of the leading causes of death in adults. The Adverse Childhood Experiences (ACE) Study. Am J Prev Med. 1998;14(4):245–58.
2. Smith SG, Zhang X, Basile KC, Merrick MT, Wang J, Kresnow M, Chen J. The National intimate partner and sexual violence survey (NISVS): 2015 data brief. Atlanta: National Center for Injury Prevention and Control, Centers for Disease Control and Prevention; 2018.
3. Polaris Project. 2017 human trafficking hotline, Washington, DC; 2018. Accessed 14 Dec 2018. Available from: https://polarisproject.org/2017statistics.
4. Miller E, Decker MR, McCauley HL, Tancredi DJ, Levenson RR, Waldman J, et al. Pregnancy coercion, intimate partner violence and unintended pregnancy. Contraception. 2010;81(4):316–22.
5. Campbell R, Greeson MR, Bybee D, Raja S. The co-occurrence of childhood sexual abuse, adult sexual assault, intimate partner violence, and sexual harassment: a mediational model of posttraumatic stress disorder and physical health outcomes. J Consult Clin Psychol. 2008;76(2):194–207.
6. Sperlich M, Seng JS, Li Y, Taylor J, Bradbury-Jones C. Integrating trauma-informed care into maternity care practice: conceptual and practical issues. J Midwifery Womens Health. 2017;62(6):661–72.
7. Ferszt GG, Palmer M, McGrane C. Where does your state stand on shackling of pregnant incarcerated women? Nurs Womens Health. 2018;22(1):17–23.
8. Bonomi AE, Thompson RS, Anderson M, Reid RJ, Carrell D, Dimer JA, et al. Intimate partner violence and women's physical, mental, and social functioning. Am J Prev Med. 2006;30(6):458–66.

9. Ottisova L, Hemmings S, Howard LM, Zimmerman C, Oram S. Prevalence and risk of violence and the mental, physical and sexual health problems associated with human trafficking: an updated systematic review. Epidemiol Psychiatr Sci. 2016;25(4):317–41.
10. Silverman JG, Decker MR, Reed E, Raj A. Intimate partner violence victimization prior to and during pregnancy among women residing in 26 U.S. states: associations with maternal and neonatal health. Am J Obstet Gynecol. 2006;195(1):140–8.
11. Williams CM, Larsen U, McCloskey LA. Intimate partner violence and women's contraceptive use. Violence Against Women. 2008;14(12):1382–96.
12. Poli-Neto OB, Tawasha KAS, Romao A, Hisano MK, Moriyama A, Candido-Dos-Reis FJ, et al. History of childhood maltreatment and symptoms of anxiety and depression in women with chronic pelvic pain. J Psychosom Obstet Gynecol. 2018;39(2):83–9.
13. Schliep KC, Mumford SL, Johnstone EB, Peterson CM, Sharp HT, Stanford JB, et al. Sexual and physical abuse and gynecologic disorders. Hum Reprod (Oxford, England). 2016;31(8):1904–12.
14. Bauer HM, Gibson P, Hernandez M, Kent C, Klausner J, Bolan G. Intimate partner violence and high-risk sexual behaviors among female patients with sexually transmitted diseases. Sex Transm Dis. 2002;29(7):411–6.
15. Stellar C, Garcia-Moreno C, Temmerman M, van der Poel S. A systematic review and narrative report of the relationship between infertility, subfertility, and intimate partner violence. Int J Gynaecol Obstet: Off Organ Int Fed Gynaecol Obstet. 2016;133(1):3–8.
16. Yost NP, Bloom SL, McIntire DD, Leveno KJ. A prospective observational study of domestic violence during pregnancy. Obstet Gynecol. 2005;106(1):61–5.
17. Alvarez-Segura M, Garcia-Esteve L, Torres A, Plaza A, Imaz ML, Hermida-Barros L, et al. Are women with a history of abuse more vulnerable to perinatal depressive symptoms? A systematic review. Arch Womens Ment Health. 2014;17(5):343–57.
18. Jasinski JL. Pregnancy and domestic violence: a review of the literature. Trauma Violence Abuse. 2004;5(1):47–64.
19. Bastos MH, Furuta M, Small R, McKenzie-McHarg K, Bick D. Debriefing interventions for the prevention of psychological trauma in women following childbirth. Cochrane Database Syst Rev. 2015;(4):Cd007194.
20. Finkelhor D, Hotaling G, Lewis IA, Smith C. Sexual abuse in a national survey of adult men and women: prevalence, characteristics, and risk factors. Child Abuse Negl. 1990;14(1):19–28.
21. Smith SG, Zhang X, Basile KC, Merrick MT, Wang J, Kresnow M, et al. The National Intimate partner and Sexual Violence Survey (NISVS): 2015 data brief – Updated Release. National Center for Injury Prevention and Control, Centers for Disease Control and Prevention, Atlanta, GA; 2018. Accessed 14 Dec 2018. Available from: https://www.cdc.gov/violenceprevention/nisvs/2015NISVSdatabrief.html.
22. Seng JS, Taylor J. Trauma informed care in the perinatal period. Edinburgh, Scotland: Dunedin Academic Press; 2015.
23. Finer LB, Zolna MR. Declines in unintended pregnancy in the United States, 2008-2011. N Engl J Med. 2016;374(9):843–52.
24. National Institute for Health and Care Excellence (NICE). Pregnancy and complex social factors: a model for service provision for pregnant women with complex social factors, Clinical guideline [CG110] London, UK; 2010, September. Accessed 14 Dec 2018. Available from: https://www.nice.org.uk/guidance/cg110.
25. Robinson K. Childhood sexual abuse. Implications for care during pregnancy and birth. Soc Obstet Gynaecol Can. 2000;22(4):303–6.
26. Simkin P, Klaus P. When survivors give birth: understanding and healing the effects of early sexual abuse on childbearing women. 1st ed. Seattle: Classic Day Publishing; 2004.
27. Seng JS, Low LK, Sperlich M, Ronis DL, Liberzon I. Prevalence, trauma history, and risk for posttraumatic stress disorder among nulliparous women in maternity care. Obstet Gynecol. 2009;114(4):839–47.

28. Seng JS, Sperlich M, Low LK. Mental health, demographic, and risk behavior profiles of pregnant survivors of childhood and adult abuse. J Midwifery Womens Health. 2008;53(6): 511–21.
29. Seng JS, Low LK, Sperlich M, Ronis DL, Liberzon I. Post-traumatic stress disorder, child abuse history, birthweight and gestational age: a prospective cohort study. BJOG. 2011;118(11):1329–39.
30. Rosen D, Seng JS, Tolman RM, Mallinger G. Intimate partner violence, depression, and posttraumatic stress disorder as additional predictors of low birth weight infants among low-income mothers. J Interpers Violence. 2007;22(10):1305–14.
31. Bryant RA, Friedman MJ, Spiegel D, Ursano R, Strain J. A review of acute stress disorder in DSM-5. Depress Anxiety. 2011;28(9):802–17.
32. Reed R, Sharman R, Inglis C. Women's descriptions of childbirth trauma relating to care provider actions and interactions. BMC Pregnancy Childbirth. 2017;17(1):21.
33. Harris R, Ayers S. What makes labour and birth traumatic? A survey of intrapartum 'hotspots'. Psychol Health. 2012;27(10):1166–77.
34. Seng JS, Sperlich M, Low LK, Ronis DL, Muzik M, Liberzon I. Childhood abuse history, post-traumatic stress disorder, postpartum mental health, and bonding: a prospective cohort study. J Midwifery Womens Health. 2013;58(1):57–68.
35. Muzik M, McGinnis EW, Bocknek E, Morelen D, Rosenblum KL, Liberzon I, et al. PTSD symptoms across pregnancy and early postpartum among women with lifetime PTSD diagnosis. Depress Anxiety. 2016;33(7):584–91.
36. Muzik M, Bocknek EL, Broderick A, Richardson P, Rosenblum KL, Thelen K, et al. Mother-infant bonding impairment across the first 6 months postpartum: the primacy of psychopathology in women with childhood abuse and neglect histories. Arch Womens Ment Health. 2013;16(1):29–38.
37. Substance Abuse and Ment Health Services Administration (SAMHSA). SAMHSA's concept of trauma and guidance for a trauma-informed approach. 2014. Accessed 14 Dec 2018. Available from: https://store.samhsa.gov/product/SAMHSA-s-Concept-of-Trauma-and-Guidance-for-a-Trauma-Informed-Approach/SMA14-4884.html.
38. National Center for Trauma-Informed Care and Alternatives to Seclusion and Restraint (NCTIC). Substance abuse and mental health services administration. 2017, September 15 (Updated). Accessed 30 June 2018. Available from: https://www.samhsa.gov/nctic.
39. Seng JS, Petersen BA. Incorporating routine screening for history of childhood sexual abuse into well-woman and maternity care. J Nurse Midwifery. 1995;40(1):26–30.
40. American College of Obstetricians and Gynecologists (ACOG). Sexual assault. Committee opinion no. 592. Obstet Gynecol. 2014;123:905–9.
41. American College of Obstetricians and Gynecologists (ACOG). Intimate partner violence: committee opinion no. 518. Washington, DC; 2012, February. Contract No.: 518.
42. Flanagan T, Alabaster A, McCaw B, Stoller N, Watson C, Young-Wolff KC. Feasibility and acceptability of screening for adverse childhood experiences in prenatal care. J Womens Health (Larchmt). 2018;27(7):903–11.
43. Nieuwenhuijze MJ, Korstjens I, de Jonge A, de Vries R, Lagro-Janssen A. On speaking terms: a Delphi study on shared decision-making in maternity care. BMC Pregnancy Childbirth. 2014;14:223.
44. National Resource Center on Domestic Violence (NRCDV). Trauma informed birth support: Survivor + Doula + Advocate. Harrisburg: National Resource Center on Domestic Violence (NRCDV); 2015.
45. Beaulieu S. Commentary: when sexual violence survivors give birth, here's what you should know. Boston: WBUR, National Public Radio; 2016. Accessed 25 June 2018. Available from: http://www.wbur.org/commonhealth/2016/01/21/sexual-violence-survivor-childbirth.
46. Rising SS. Centering pregnancy. An interdisciplinary model of empowerment. J Nurse Midwifery. 1998;43(1):46–54.

47. Chen L, Crockett AH, Covington-Kolb S, Heberlein E, Zhang L, Sun X. Centering and racial disparities (CRADLE study): rationale and design of a randomized controlled trial of centering pregnancy and birth outcomes. BMC Pregnancy Childbirth. 2017;17(1):118.
48. Mazzoni SE, Carter EB. Group prenatal care. Am J Obstet Gynecol. 2017;216(6):552–6.
49. DeCesare JZ, Jackson JR. Centering pregnancy: practical tips for your practice. Arch Gynecol Obstet. 2015;291(3):499–507.
50. Humphrey T, Tucker JS, de Labrusse C. Does women's contribution to co-constructed hand-held maternity records support patient-centered care? Int J Childbirth. 2013;3(2):117–27.
51. Hawley G, Hepworth J, Wilkinson SA, Jackson C. From maternity paper hand-held records to electronic health records: what do women tell us about their use? Aust J Prim Health. 2016;22(4):339–48.
52. Say R, Robson S, Thomson R. Helping pregnant women make better decisions: a systematic review of the benefits of patient decision aids in obstetrics. BMJ Open. 2011;1(2):e000261.
53. Vlemmix F, Warendorf JK, Rosman AN, Kok M, Mol BW, Morris JM, et al. Decision aids to improve informed decision-making in pregnancy care: a systematic review. BJOG. 2013;120(3):257–66.
54. Ledford CJW, Womack JJ, Rider HA, Seehusen AB, Conner SJ, Lauters RA, et al. Unexpected effects of a system-distributed Mobile application in maternity care: a randomized controlled trial. Health Educ Behav. 2018;45(3):323–30.
55. Gruber KJ, Cupito SH, Dobson CF. Impact of doulas on healthy birth outcomes. J Perinat Educ. 2013;22(1):49–58.
56. Seng JS, Sperlich M, Rowe H, Cameron H, Harris A, Rauch SAM, et al. The survivor moms' companion: open pilot of a posttraumatic stress specific psychoeducation program for pregnant survivors of childhood maltreatment and sexual trauma. Int J Childbirth. 2011;1(2):112–20.
57. Sperlich M, Seng JS, Rowe H, Cameron H, Harris A, McCracken A, et al. The survivor mom's companion: feasibility, safety, and acceptability of a posttraumatic stress specific psychoeducation program for pregnant survivors of childhood maltreatment and sexual trauma. Int J Childbirth. 2011;1(2):122–33.
58. Tuck SG, Summers AC, Bowie J, Fife-Stallworth D, Alston C, Hayes S, et al. B'More fit for healthy babies: using trauma-informed care policies to improve maternal health in Baltimore City. Womens Health Issues. 2017;27(Suppl 1):S38–45.
59. Kiser LJ, Medoff DR, Black MM. The role of family processes in childhood traumatic stress reactions for youths living in urban poverty. Traumatology. 2010;26(2):33–42.
60. Shields SG, Candib LME. Women-centered care in pregnancy and childbirth. Oxford: Radcliffe Publishing Ltd; 2010.
61. Bailey JM, Crane P, Nugent CE. Childbirth education and birth plans. Obstet Gynecol Clin N Am. 2008;35(3):497–509. ix
62. Maher S, Crawford-Carr A, Neidigh K. The role of the interpreter/doula in the maternity setting. Nurs Womens Health. 2012;16(6):472–81.
63. Sobel L, O'Rourke-Suchoff D, Holland E, Remis K, Resnick K, Perkins R, et al. Pregnancy and childbirth after sexual trauma: patient perspectives and care preferences. Obstet Gynecol. 2018;132(6):1461–8.

# Chapter 9
# Trauma-Informed Pediatrics: Organizational and Clinical Practices for Change, Healing, and Resilience

Emily B. Gerber, Briana Loomis, Cherie Falvey, Petra H. Steinbuchel, Jennifer Leland, and Kenneth Epstein

## Introduction

While this volume has primarily focused on care of adults, we thought it important to include a discussion of the care of children and adolescents in part to meet the needs of Family Medicine clinicians but also to acknowledge that trauma, by its very nature, does not respect the boundaries of age and impacts generations of families and communities. When unaddressed, adverse childhood experiences (ACEs), can result in lifelong consequences; this chapter provides strategies and tools for pediatricians and other child practitioners to head off these effects before they develop and persist as chronic physical and behavioral problems for adults. The authors explore creation of trauma-informed *systems* of care, a topic that is relevant to all healthcare teams, administrators and leaders.

---

E. B. Gerber (✉)
Kaiser Permanente, San Rafael, CA, USA

B. Loomis
San Francisco Department of Public Health, San Francisco, CA, USA

C. Falvey · J. Leland
Trauma Transformed, East Bay Agency for Children, Oakland, CA, USA

P. H. Steinbuchel · K. Epstein
UCSF Department of Psychiatry, University of California, San Francisco, San Francisco, CA, USA

© Springer Nature Switzerland AG 2019
M. R. Gerber (ed.), *Trauma-Informed Healthcare Approaches*,
https://doi.org/10.1007/978-3-030-04342-1_9

# A Trauma-Organized Clinic: You Can't Provide What You Don't Have

*You are a PGY-2 pediatric resident waiting for your attending to arrive in a busy primary care clinic at a community health center that primarily serves patients insured by Medicaid and is located in East Oakland, an under-resourced urban community where many Black and Latino families reside. You are sitting in the waiting room, when your first scheduled patient arrives, 20 min late, for a 15-min scheduled well-child check. M is a 5-year-old boy with "behavior problems" whose mother frantically checks in at the front desk. The receptionist greets her and then firmly says, "Since you are late, the doctor may not be able to see you." The mother looks overwhelmed, carrying three bags and pushing a baby stroller with M's baby half-sister, who just woke up and is crying loudly; she responds to the receptionist, "Who do you think you are, talking to me like that? I made this appointment 3 months ago, and my son needs his checkup and shots so he can go to school! I'm not leaving until you get me back there to see the doctor!" She then turns to M's sister and shouts, "Stop crying!" and shoves a bottle into her hands.*

*M has been staring at his mother with a faraway look in his eye, not really moving nor speaking. M suddenly darts off heads straight for the toys, yanks them all off the shelf, and disrupts the play of two other children, saying "you are bad. I'm gonna kill you dead" throwing the "dead" toy soldiers across the room at the other waiting parents. The receptionist, now standing up, points at M and tells the mother in an authoritarian tone she needs to take charge of her son. "You need to quiet down, or I will call security!" The receptionist storms off into a back room to "take a break" and tearfully tells her coworkers what just happened. Meanwhile the mother is shushing and vigorously rocking her baby, in between yelling at M to "calm down." You pause to notice that your own heart rate seems to be elevated, your breathing is quicker, and you find yourself wanting to disappear into the wall or run out the door. You think about how you would rather be going home to your family and all the clinical notes you will be writing until midnight after you get your kids into bed. You wonder where in the world your attending is, but you know through the grapevine that she is likely in a meeting about productivity and budget cuts. You are exhausted to the core both physically and emotionally from last night's PICU where your 15-year-old patient with a gunshot wound died. The patient's mother crying and the nurse trying to comfort her are received by you with distance and detachment as you prepare to see M, your next patient. Relying on a calming technique you were taught, you close your eyes, take three deep breaths, and calmly introduce yourself to the mother and tell her you will see what can be done to help.*

## Understanding Trauma

As described in the case of M, pediatricians are usually first responders in exposure to the developmental and behavioral concerns in children. Children, youth, and families are experiencing greater levels of toxic stress as evidenced by the nearly threefold increase of patients in acute psychiatric crisis presenting in our pediatric emergency departments [1]. With trauma awareness and understanding, the interactions and experiences described above could have unfolded in a more compassionate way. We know from the Centers for Disease Control (CDC)-Kaiser Permanente Adverse Childhood Events (ACEs) Study [2] and a very large body of subsequent work that trauma experienced by children like M can harm development and increase risks for poor physical, emotional, behavioral, social, and cognitive outcomes across the life span [2]. The scene that unfolded above in the East Oakland Clinic with dysregulated patients and staff is all too common and repeats itself every day in healthcare organizations across the country; it is now apparent that trauma impacts healthcare organizations and clinics and the people who provide services to children and families experiencing trauma.

Yet the difference between what we know works (science) and how we respond (practice) remains. It turns out that trauma is a barrier that can impede our ability to take the steps necessary for healing to take place [3]. Pediatric leaders and providers experience this paradox each and every day. While medical advances and increasing specialization have strengthened an already well-trained and experienced healthcare workforce, our providers are simultaneously operating in a delivery system that is overly stressed by reimbursement structures and technological and regulatory obligations that decrease their capacity to listen, understand, prevent, coordinate, and reflect on their relationship with the patient. Meanwhile, sociocultural stressors such as poverty, discrimination, and disenfranchisement have contributed to increased health disparities, including chronic disease, in the children, youth, and families they are serving [4].

To improve care for families like M's, this chapter is both a guide and a call to action for pediatric healthcare leaders, providers, and their organizations to better understand the impact of trauma on their work and cocreate meaningful strategies and transform from a trauma-organized (reactive) organization/system to a healing and resilient one uniquely equipped to counter the toxic effects adversity has on the health of children, youth, and families. This process can improve lives, quality of care, and organizational performance [5, 6]. We will present a trauma-informed systems (TISs) framework for leaders and practitioners, recommend strategies and tools and ways to measure progress, and share some examples from early adopter systems and agencies.

## Adverse Childhood Experiences: Understanding the Impact

The ACEs Study was one of the largest investigations of childhood abuse and neglect and later-life health and well-being. Seven categories of adverse childhood experiences were studied: psychological, physical, or sexual abuse, violence against mother, or living with household members who were substance abusers, mentally ill or suicidal, or ever imprisoned [2].

The number of categories endorsed by patients was then compared to measures of adult risk behavior, health status, and disease. Strikingly, results found that ACEs are strongly related to development of risk factors for disease—like smoking, drug and alcohol abuse, risky sexual behavior, and physical inactivity—and also a number of behavioral and physical health conditions including depression, cardiovascular disease, cancer, stroke, and broken bones, as well as reduced socioeconomic status and early death [7].

Subsequent work has found that that ACEs are incredibly common, and most will experience at least one or more in childhood, affecting nearly 35 million out of 74 million, or 47% of the children in the United States, regardless of socioeconomic status [8]. For Black and Brown families like M's experiencing poverty in under-resourced communities, children and youth are exposed to multiple ACEs. Prevalence rates for categories of traumatic experiences in children and youth under 18 have been estimated as follows: 8–12% have experienced sexual abuse/assault, 9–19% have experienced physical abuse or assault, 38–70% have witnessed community violence, 10% have witnessed caregiver violence, and 20–25% have been exposed to a man-made or natural disaster [9]. In addition, the mechanisms through which ACEs have their effects include brain development, hormonal and immune systems and even DNA; in turn, these changes can contribute to behavioral problems, learning difficulties, and physical health issues that can lead to significant and chronic health issues with lasting consequences and shorter life span [5].

## Posttraumatic Stress Disorder (PTSD)

Despite the potential for effects that last over the life course, not all adverse experiences develop into posttraumatic stress disorder (PTSD). The Diagnostic and Statistical Manual of Mental Disorders [10] defines trauma as "exposure to actual or threatened death, serious injury, or sexual violence in one (or more) of the following ways: directly experiencing the traumatic event(s); witnessing, in person, the traumatic event(s) as it occurred to others; learning that the traumatic event(s) occurred to a close family member or close friend (in case of actual or threatened death of a family member or friend, the event(s) must have been violent or accidental); or experiencing repeated or extreme exposure to aversive details of the traumatic event(s)". This is an important expansion that includes secondary or vicarious traumatization to persons close to the victim.

While nearly half of persons under 18 have experienced at least one significant trauma [8], the prevalence of PTSD among adolescents is about 4–8% [9]. Many persons who experience significant trauma may develop symptoms of acute stress disorder, marked by symptoms of dissociation, arousal, re-experiencing, and avoidance for up to 4 weeks after the trauma. If these symptoms last longer than 4 weeks, it is considered PTSD. If symptoms persist longer than 6 months, PTSD is more likely to become chronic, with long-term impact on overall functioning. Trauma can take on various forms, including major, often recent, life events that have a significant impact, sometimes referred to as acute "Type 1" or "T" traumas, but repeated, cumulative trauma over a life span may also be referred to as "complex trauma" [11], "Type 2 trauma," or "t" trauma.

Acute trauma affects neurobiology in several important ways. Core trauma symptoms are experienced in the brainstem and involve the autonomic nervous system

(ANS). During an acute traumatic event, the brain's natural response is to alert, flight, fight, or freeze and not always in this order [12]; our brains first signal to become extra alert and take in everything around us, in order to help us properly assess the threat. Fight or flight responses are activated when increased sympathetic activation of acetylcholine release from the adrenal medulla signals skeletal muscles to take action, accompanied by increased heart rate, quickened breathing, and dry mouth. A "freeze" signal, sometimes called collapsible immobility, may be protective in animals and may be related to a complete overwhelm of the nervous system and an extension of the fight or flight response. In the developing brain, chronic trauma can lead to a state of fear-related activation with adaptive changes in emotional, behavioral, and cognitive functioning; however, with repeated activation, it can lead to a maladaptive and persistent state of fear even after a threat has passed. What was once an adaptive and reflexive fear response critical to our ancestors' survival can go awry [13].

The term historical trauma or transgenerational trauma was initially developed to describe the residual impact of trauma on children of Holocaust survivors and is defined as "the cumulative emotional and psychological wounding, as a result of group traumatic experiences, which is transmitted across generations within a community" [14]. The intergenerational experience of racism on indigenous peoples of the Americas and its continuing impact on Black Americans [14] also falls in this category and can also be experienced in the present as chronic racism-based trauma due to ongoing violence and discrimination.

Vicarious traumatization is a term used to describe the impact on those who treat persons with trauma, and results from empathic engagement with traumatized persons and their reports of traumatic experiences. As illustrated by the opening vignette, as clinicians, our experiences of autonomic hyperarousal, marked by increased heart and respiratory rates, emotional numbing, and a desire to get away from the situation, are symptoms of vicarious trauma related to the cumulative effect of caring for patients with multiple types of trauma; this can lead to staff disengagement and/or burnout, turnover, and patient safety concerns and medical errors [14]. In turn, cumulative vicarious trauma spreads like an epidemic taking its toll not only on individuals but also on organizations.

## Trauma-Informed System Practices: Responding to the Impact

This triple threat of overburdened individuals, communities, staff, and bureaucracies induces collective stress in patients, staff, and organizations and complicates the goal of facilitating healing and recovery. Sandra Bloom, MD, who developed the Sanctuary Model (http://www.sanctuaryweb.com/Home.aspx) has stated that like families and communities, organizations and agencies are "interconnected living systems subject to the stresses, strains and trauma of being alive" [15]. As a result, as we saw in the East Oakland Clinic, individuals and our entire healthcare delivery systems can become trauma organized, inducing rather than reducing stress in patients, staff, and administrators; however, there is hope. Brains and systems are plastic, which means that they are capable of change and healing (Fig. 9.1). The prescribed antidote to individual, community, and organizational trauma is to take a comprehensive and relationship-based approach.

Trauma-informed systems (TIS) provide an approach to understanding the impact of trauma on our staff, services, and patients and provide a way back to reflective and relationship-based care. As Bloom and Farragher discuss in *Restoring Sanctuary: A New Operating System for Trauma-Informed Systems of Care*, [16]

| Trauma organized | Trauma informed | Healing organization |
|---|---|---|
| Organizations impacted by stress, operating in silos, avoidant of issues and isolated in their practises or services delivery. These organizations can be trauma inducing. | These are organizations that develop a shared language to define, normalize and address the impact of trauma on clients and workforce. They operate from a foundational understanding of the nature and impact of trauma. | Organizations where staff policies, procedures, services and treatment models apply an understanding of trauma embedded within them. Their approaches to providing services are trauma-shielding or trauma-reducing. |
| • Reactive<br>• Reliving/retelling<br>• Avoiding/numbing<br>• Fragmented<br>• Us vs. them<br>• Inequity<br>• Authoritarian leadership | • Understanding of the nature and impact of trauma and recovery<br>• Shared language<br>• Recognizing socio-cultural trauma and structural oppression | • Reflective<br>• Making meaning out of the past<br>• Growth and prevention-oriented<br>• Collaborative<br>• Equity and accountability<br>• Relational leadership |

**From trauma-inducing to trauma-reducing**

**Fig. 9.1** Trauma-informed systems and healing

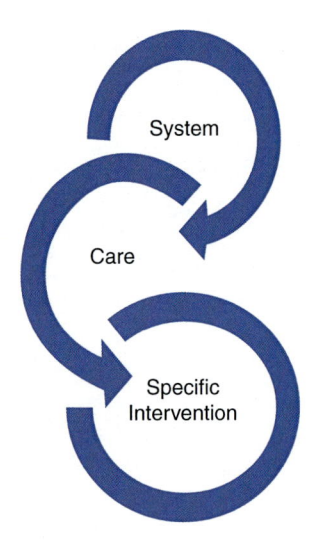

**Fig. 9.2** Three levels of a trauma-informed system

this means "becoming sensitive to the ways in which managers, staff, groups, and systems are impacted by individual and collective exposure to overwhelming and toxic stress and how they adapt (or not) to these stressors."

There are three levels that build a trauma-informed system: (1) trauma-reducing/healing organizational practices, (2) trauma-informed service delivery or care, and (3) trauma-specific clinical assessment and intervention (Fig. 9.2).

A trauma-informed system (TIS) recognizes the impact of trauma and incorporates specific values into organizational interactions and infrastructure to buffer staff and patients; this requires taking steps to heal broken systems, while we are also working to heal patients, families, and communities from the impact of trauma. Trauma-informed care (TIC) applies knowledge about trauma across all aspects of service delivery; however, it is not specifically designed to treat symptoms or syndromes related to trauma.

Trauma-specific (or trauma-focused) assessment, screening, and treatment, on the other hand, is evidence-based and provides best practice treatment models that have been proven to facilitate recovery from trauma. Trauma-specific treatments directly address the impact of trauma on an individual's life and facilitate trauma recovery; they are designed to treat the actual consequences of trauma. First, however, providing the organizational foundation to support these trauma-informed and specific practices is fundamental to implementing and sustaining change on all TIS levels.

## Taking Steps Toward a Trauma-Informed System

> Trauma Informed Systems principles and practices support reflection in place of reaction, curiosity in lieu of numbing, self-care instead of self-sacrifice and collective impact rather than siloed structures [17].

For lasting change, a new response is needed – a comprehensive, multilevel public health approach to devastating effects of trauma on individuals, families, and communities. This framework for organizational change will scaffold leaders and providers to respond as a learning healthcare system with the flexibility to incorporate specific values into interactions and operations. This includes both organizational and clinical practices like support for staff engagement and wellness at work, universal and early identification systems, as well as staff training to increase access to trauma-specific interventions and trauma-informed care for those who need it. Interventions that prevent trauma from occurring and promote health and well-being are also included.

TIS organizational practices aim to create safe physical, social, and emotional environments so everyone in the system has the resources and supports to achieve their full potential. Like individuals, resilient organizations are ones that can bounce back after distress and trauma; however, without awareness of what is happening, overstressed agencies and teams experience a gravitational pull toward disintegration and disorganization. Symptoms of trauma-organized settings manifest in leader and staff behaviors that include mistrust, scapegoating, blaming, bullying, "emotional flashbacks," or responses that are out of proportion to an event or environ-

**Growing a trauma-informed system**

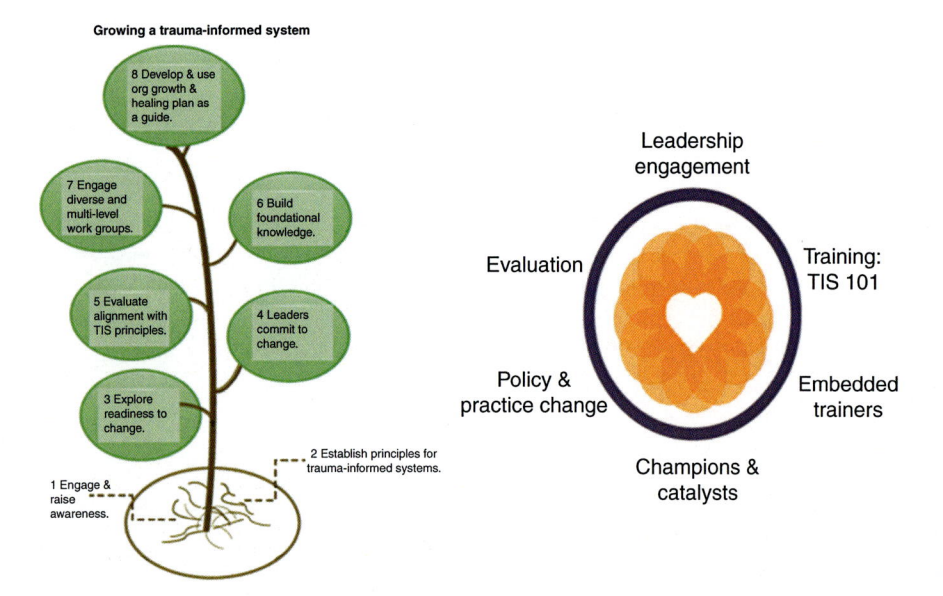

- 8 Develop & use org growth & healing plan as a guide.
- 7 Engage diverse and multi-level work groups.
- 6 Build foundational knowledge.
- 5 Evaluate alignment with TIS principles.
- 4 Leaders commit to change.
- 3 Explore readiness to change.
- 2 Establish principles for trauma-informed systems.
- 1 Engage & raise awareness.

Leadership engagement
Evaluation
Training: TIS 101
Policy & practice change
Embedded trainers
Champions & catalysts

**Fig. 9.3** TIS steps and components

ment. Leaders may default to an authoritarian instead of a relational style, engaging in misuse of power and silencing of dissent. There may be a pervasive over-focus on threat reduction, risk mitigation, or compliance at the expense of reflection, planning, and creativity. Authoritarian top-down decision-making processes are used rather than participatory ones that can aid agency and "voice and choice," which are key ingredients in a TIS. Continuous demands for improvement and transformation and widespread fatigue with multiple and seemingly disconnected initiatives are markers of a trauma-organized system.

Becoming trauma-informed is not just another initiative; instead it is an approach to understanding, organizing, interacting, and responding in a way that brings coherence to and aligns with and reduces competing demands. Figure 9.3 illustrates what we view as the essential steps toward, and components of this work; the order in which these steps unfold is largely determined by agency leadership and staff readiness. We explore some of these steps in more detail below.

## Raising Awareness

While your agency and staff may already be experiencing symptoms of a trauma-organized system and feel that something is wrong, an understanding about how and why it is affecting them may be absent. An initial step in the TIS process involves getting buy-in and selling the approach as a shift that can decrease their workplace stress, improve morale, and promote wellness. Building a shared language is done with introductory trainings, educational resources, and integrating concepts into daily communications. For example, the San Francisco Department of Public Health has trained its entire workforce with Trauma-Informed Systems (TISs) 101, a half-day program geared toward staff across all different positions and levels from the front desk and cafeteria to facilities, exam rooms, and the boardroom [17]. It blends didactic approaches with group discussions, role plays and exercises, as well as a unique commitment to change component. If all the leaders and staff in M's pediatric clinic were trauma aware, the setting and interactions with staff could have regulated rather than reinforced the family's trauma reactions [18]. It is up to pediatric leaders and staff to plant and nurture these seeds so that M and other children and families like his find healing rather than hurt in their care experiences.

## The Role of Leaders: Walking the Talk

As a leader, you must be the first to engage in and model change in your communication and behaviors; disaffected staff and patients will not engage in a process where leadership is absent and entreaties for change feel top-down and inauthentic. Your values must be visible and lived. On your part, this includes active listening and responsiveness to staff and patient and family needs and an ability to welcome and incorporate a diversity of perspectives in decision-making. For example, your training director and residents could ask you to meet with them regularly to explore and try different strategies to improve relative value unit (RVU) benchmarks rather than meetings which happen after the close of the quarter and feel punitive. Or M's mother would have a way to provide feedback to you about what prevents her from arriving on time.

As a leader, you must also be open to engaging in "meaning making" that shows a willingness to learn from successes and failures. Exploring your individual and organizational readiness, preparation and capacity for change is important as you and your staff undertake the intentional work required to become a TIS. This includes obtaining supports and resources for training, implementation, and ongoing evaluation, as well as committing to a participatory process of ongoing reflection, decision-making, and adaptation to the changing needs of your agency as it transforms [19]. For example, in order to sustain and spread its TIS 101 training to other agencies and locales, the San Francisco Department of Public Health (SF DPH) created a "train the trainer" model to help other child-serving agencies and other Bay Area counties develop the capacity to raise awareness and establish a shared language and understanding of trauma, the first step in developing a TIS [17]. This requires an ongoing, dynamic process with no expiration date that involves establishing a culture of ongoing learning, positive relationships in the workplace, and collaboration and empowerment at all levels [11, 20]. Key components in creating this culture include leadership engagement, organizational evaluation, staff participation in the change process, alignment of TIS principles to practices and policies, communication, and accountability to implementation goals.

Once you and your staff decide to move forward in implementing TIS, a vision and framework to direct and guide efforts should be developed. This vision starts with "the why" for the change, some proposed approaches, and what will be accomplished if everyone takes action and the change is successful. This allows everyone in the system to recognize how present efforts connect to future outcomes and ways in which they can work together to make their vision a reality. However, in order to create a vision for change, it's essential to first ground your efforts in and live your core principles.

## TIS Core Principles and Practices

Trauma is unpredictable, which can lead to feelings of fear, instability, loss of trust, devaluation, powerlessness, and distress. Building a TIS should be based on a shared set of core principles and competencies that counteract the negative impacts of trauma and strengthen those factors that contribute to healing and resilience.

Leaders can do this by working with their champions and staff to understand and develop ways to translate and align trauma-informed care principles into all organizational policies, infrastructure, and operations of the organization. The objective is to make trauma-informed principles and competencies actionable in what we do and how we interact with one another and our staff and how we provide care to our patients. Regardless of whether or not you know the individual trauma histories of your patients in your pediatric setting, grounding your organizational and clinical practices in these principles will improve the care provided to all.

For the purposes of this discussion, we will employ the six TIS principles (Fig. 9.4) developed as part of the SF Department of Public Health (SF DPH) TIS Initiative [17] and briefly present some ideas about how to translate them into work policies and practices.

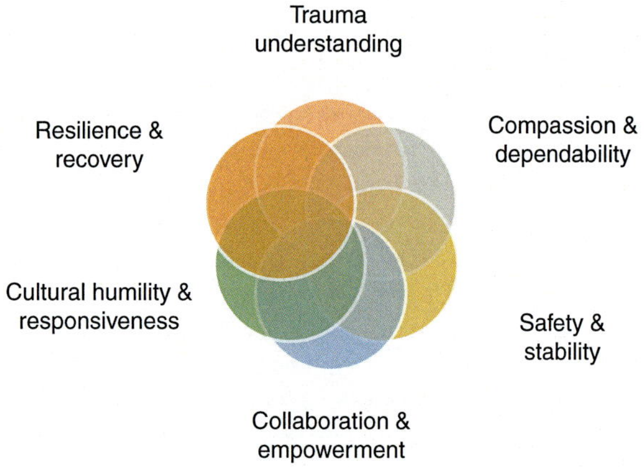

**Fig. 9.4** Six principles of trauma-informed systems

- Trauma understanding
- Compassion & dependability
- Safety & stability
- Collaboration & empowerment
- Cultural humility & responsiveness
- Resilience & recovery

## Trauma Understanding

Trauma understanding involves building knowledge and increasing awareness of the multilevel impacts of and varying responses to trauma. This awareness shifts perspectives to view behaviors as adaptations instead of pathologies and changes the conversation from "what's wrong with you?" to "what happened to you?" This awareness will help you and your staff take a step back to understand behavior in the context of trauma as M's pediatric resident did. Understanding trauma is a stress reducer and could have helped the receptionist to be present and not react to the mother's frustration and anger. If M's mother had a cast on her arm, we would be able to see it and avoid bumping into it. But trauma is invisible, and without awareness, we can react in ways that harm rather than heal.

It is also important to demonstrate trauma understanding to staff and patients and their families by providing easy-to-read, destigmatizing information on trauma as a health issue and creating welcoming, stress-reducing environments that minimize re-traumatization. For example, signage is clear, making it easy to get in and out of parking lots; ramps provide easy access to patients and families with disabilities; waiting rooms are welcoming, calming, comfortable, and not overstimulating; signs are in multiple languages; and lights around the clinic are in working order at night.

## Compassion and Dependability

Trauma can leave us feeling isolated or betrayed, which makes it difficult to trust or accept support. Consider M's mother and how betrayed she felt by staff who were "just following a routine procedure." Counter this with compassionate and dependable relationships and communication that include authentic expression of concern and support. For example, when you ask your patients or staff "how are you today?" as you go through the work day, this demonstrates that you have genuine interest in and commitment to their health and well-being. Leaving time for questions and/or holding regular times for consultation and feedback with patients and/or staff meetings and supervision is also essential.

## Safety and Stability

Trauma unpredictably violates our physical, social, and emotional safety resulting in a sense of threat and need to manage risks. Increasing stability in our daily lives and having these core safety needs met can minimize our stress reactions and allow us to focus our resources on wellness. This includes regularly monitoring the physical clinic and workspace environment for universal precautions, security measures, appropriate lighting, access to the building for patients with disabilities, and exits that are clearly labeled. Provide comfortable seating arrangements that give patients and families options for privacy or sitting with others. A play nook for M could have helped him to feel more secure and prevented the barrage of toy soldiers thrown at other waiting patients and families.

Also, make sure your staff have the resources they need to do their jobs (we know one TIS leader who each month gathered information about broken equipment and needed facility repairs for a spreadsheet, which he brought regularly to executive-level meetings). TIS have policies and procedures that are transparent, easily understood, and consistently followed. Clear and well-rehearsed communication protocols and procedures are essential when critical incidents do occur (examples include staff injury or a patient threatening self-harm).

## Collaboration and Empowerment

Trauma involves a loss of power and control that can make us feel helpless; providing information, preparation, and real opportunities to make choices can help staff and patients to feel empowered and can enhance wellness. Involve all those affected by a policy, practice, or treatment in decision-making processes, including the communities in which your organization or practice is located, patients and families, and staff at all levels of the system. Given this opportunity, M's mother and other families served in the East Oakland Clinic could have helped staff understand the causes behind perennial problems with late arrivals, for example, broken-down buses and trains. The team could then brainstorm other transportation options and develop a lateness policy for the clinic, increasing understanding and shared responsibility.

Accessible information is also empowering for patients and staff. Provide orientation and training and easy access to user-friendly patient health information, and choose electronic health record (EHR) and flexible information management systems that allow staff to adapt functions and reports to make them simpler, less burdensome, and useful. Give both patients and staff correct information and choices for communicating concerns. Knowing when to pick up a phone or talk face-to-face to solve a problem is also critical. Meeting agendas should be realistic and balanced between items focused on building relationship and supporting agency productivity.

## Cultural and Racial Humility

Appreciate and respect the diverse social and cultural backgrounds that influence how we see and respond to the world, as well as how the world sees and responds to us. In a TIS, cultural, social, and antiracist considerations are incorporated into discussions, thinking, and implementation and as a fundamental frame for patient experience and care [21]. Policies and tools for addressing differences and conflict, which understandably will arise, are readily understood and available. In addition, personnel practices—hiring, onboarding, performance appraisal and disciplinary practices, and talent retention practices—should highlight and promote a workforce that reflects the patient community, and policies and practices are regularly audited for equity and alignment to TIS principles. Providers are informed and can link patients to cultural healers, mental wellness professionals, indigenous healers, and support networks.

## Resilience and Recovery

Trauma can have a long-lasting and broad impact on our lives that may create a feeling of hopelessness. Yet, when we focus on our strengths, and clear steps we can take toward wellness, we are more likely to be resilient and recover. Given more trauma-informed supports, M's receptionist would have been able to understand, express more empathy, and respond more flexibly, communication would have remained open, and a plan could have been developed keeping patient appointments on track and providing doable alternatives, so M received his vaccines on time.

While healthcare delivery systems are mandated to identify only pathology and impairments for payment, holding resilience as a foundation for healing and using a strengths-based approach to uncover and acknowledge existing assets is a powerful way to support patient treatment and healing. Trauma-informed organizations provide professional development opportunities that reflect a commitment to TIS and the diversity of patients and staff including nonviolent communication or de-escalation training and workforce wellness practices. In addition to training, wellness activities and opportunities can be integrated into the work day.

## Evaluating Your Organizational Baseline

How do you know what your organization or clinic needs? An essential next step is an assessment that can help you understand the ways in which your organization is aligned with the trauma-informed principles and practices presented above. This will uncover areas of strength and challenges. Ideally this should take place at the start of TIS implementation and at regular intervals thereafter. There are a number of organizational assessments available, such as the Trauma-Informed Agency Assessment [22], the Tool for a Trauma Informed Work Life [23, 24], or the Trauma-Informed Program Self-Assessment Scale (TIPS) [25]. For additional resources, please see http://traumatransformed.org/resource-grid/. The majority of currently developed assessments focus on structural components of trauma-informed care, such as specific practices or policies that speak to a concrete issue related to trauma-informed care. Once baseline results are available, explore with staff at all levels how much the social and emotional culture of the organization has been impacted by stress and trauma and what factors may be supporting healing and resilience.

## Engaging Champions and Developing a Plan

Recruit champions to participate in a reflective workgroup that acts as the implementation team and will significantly increase the likelihood that TIS implementation will be successful and sustainable [26]. Include staff from all levels of the organization so that multiple perspectives are included. Leadership should be responsive and supportive of this workgroup, but not drive the agenda. Workgroup tasks include interpreting results from organizational assessments, incorporating staff feedback into planning and development of TIS strategies, and developing an organizational healing and growth plan that targets the assessed areas of TIS that need strengthening; this will in turn guide efforts and help to communicate progress.

Strategies that the workgroup might help lead or guide include those focused on supporting staff wellness, aligning current patient care policies and practices with TIS principles, or developing procedures to respond to the emotional needs of staff in response to anticipated or common traumatic events experienced. The workgroup can also serve as a model for behaviors and practices that support trauma-informed principles. Information on TIS should be clear and transparent and communicated through a variety of modalities (e.g., verbally during staff meetings and in written communication such as through emails, newsletters, and flyers) to ensure everyone in the system receives updates and feels included in the change process. This further sustains TIS by keeping staff informed on what is going on and how they can continue to support TIS, as well as maintaining participation in the change process by creating transparency and accountability around how ideas are put into place.

## Trauma-Specific Interventions: The Role of Pediatric Providers

Once organizational work has established the foundation and the practice of TIS principles within a system, trauma-informed care and trauma-specific practices can be implemented more effectively and sustainably. Pediatricians within a TIS are critically influential through their commitment to embrace and embed trauma screening, to be trusted as partners and change agents by parents and caregivers, to be knowledgeable about treatment options, and to refer and follow families through treatment [27]. For those working in vulnerable communities, the public health impact could be significant for children and youth like M, their development, well-being, and for the prevention of chronic disease over their lifetimes.

## Screening: What You See Can Be Treated

Screening and psychoeducation are a routine part of pediatric care, and pediatricians have a responsibility to regularly screen and identify patients in need of mental health services [28]. As discussed earlier, there is compelling evidence that the effects of trauma may emerge from exposure to even a single event or, slowly, accumulating over time from collective exposure. Screening methods must identify those who are suffering currently or who are at risk for future distress and impairment by measuring three interrelated factors: trauma exposure, traumatic stress, and related symptoms.

Given the scarcity of appropriate pediatric screening methods, a two-step screening process—a trauma exposure inventory followed by a symptom screen—may provide the most utility. The UCLA-PTSD-Reaction Index (RI) is one of the few psychometrically validated measures to assess for both trauma exposure and traumatic stress with a minimal time burden (20 min) [29].

Two brief measures developed by and for pediatric practitioners are also good and brief screening options; these measures expand traditional definitions of traumatic events (e.g., child abuse) to recognize the impact of other adverse childhood experiences in the assessment of risk. The first is the Loma Linda Whole Child Assessment (WCA), which embeds trauma exposure screening items within the broader context of a lifestyle questionnaire that assesses multiple health risks. In addition to potentially traumatic events (e.g., intimate partner violence, child abuse, divorce), it asks about factors such as environmental risks, caregiver mental health, child development concerns, nutrition, etc. The WCA has also been approved for use by Medicaid providers in the state of California [30]. The second instrument is the Center for Youth Wellness (CYW) Adverse Childhood Experiences Questionnaire developed by the Bayview Child Health Partnership [31]. This tool expands the concept of trauma exposure to include traumatic grief, medical trauma, discrimination, bullying, and involvement in the child welfare and juvenile justice systems. The CYW ACE-Q uniquely allows the reporter to endorse exposure(s) without divulging the actual experience(s) which may reduce the distress and sense of vulnerability associated with disclosing specific traumatic events [31].

Regardless of the screening tool used, it is essential to be attuned to patients throughout and be prepared for the possibility that asking about trauma may evoke intense emotions in some. If this does occur, it's an opportunity to educate and reassure by recognizing this as a normal response to trauma. It is also not necessary to press for more details, as that can be done in a comprehensive assessment as part of ongoing therapy with a behavioral health provider.

Regularly employing a trauma exposure screen, such as those described above, during well-child or periodic health visits can allow for the identification of both new and cumulative trauma exposure which may indicate that a patient should proceed to a secondary screen for symptoms and/or treatment. You can embrace this next step by advancing and maintaining your knowledge on evidence-based trauma-specific interventions.

## Treatment Knowledge

Patients and communities instill a high degree of faith in their pediatric providers, and that trust must be met with recommendations that recognize best standards for quality care, particularly when connecting families to trauma-specific services. Fortunately, trauma-specific treatments have evolved with a strong and growing evidence base that reflect TIS principles across multiple treatment modalities. To consolidate existing knowledge from the burgeoning treatment literature, Strand, Hansen, and Courtney [32] coded eight evidence-based trauma treatment manuals and from their work generated nine components common to effective trauma treatments for children and families:

1. Trauma Assessment: Activities that assess the presence and impact of trauma.
2. Safety: Activities that reduce potential for harm and increase socio-environmental stability.
3. Engagement: Activities that foster therapeutic alliance and client motivation, provide psychoeducation, or identify obstacles.
4. Attachment/Strengthening Relationships: Activities that strengthen relationships, particularly with caregivers.
5. Core Treatment Interventions: Culturally appropriate interventions that reduce symptoms and enhance coping.
6. Attention to the Social Context: Collaborative treatment planning, advocacy, or case management to address socio-environmental adversities.
7. Trauma Processing: Activities that focus on processing and integrating traumatic experience.
8. Consolidation/Post-trauma Growth: Activities that make meaning out of the trauma and promote adaptive functioning.
9. Therapist Self-care: Interventions that anticipate and manage therapist vicarious or secondary traumatic stress.

These common elements for effective treatment share practice overlap and mission with the TIS principles discussed earlier. You will also recognize the TIS principles embodied in the treatment modalities provided by partnering behavioral health providers.

Evidence-based trauma treatments for children and youth have burgeoned in recent years, and though the evidence base is still developing, cognitive behavioral therapy (CBT) currently offers the most solid evidence for resolving traumatic stress, but not to the exclusion of other complementary or integrative methods. Several promising and established evidence-based practices have been designed across the span of childhood that recognize the developmental stages of children and families impacted by trauma. From infancy to late adolescence, these interventions alleviate the impact of trauma through cognitive behavioral methods, relationship building, and coping skills, such as mindfulness. For a more exhaustive review of evidence-based trauma treatments, please consult the National Child Traumatic Stress Network (NCTSN; https://www.nctsn.org), the National Registry of Evidence-Based Programs and Practices (NREPP; https://nrepp-learning.samhsa.gov), or the California Evidence-Based Clearinghouse for Child Welfare (CEBC;

http://www.cebc4cw.org), each of which details different evidence-based treatments for trauma.

## Capacity Building

The movement toward integrating behavioral health into pediatric care practice, particularly among pediatric care networks, is not new, and efforts to adopt integrated care models are gaining traction, slowly. The associations between trauma and physical and behavioral health outcomes across the life span underscore the need for adequate care capacity that is well-coordinated and collaborative. Many healthcare programs are adopting internal capacity building methods, while others are establishing or re-envisioning collaborative partnerships with external providers.

Expanding capacity for treating trauma requires adopting new service delivery approaches to integrated physical and behavioral health. Many major healthcare and public health networks are now employing providers to bridge the gap between physical and behavioral healthcare needs and coordination [33]. Often titled as Behaviorists, Behavioral Health Specialists/Consultants, or Integrated Behavioral Health Providers, these collaborative care teams typically operate within the traditional healthcare model to provide colocated expertise and services [34].

Over time, these integrated providers develop relationships with both their pediatric colleagues and the families served, allowing for the establishment of trust and alliance across the health team or medical home. They are well-positioned to screen for traumatic stress and/or related impairment, offer brief interventions, (e.g., cognitive behavioral techniques) to alleviate mild to moderate distress, to monitor symptom severity over time, and to connect patients with more intensive specialty behavioral health care when needed. These providers may also be a valuable resource shortly after a traumatic experience by providing preventive or supportive care, such as Psychological First Aid (PFA) or Skills for Psychological Recovery (SPR). *PFA and SPR were* developed by the National Child Traumatic Stress Network and the National Center for PTSD (https://www.ptsd.va.gov) as an evidence-informed approach to supporting individual and families in the days, weeks, and months following a disaster or trauma [35].

As an alternative or supplement to the integrated behavioral health providers, pediatric care systems may annex or embed their own behavioral health outpatient programming. Utilizing a traditional behavioral health model can provide the benefits of evidence-based trauma treatments, which are typically administered an hour or more per week over the course of weeks or even months, while partnering pediatric primary care and behavioral health providers within the same health system.

However, for many pediatric healthcare systems, it may not be feasible to focus on internal capacity building; instead TIS pediatric providers identify collaborations that can provide their patients with high quality, evidence-based care. These partnerships are most likely to take place within the networks of behavioral health providers that exist across community-based organizations, public health programs, and the school system. Indeed, many school systems have taken a proactive approach to creating TIS programming, including the integration of evidence-based trauma treatments such as Cognitive Behavioral Intervention for Trauma in Schools (CBITS) [36]. CBITS is a brief, skills-based group intervention for children, ages 10–15. The treatment focuses on alleviating traumatic stress, depression, and general anxiety. The impact of such treatment options may be heightened when school systems also embrace a TIS model, such as the University of California at San Francisco's Healthy Environments and Response to Trauma in Schools (HEARTS) program [37] which found improvements in student symptoms and observed that school disciplinary actions were reduced when on-site trauma treatment was embedded within a TIS model.

## TIS Early Adopter Systems and Agencies

Even before the ACE study and prior to the formal recognition of children's mental health problems as different than adult ones, pediatricians have been at the forefront of identifying and responding to behavioral health problems in their pediatric patients and families. Across the United States, clinics are also embodying the cultures of trauma-informed care through transforming environments to be educational, nurturing, and soothing, expanding clinic hours and wellness definitions to align to the cultures and priorities of patients, and attending to the secondary stress of the workforce so that our delivery systems, our staff, are sustainably equipped to attend to patient trauma. As mentioned above, some have successfully linked to, employed, colocated, and collaborated with behavioral health professionals to provide services for children under their care. While some have been successful, others have been challenged by ongoing and chronic shortages of child behavioral health professionals, barriers to access, and the fragmentation of systems and services.

With the now well-established evidence that ACEs and physical health are interconnected and that trauma impacts individuals, communities, and agencies, child-serving systems and healthcare organizations across the country are responding with TIS initiatives and programs. In general, initiatives tend to either start with organizational practices or with direct clinical care. From our experience and as we have shared, to be successful, both organizational and clinical practices need to be addressed.

## Care-Focused Initiatives

Below we describe several initiatives with the shared goals of improving identification of children, youth, and families who are experiencing trauma and increasing the availability of and linkages to trauma-specific interventions.

*The Bayview Child Health Center (BCHC)-Center for Youth Wellness (CYW)* [31]. The Center for Youth Wellness is located in the Bayview Hunters Point Neighborhood of San Francisco, a section of the city with communities of color impacted by racism, high rates of poverty, community violence, pollution, and crime. CYW has led the effort to use ACE science to transform pediatric understanding and practice for children exposed to early adversities and their families. CYF developed the Adverse Childhood Experience Questionnaire (ACE-Q) and User Guide for routine use by pediatric care providers (https://centerforyouthwellness.org/cyw-aceq/). In addition, for children exposed to four or more ACEs, CYW offers care coordination, psychiatry, biofeedback training, and linkage to multidisciplinary evidence-based interventions to help children and families heal from the effects of repeated toxic stress. In partnership with UCSF Benioff Children's Hospitals, it has launched a study of biomarkers of adversity and children's health to further inform the development of effective interventions to prevent immediate and long-term health risks and problems.

*Children's Hospital Philadelphia (CHOP)* The National Child Traumatic Stress Network (NCTSN)-funded CHOP Center for Traumatic Pediatric Stress addresses medical trauma in the lives of children and families due to pediatric illness and injury. CPTS is an interdisciplinary effort with partners from psychology, critical care medicine, emergency medicine, nursing, oncology, primary care, psychiatry, and surgery. The goal is to prevent and treat medical traumatic stress in healthcare settings. "Helping parents to help their kids recover." Strategies include providing information and resources to medical and mental health professionals and partnering with national healthcare provider organizations to promote trauma-informed care and best practices in preventing and treating medical trauma. https://www.chop.edu/centers-programs/center-pediatric-traumatic-stress.

*Massachusetts Child Trauma Project (MCTP)* MCTP is a state-wide initiative and partnership between the behavioral health and child welfare systems to improve identification through screening and assessment of children with complex trauma. MCTP fosters trauma awareness and informed practices among child-serving agencies and caregivers, increases the number of providers delivering evidence-based trauma interventions, and ensures more appropriate linkages to effective treatments. https://www.luk.org/services/counseling-mainmenu-396/mctp-mainmenu.

*Philadelphia Alliance for Child Trauma Services (PACTS)* The goal of this initiative is to create a publicly funded trauma-informed behavioral health system by building a coordinated network of providers trained in evidence-based trauma screening, assessment and trauma-focused CBT. Elements include relationship building, planning and problem-solving implementation, along with education, training, and coaching strategies to change knowledge and practice and financial incentives for agencies implementing trauma-focused CBT (TF-CBT). http://www.philadelphiapacts.org.

## Systems-Focused Initiatives

Below we describe several initiatives with the shared goals of improving organizational practices in systems and agencies providing services to youth and families who have or are experiencing trauma.

**Maine Thrive** (http://thriveinitiative.org) began as a SAMHSA-funded statewide system of care to meet the needs of children and youth with serious emotional and behavioral health challenges and their families. Now a nonprofit, Thrive is a training and technical assistance partner to implement trauma-informed principles, practices, and assessments in all state-contracted mental health agencies, family partner organizations, and juvenile justice services.

**Montefiore HealthySteps** [38] is part of a behavioral health integration program at Montefiore Children's Hospital in Bronx, NY (http://www.cham.org/programs-centers/healthy-steps) [37]. It is a unique, evidence-based pediatric primary care program designed to address both organizational and care practices to impact healthy early childhood development and effective parenting so that all children are ready for school and success in life. Over 120 pediatric and family medicine practices across the country have implemented HealthySteps and have reached more than 37,000 children ages 0–3, their parents, and caregivers.

**The Sanctuary Movement** was launched in the ealy 1980's by Dr. Sandra Bloom and her team of clinicians on an adult inpatient psychiatric unit; they developed the Sanctuary Model as a response to the negative impact of trauma on patients and the people and systems who provide treatment [16]. As mentioned earlier in this chapter, Sanctuary is a blueprint for change at both the clinical and organizational levels.

Recognizing the need for a shared approach to organize a response, Bloom developed the Sanctuary Commitments (similar to SF DPH's principles and competencies) and the SELF rubric, *s*afety, *e*motion management, *l*oss, and *f*uture. These four elements are the basis for how providers conduct community and team meetings, treatment planning, and collaborative decision-making and support a focus on the most important aspects of helping people heal from trauma in a simple and accessible way. Sanctuary has been used to develop safe and healing environments for children, families, and adults who have experienced chronic stress and adversity in residential treatment, juvenile justice, child welfare, drug and alcohol treatment, school and community-based programs, partial hospitals, domestic violence, and homeless shelters.

**The San Francisco Department of Public Health (SF DPH) TIS Initiative** [17] is led by the Children, Youth and Families System of Care (children's behavioral health services in San Francisco, CA) and is the largest public systems effort of its kind in the United States. For context, SF DPH is the largest agency in the city and county of San Francisco made up of three divisions, hospital, ambulatory, and community health services. As described in a Center for Healthcare Strategies Report and as discussed above, it developed a TIS 101 training and trained 9000 employees at all levels in trauma knowledge and understanding to establish a common language and framework in which to anchor organizational practice change [40]. Related efforts include the development and testing of a trauma-informed leadership and champions model to initiate and sustain organizational practice change (https://www.chcs.org/resource/implementing-trauma-informed-practices-throughout-the-san-francisco-department-of-public-health/) and Trauma Transformed (http://traumatransformed.org), a SAMHSA-funded partnership among seven SF Bay Area counties led by children, youth, and families served in these systems, San Francisco County, and the East Bay Agency for Children (EBAC; http://www.ebac.org) to develop a trauma-informed regional system of care to ensure continuous and seamless care coordination and provision across county lines and to establish a common TIS language, framework, and practices across SF Bay child-serving systems, i.e., child welfare, school districts, behavioral health, and juvenile justice.

## Conclusion

> If you don't transform it, you transmit it.
> ~ Youth leader, Trauma Transformed

Trauma is a part of our human experience. It is not easily measured and not always visible. Youth and families experiencing trauma have told us that how we deliver care is just as important as what type of care is provided. When we as pediatric leaders and providers are aware, understand trauma, commit to TIS principles and change, implement the TIS components, and infuse day-to-day work with the tools and practices presented in this chapter, there will be small steps and little epiphanies that eventually add up to a transformation in care teams and a revolution in our patient care. By doing so, we can restore authentic connection between leaders, staff and patients, and address the conditions in our health systems and agencies that deepen trauma's existing wounds and undermine health and wellness. In responding to the triple threat of overburdened individuals, communities, staff, and bureaucracies with TIS, we help to heal not only our patients like M but ourselves and the organizations in which we provide care.

## References

1. Plemmons G, Hall M, Doupnik S, Gray J, Brown C, Browning W, Casey R, Freundlich K, Johnson DP, Lind C, Rehm K, Thomas S, Williams D. Hospitalization for suicide ideation or attempt: 2018–2015. Pediatrics. 2018;141(6):e20172426.
2. Felitti V, Anda R, Nordenberg, D, Williamson D, Spitz A, Marks J, et al. Relationship of childhood abuse and household dysfunction to many of the leading causes of death in adults: the Adverse Childhood Experiences (ACE) study. Am J Prev Med. 1998;14(4):245–258.
3. Epstein K, Gerber EB. Healing the healer: changing the way we understand and respond to trauma. J SF Med Soc. 2016;89(4):25. Accessed 20 May 2018. Available from: https://issuu.com/sfmedsociety/docs/may-16/25

4. Aragon TJ, Lichtensztajn DY, Katcher BS, Reiter R, Katz MH. Calculating expected years of life lost for assessing local ethnic disparities in causes of premature death. BMC Public Health. 2008;8:116.
5. Burke Harris N, Silvério Marques S, Oh D, Bucci M, Cloutier M. Prevent, screen, heal: collective action to fight the toxic effects of early life adversity. Acad Pediatr. 2017;17(7S):S14–S15.
6. Oh D, Jerman P, Silvério Marques S, Koita K, Purewal Boparai S, Bucci M, et al. Systematic review of pediatric health outcomes associated with childhood adversity. BMC Pediatr. 2018;18(1):83.
7. McFarlane AC. The long-term costs of traumatic stress: intertwined physical and psychological consequences. World Psychiatry. 2010;9(1):3–10.
8. U.S. Department of Health and Human Services, Health Resources and Services Administration (HRSA), Maternal and Child Health Bureau (MCHB). Child and adolescent health measurement initiative: overview of adverse child and family experiences among US children. [Internet] 2013. Accessed 20 May 2018. Available from: www.childhealthdata.org
9. Saunders B, Adams Z. Epidemiology of traumatic experiences in childhood. Child Adolesc Psychiatr Clin N Am. 2014;23(2):167–184.
10. American Psychiatric Association. Diagnostic and statistical manual of mental disorders: DSM-5. Arlington, VA: American Psychiatric Publishing; 2013. p. 265–90.
11. Substance Abuse and Mental Health Services Administration. Trauma-informed care in behavioral health services. Rockville, MD: Treatment improvement protocol (TIP) series 57. HHS publication no. (SMA) 13-4801.
12. Bracha HS. Freeze, flight, fight, fright, faint: adaptationist perspectives on the acute stress response spectrum. CNS Spectr. 2004;9(9):679–85.
13. Baldwin DV. Primitive mechanisms of trauma response: an evolutionary perspective on trauma-related disorders. Neurosci Biobehav Rev. 2013;37:1549–66.
14. Substance Abuse and Mental Health Services Administration. SAMHSA's concept of trauma and guidance for a trauma-informed approach. Rockville, MD: 2014.
15. Hall LH, Johnson J, Watt I, Tsipa A, O'Connor DB. Healthcare staff wellbeing, burnout, and patient safety: a systematic review. Harris F, editor. PLoS One. 2016;11(7):e0159015. https://doi.org/10.1371/journal.pone.0159015.
16. Bloom SL, Farragher B. Restoring sanctuary: a new operating system for trauma-informed systems of care. New York, NY: Oxford University Press; 2013.
17. Epstein K, Speziale K, Gerber E, Loomis B. Trauma informed systems initiative: 2014 year in review. San Francisco, CA: San Francisco Department of Public Health; 2014.
18. Leitch L. Action steps using and trauma-informed care: a resilience model. Health Justice. 2017;5:5.
19. Kaner S. Facilitator's guide to participatory decision-making. 3rd ed. San Francisco, CA: Jossey-Bass; 2014.
20. Bowers C, Kreutzer C, Cannon-Bowers J, Lamb J. Team resilience as a second-order emergent state: a theoretical model and research directions. Front Psychol. 2017;8:1360.
21. Hardy K. Antiracist approaches for shaping theoretical and practice paradigms. In: Carten AJ, Siskind AB, Greene MP, editors. Strategies for deconstructing racism in the health and human services. New York: Oxford University Press; 2016. p. 125–39.
22. Maine Department of Health and Human Services. Trauma-Informed Agency Assessment (TIAA). 2012. Accessed 28 May 2018. Available from: http://thriveinitiative.org/wp-content/uploads/2015/07/Copy-of-TIAA-Manual-7-9-12-FINAL.pdf
23. Loomis B. Tool for a trauma informed worklife (TTIW). Unpublished measure.
24. Loomis B, Falvey C. Leveraging knowledge of worklife experiences to create Trauma Informed Systems change. Paper presented at: the 32nd Annual International Society for Traumatic Stress Studies Meeting, Dallas, TX. Nov 10–12, 2016.
25. Fallott RD, Harris M. Creating cultures of trauma-informed care (CCTIC): a self-assessment and planning tool [Internet]. 2009. Accessed 28 May 2018. Available from: https://www.healthcare.uiowa.edu/icmh/documents/CCTICSelf-AssessmentandPlanningProtocol0709.pdf

26. Fixsen DL, Naoom SF, Blasé KA, Friedman RM, Wallace F. Implementation research: a synthesis of the literature [Internet]. 2005. Available from: http://nirn.fpg.unc.edu/sites/nirn.fpg.unc.edu/files/resources/NIRN-MonographFull-01-2005.pdf
27. Conn A, Szilagyi M, Jee S, Manly J, Briggs R, Szilagyi P. Parental perspectives of screening for adverse childhood experiences in pediatric primary care. Fam Syst Health. 2018;36(1):62–72.
28. Heneghan A, Garner A, Storefer-Isser A, Kortepeter K, Stein REK, Horowitz SM. Pediatricians role in providing mental health care for children and adolescents: do pediatricians and child and adolescent psychiatrists agree? J Dev Behav Pediatr. 2008;29(4):262–9.
29. Steinberg AM, Brymer MJ, Kim S, Ghosh C, Ostrowski SA, Gulley K, Briggs EC, Pynoos RS. Psychometric properties of the UCLA PTSD reaction index: part 1. J Trauma Stress. 2013;26:1–9.
30. Marie-Mitchell A, O'Connor TG. Adverse childhood experiences: translating knowledge into identification of children at risk for poor outcomes. Acad Pediatr. 2013;13(1):14–9.
31. Burke Harris N, Renschler T. Center for Youth Wellness ACE-Questionnaire (CYW ACE-Q Child, Teen, Teen SR). San Francisco, CA: Center for Youth Wellness; 2015.
32. Strand VC, Hansen S, Courtney D. Common elements across evidence-based trauma treatment: discovery and implications. Adv Soc Work. 2013;14(2):334–54.
33. Tyler ET, Hulkower RL, Kaminski J. Behavioral health integration in pediatric primary care: considerations and opportunities for policymakers, planners and providers. Milbank Memorial Fund. 2017. Available from: https://www.milbank.org/wp-content/uploads/2017/03/MMF_BHI_REPORT_FINAL.pdf
34. Talmi A, Muther EF, Margolis K, Buchholz M, Asherin R, Bunik M. The scope of behavioral health integration in a pediatric primary care setting. J Pediatr Psychol. 2016;41(10):1120–32.
35. Brymer M, Layne C, Jacobs A, Pynoos R, Ruzek J, Steinberg A, Vernberg E, Watson P. Psychological first aid field operations guide. 2nd ed: National Child Traumatic Stress Network; 2006. Accessed 16 December 2018. Available from: https://www.nctsn.org/resources/psychological-first-aid-pfa-field-operations-guide-2nd-edition
36. Nadeem E, Jaycox LH, Kataoka SH, Langley AK, Stein BD. Going to scale: experiences implementing a school-based trauma intervention. School Psych Rev. 2011;40(4):549–68.
37. Dorado JS, Martinez M, McArthur LE, Leibovitz T. Healthy environments and response to trauma in schools (HEARTS): a whole-school, multi-level, prevention and intervention program for creating trauma-informed, safe and supportive schools. Sch Ment Heal. 2016;8(1):163–76. Available from: https://doi.org/10.1007/s12310-016-9177-0
38. Briggs RD, Hershberg RS, Germán M. Healthy steps at Montefiore: our journey from start up to scale. In: Briggs R, editor. Integrated early childhood behavioral health in primary care. Cham: Springer; 2016. p. 105–16.
39. Elwyn LJ, Esaki N, Smith CA. Importance of leadership and employee engagement in trauma-informed organizational change at a girls' juvenile justice facility. Hum Ser Organ Manag Leadersh Gov. 2017;41(2):106–18.
40. Center for Healthcare Strategies. Trauma informed care in action profile: implementing Trauma-Informed Practices throughout the San Francisco Department of Public Health. 2018 Accessed 1 June 2018. Available from: https://www.chcs.org/resource/implementing-trauma-informed-practices-throughout-the-san-francisco-department-of-public-health/

# Chapter 10
# Trauma-Informed Nursing Care

**Jay Ellen Barrett**

## Introduction

The nurse is often the first healthcare professional to assess the patient in any care setting. Due to the considerable prevalence of physical and psychological violence in our society, nurses frequently care for the victims, the perpetrators, and the witnesses of physical and psychological violence [1]. As members of the largest group of healthcare professionals, nurses must be aware of assessment methods and nursing interventions that will interrupt the cycle of violence and promote healing [1, 2]; they are critical to providing trauma-informed, person-centered care. Recognition that past trauma can impact the patient's engagement in their own healthcare [2] can serve to facilitate creation of a safe environment, free of judgment and preconceptions about the patient's adherence, or lack thereof, to medical recommendations. Understanding trauma histories and engaging the patient in care addresses both the mental health effects of trauma, and the resulting chronic disease issues and adverse health behaviors that ensue [3]. Most of the extant literature on trauma-informed nursing care focuses on mental health [4] and pediatric care [5, 6]; this chapter will review trauma-informed nursing care in adult medical settings in order to begin to address this gap. Engaging patients through a trauma-informed nursing approach, can improve health outcomes and potentially decrease care utilization and costs [7]. In essence, nurses are ideally situated to respond to identity and context by addressing the potential ways in which the physical environment and staff interactions can create a welcoming environment for survivors.

The healthcare environment is often a difficult setting for trauma-exposed persons. Many patients have had negative experiences with healthcare, either personally or through a friend or loved one. Any medical encounter regardless of the setting (primary or specialty care, emergency department or inpatient ward) can

---

J. E. Barrett, RN, BSN, MBA (✉)
US Army Nurse Corps, LTC (Ret), Veterans Affairs (VA) Boston Healthcare System, Boston, MA, USA

© Springer Nature Switzerland AG 2019
M. R. Gerber (ed.), *Trauma-Informed Healthcare Approaches*,
https://doi.org/10.1007/978-3-030-04342-1_10

trigger disturbing memories that may intrude on the current visit and interfere with its goals. The common thread uniting nurses who work in varied fields is the nursing process—the essential core of practice for the delivery of holistic, patient-focused care [8]. The Nursing Process (Assess, Diagnose, Plan, Implement, Evaluate) [9] is the ideal foundation upon which to deliver TIC.

In the trauma-informed nursing process, Assessment includes inquiry into the patient's past experiences of physical, emotional, and sexual traumas as well as traumatic experiences within the healthcare system; nurses can use validated screening measures [10] or develop questions of their own to accomplish this. Recognition of the signs and symptoms of a possible trauma reaction is a first step in assessing the patient. Signs like elevated blood pressure, heart rate, sweating, nervous tics, or behaviors, like anger, anxiety, avoidance of eye contact, coupled with a history of behaviors such as "no shows" or late arrival to appointments, and non-adherence to medical regimes [7], are clues that can indicate a response to a prior trauma (within healthcare or outside of it). The presence of these characteristic features may lead a trauma-informed nurse to identify (Diagnose) a patient as trauma-exposed.

The next step in the process is Planning. In the TIC nursing process, when possible, advanced preparation for the patient encounter [2] is important to identify potential for the ability of the patient to engage in evaluation and goal setting and to avoid unintended re-traumatization. The medical home model, or patient aligned care team (PACT) as it is called in the Veterans Health Administration (VA), offers examples for nursing-directed preplanning, daily huddles, and population management of panels of patients [11–13], all of which are ideal conduits for implementing trauma-informed nursing care.

Next, Implementing and Evaluating are critical to delivery of TIC. Nursing implementation of TIC includes creating a safe and collaborative care environment [14], critical for the patient to engage. When TIC is implemented, patients can feel that they are not being judged for their behavior, share their experiences and feelings without negative verbal or non-verbal responses, and sense empathy and understanding from the care team. Evaluation can include assessing patient comfort, satisfaction with care, or using process improvement methods to identify areas of strengths and weakness in the practice.

Recognition that nursing staff may have their own trauma histories is also essential to caring for patients in a trauma-informed manner [15–17]. Nurses may have personal trauma experiences similar to that of the patient, or with the event that led to the visit or hospitalization. They may have had a previous negative encounter with a particular patient who had a prior difficult presentation. When possible, planning who will care for the patient and understanding the underlying (often unspoken) expectations of the encounter (*will the patient come, be on time, have a positive attitude, be willing or able to engage?*) will ensure that the interaction will be as therapeutic as possible for the patient and the staff, and reduce the occurrence of re-traumatization for both. Knowing the available resources (referral sources, educational interventions) within the healthcare setting is critical to responding to a strong patient reaction and is a priority in preparation for any patient encounter.

Trauma-exposed patients are commonly seen throughout the healthcare system, [18, 19] and nurses are ideal change agents in implementing TIC. This chapter will review trauma-informed nursing care of the adult medical and surgical patient.

## Safety and Connections: A Positive Environment of Care

Nursing can play a key role in implementing the core principles of TIC which include [14] physical and psychological safety, trustworthiness, collaboration, empowerment, and appreciation of the patient's cultural, historical, and gender issues. Nursing fundamentally recognizes that healing happens in relationships and in the meaningful sharing of control and decision-making. This includes recognition of resilience and in the ability of individuals, organizations, and communities to heal and promote recovery from trauma [14]. Research has linked exposure to trauma with significantly higher rates of healthcare utilization and physical and mental disorders [18, 19]. For this reason, it is recommended that all patients be approached as if they have experienced trauma, a form of "universal trauma precautions" [20, 21]. This follows the concept of patient-centered care that is at the core of nursing.

Patients, especially those who have experienced trauma, need to feel safe within the healthcare environment to achieve any level of engagement in their care and to begin to foster trust. This begins with a welcoming and warm environment where all staff addresses the patient using non-judgmental positive and professional language. This sets the tone for the entire experience. The message should be one of caring and accurate communication beginning with reception and progressing through the entire encounter.

Privacy is one of the most important elements in establishing safety for the patient with a trauma history. Ensuring privacy during the nursing assessment provides a sense of security and is critical to creating an environment of trust in initial interviews and contacts with the patient. This is not always easy to accomplish in busy emergency departments (ED) or urgent care settings, or in multiple bed inpatient rooms, but must be considered to create the sense of safety the patient needs to potentially disclose current or past trauma. A patient cannot be expected to share personal history in an area where others will hear, this can result in fear of judgement or shame [22]. Auditory privacy can be created with private rooms with a closed door or with a white noise sound machine. Whatever is used to produce a confidential atmosphere should be tested in advance to allow the nurse to reassure the patient that there is a private and safe milieu.

Privacy for the examination is another area of concern for any patient. Depending on the trauma history, assurance that there will be no unexpected interruptions by providing a lock on the door, privacy curtains in front of the door, or someone to "guard" the entrance is supportive and demonstrates understanding of the patient's possible fears. Assessing each individual patient's preferences is important, as for some patients a closed/locked door could feel frightening [23]. Privacy curtains are essential in all settings and installation is neither complicated nor expensive, portable screens can be used when curtains are not available. Examination tables should always be positioned facing away from the door so that patients receiving sensitive examinations (e.g., pelvic or genitourinary), in particular, do not anticipate or fear entry by another person. Use of window coverings that completely obscure the outside is also essential.

Other simple trauma-informed nursing interventions include requesting permission for the exam and for the presence of additional healthcare personnel in the room. Additional personnel in the room should always be identified by role and introduced. The nurse can ask the patient "is there anything we can do to make this encounter/examination more comfortable for you?" This is more difficult in an urgent care or ED but needs to be considered as an accommodation for the patient with a trauma history. Some healthcare settings dedicate rooms specifically for patients with trauma histories, and the ability to respect a person's anxiety can make the physical examination a less disturbing event and prevent re-traumatization. These considerations are particularly important for the patient with a history of sexual assault.

Consideration should also be given to the inclusion of family or friends or associates and whether this will provide support for the patient, create a distraction to care, or prevent disclosure of information. A patient should ideally be alone when asked if the presence of others (family, friends, associates) in the room is desired. Assessing this aspect of care should be done with confidentiality. Adaptation of nursing care in specific medical environments will be discussed next.

## TIC in Primary Care

The primary care setting should be designed to reduce trauma-related triggers and promote healing. The physical space should be set up to provide for privacy, confidentiality, and community (areas for group treatment, support meetings). Whenever possible, space should be allocated to interdisciplinary, extended team members from behavioral health, mental health, social work, pharmacy, and integrative health to ensure consistent, coordinated care.

An important feature of TIC in primary care nursing is building resilience and helping patients find their strengths to promote health and healing through improved self-care and lifestyle changes. The concept of "holistic nursing" appreciates the wholeness of human beings and holds great promise in supporting the TIC approach and helping survivors of trauma heal [24, 25]. The concepts of patient-centered care and "whole health" acknowledge that all people exist in a community, have multiple factors influencing their health, and have control over their own engagement with each factor [26]. These factors—sleep and recovery, energy and flexibility, nourishment and fuel, personal life and work life, relationships, spirit and growth, physical and emotional surroundings, and strengthening and listening to the mind—can be used to help the patient find resources, make choices for health goals, and foster healing and resilience. Nurses play a central role in implementing this personalized, or whole health, approach which was initially developed at Duke University Health System in 1998 [27] and is being widely disseminated nationally, including in VA settings [26]. This holistic approach to care holds great promise for fostering resilience and health among trauma-exposed patients. Collaborating with a patient and enabling that person to set goals for the encounter, and beyond, can help that individual regain a sense of control, achieve a satisfying outcome, and improve the odds of success in future healthcare encounters.

## Preparing for the Visit

In the patient-centered medical home [11], or PACT [12], nurses often take the lead in ensuring that patients have access to care when needed and in preparing for the medical visit. Advance preplanning [28] for scheduled patients is often led by the nurse care manager and should include review of medical records to identify not only needed preventive interventions or testing to monitor chronic disease, but any past experiences that will potentially impact the appointment and can facilitate minimizing re-traumatization. This review includes past primary care visits, consultations, imaging and lab data, recent hospitalization, and even a history of multiple missed or cancelled appointments that would indicate the patient may need additional outreach and assistance to attend the upcoming appointment. Including all care team members in this process prepares staff and allows for input from all; each can contribute different perspectives and experiences with the patient. This process also has potential to support all team members who may have experienced trauma themselves or may be experiencing vicarious traumatization (discussed in prior chapters). The staff can express concerns or empathy within a safe environment and make recommendations that are therapeutic for the patient and facilitative for the encounter. Preplanning also allows for pre-visit collaboration with extended team members, such as behavioral health, who may have had a previous contact with the patient or may be available for a warm hand-off at the end of the visit. Inclusion of behavioral health further allows staff members to share their prior experiences with the patient, or their own trauma, and develop a strategy for working effectively with the patient.

Because trauma can result in a wide range of responses, including feelings of fear, loss of trust in others, decreased sense of personal safety, guilt, and shame [22], patients may avoid contact with medical care and recurrently cancel or miss appointments [7]. These patients may also present frequently on a "walk-in" basis or in crisis, and the nurse is commonly the first staff person to see them. Trauma-exposed individuals can often present as irritable, hostile, or angry; they often seek help in primary care settings, presenting with physical symptoms, rather than going to mental health services, and may not even be aware that their physical complaints are connected to past (or current) traumas [29, 30]. Nurses should be aware of these presentations and always keep in mind that the patient may find even very routine examinations or procedures distressing. In particular, gender-specific examinations (i.e., pelvic and breast exams) and invasive procedures are causes for the patient to feel vulnerable and not in control. As mentioned above, this is especially true for survivors of sexual assault. Advanced planning for visits facilitates trauma-informed nursing care.

## During the Visit

Nursing assessment is the first step in the process. Research suggests that most patients with a trauma history do not object to being asked about these experiences in a primary care visit, but will not typically disclose information unless asked directly in a safe, supportive manner [6, 31]. It may be beneficial to send patients any questionnaires or forms that inquire about sensitive information ahead of the visit to foster feelings of safety and security; conversely some will not feel (or be) safe answering sensitive questions when an abusive partner or family member might be able to see the answers. A trauma-informed holistic nursing approach replaces "what is wrong with you?" with "what happened to you?" and considers "who are you?" [14, 32]. This approach parallels the holistic, or "whole health," process of asking patients, "what really matters to you?" and "what do you need to be healthy for?" [26, 33].

Creating a safe space to talk with the patient may enable discussion of prior trauma; this is done through a validating trauma-informed approach that builds collaboration. Simple introduction of name and role is an important form of collaboration and information-sharing that lets the patient know the reason for inquiries and begins establishing a relationship based on trust. The patient may or may not be ready to share traumatic experiences; the best approach is meeting the person where they are at that moment in time. In a trauma-informed holistic approach, nurses can routinely assess the patient's knowledge, coping skills, emotional status, and readiness for goal setting while eliciting the patient's health history and physical complaints. As important as vital signs are to the diagnosing of illness, identifying the possibility of a patient's past trauma through screening is helpful in fully understanding the patient's current and chronic needs. On the day of the patient's visit to primary care, a care team huddle [34] will serve to identify the need for invasive examinations or other difficult interactions, creating opportunity to avoid re-traumatization. Trauma-informed preparation and precautions, especially around expected physical examinations, can inform room preparation, staff assignment, potential extended team involvement or warm hand-off, and safety needs.

The medical visit is critically important, but potentially difficult for patients with traumatic pasts. Anxiety and fear can interfere with what the patient experiences, hears, and remembers. If the patient shares their story in response to careful and empathic questions, the nurse must respond with validation of the experience, it is that person's experience and is defined by that person. This means being present both mentally and physically which can be challenging in typical high-volume healthcare settings.

In traditional approaches to care, there are often labels and preconceptions assigned to patients (labeling a patient by a diagnosis), for example, a patient who seeks help for anxiety has the identity in a clinic as a person with anxiety symptoms. An appreciation of the whole person is obstructed by the importance of the single diagnosis [35]. In a holistic, trauma-informed approach, the nurse is in a position to emphasize the strengths of the patient in surviving the trauma, rather than dwell on the victimization and isolated diagnoses. This leads to a relationship where the patient is comfortable expressing fears and anxieties, identifying triggers, past coping measures, and expectations. Applying the concepts of patient-centered care and whole health [26] can assist the patient in seeing the various areas where they have strengths and opportunities. Coaching the patient in setting SMART (Specific, Measurable, Achievable, Realistic, and Time-bound) goals [36] will aid in the strengthening of self-compassion and enhanced health behaviors. The primary care nurse is in a position to partner with, and coach, patients over time in reaching health goals, reinforcing their ability to take control of their health and well-being. Trauma survivors need to believe their behavior makes sense and can be brought under their control [35]; for example, applying this paradigm a patient using substances can learn that this is a coping mechanism and not simply "self-defeating" behavior.

## Between Visits

Preparation for care does not end with the visit. A team, or panel, population management meeting [37] is the time to communicate recent disclosures to all staff and ideally includes mental health and behavioral health professionals. It provides the opportunity to learn more about TIC and the impact on medical issues. Ideally, a champion can be selected to become the content expert and share the knowledge with all staff. It is also a chance to share information about community resources and review referrals and the completion of consults by patients. Staff can also share their own experiences with the patient encounter, the impact it had on them and share or solicit helpful strategies or lessons learned. Vicarious traumatization, as discussed in previous chapters, can lead to burnout and lack of empathy for patients [38]. Holding open team discussions in a safe environment among colleagues can serve to identify staff concerns and address them, consistent with the TIC principle of peer support and mutual self-help [14]. Including behavioral health colleagues in these discussions can enhance nursing understanding and preparation for ongoing care management and future visits.

Trauma-exposed patients commonly access primary care clinics [39]. For this reason, it is imperative that care teams recognize symptoms of trauma and provide care with an awareness of the impact that trauma has on chronic disease, chronic pain, and emotional health. Often these patients will avoid important but invasive screening tests like pap smears, mammograms, and colonoscopies due to fear of re-traumatization. Understanding how trauma affects the patient's ability to complete these examinations will give the nurse clues to how they can assist the patient in finding the strength and tools to cope with fear and anxiety. Health coaching [40] is extremely important in this phase of care because patients may experience increased anxiety as the event nears. Nurses can facilitate, or manage, health care and play a critical role in helping patients see the importance of tests/procedures and can provide coaching for follow-through.

The nurse care manager, or population care coordinator (PCC), role is especially critical for patients with trauma histories who may have difficulty navigating systems of care. Research demonstrates that patients, especially those with chronic disease, report feeling more supported and encouraged by their nurse in self-management skills than by their primary care provider (PCP) [41]. By following patient experience across the health system, nurses will learn which extended care members and specialists, have the greatest skill and success with trauma patients. Maintaining contact with the patient to coach continuation with care, foster self-efficacy and provide ongoing support will aid the patient in seeing the benefits of treatment. Each practice, health system and community has a variety of resources available to work with patients to address the trauma and to find new behaviors and coping mechanisms. Serving in a care manager, or PCC, role, the nurse can collaborate with social work to maintain a file of available trauma-relevant resources as reference for the care team.

## Trauma-Informed Care Considerations for Emergency Department/Urgent Care Nursing

While the principles described for trauma-informed primary care nursing apply to all settings, some adaptations are needed for other practice environments. Emergency department (ED) and often urgent care centers (UCC) are anxiety-producing locations at any time for anyone, and implementing TIC is challenging in this setting. For the patient with a trauma history, this is a particularly distressing environment as the sights and sounds of this environment can be disturbing and reminiscent of the trauma. The critical nature and urgency of the physical and emotional needs of persons who present in ED due to medical, surgical, or mental health needs, are often met with a *find it/ fix it* model. Turnover of patients is rapid, and staff are faced with many different presenting complaints and competing demands. This setting often appears chaotic, and it seldom allows for intensive emotional assessment. For this reason, it is an area where nurses can have a positive impact. Recognizing the patient who is exhibiting signs of acute anxiety and assessing the past ED history can have a major effect on the outcome. Before patients can be assessed, they must feel safe and they must trust the caregiver. Past traumatic experiences in the ED will influence the outcome of the current episode unless they are suspected and recognized. Application of the TIC approach will facilitate this and allow the nurse to establish trust and a therapeutic rapport. This discussion will not cover nursing care of patients after acute sexual assault or other trauma, its focus is on adopting a trauma-informed approach toward all patient presentations.

The ED is often the entry point for many people into the healthcare system. It can also be a source for meeting acute needs between primary care visits, a place for immediate relief of pain and suffering. As in primary care, the simple act of introduction of staff names and roles helps to create a sense of trust. Nothing is more disconcerting to the patient than to wonder who is treating them or what is the expertise they bring to the encounter. All staff should have name tags that also identify their roles, since there are often multiple staff members caring for one patient. Transitions of care can be challenging for trauma-exposed patients and when possible, one nurse should be assigned to the patient, to increase the likelihood of providing a safe environment.

Communication between staff will enhance the patient-centered aspects of care. The patient should not have to tell their story multiple times to a variety of people. In a chaotic ED, this may be difficult but a satisfactory outcome will depend on thorough interdisciplinary communication. The nurse can assist the patient in identifying goals for the ED visit and for care following the encounter. Written information, or an after-visit summary, should always be provided and reviewed with the patient prior to discharge.

In the ED, patients arriving in acute, emotional distress will need to be recognized immediately and preferentially should be moved to a quiet and secure environment to lessen the impact of re-traumatization during this episode of care. Often, disruptive patients are seen as an annoyance by ED staff. Research has shown that understanding the role of trauma on the health and neurobiological development of patients can positively influence staff attitudes toward challenging behaviors [42]. Application of TIC in the ED can reduce the use of restraints with patients who arrive with aggressive or dysregulated behavior. Often the patient who is under the influence of substances or brought to the ED by police may not be an appropriate subject for this approach and safety takes precedence.

At the conclusion of the encounter, it is important that the appropriate follow-up referrals to colleagues be made. Ideally warm hand-offs can occur to increase the likelihood of patient follow-through. The ED/UCC nurse can help facilitate the patient's completion of needed referrals by providing phone numbers to make appointments. Communication between the future primary or specialty care teams concerning the visit will provide consistency and apprise the receiving teams of the potential for re-traumatization. It will also ensure that all caregivers are working toward the same goals identified in tandem with the patient.

## Trauma-Informed Care Considerations for Inpatient Care

Non-psychiatric medical and surgical inpatient units can be traumatic environments in and of themselves. There is loss of control over all aspects of care and daily activities. There is little privacy, frequent disturbances, fear of pain and the unknown, multiple handoffs, and reliance on strangers who are suddenly responsible for the patient's comfort and communication [43]. A history of trauma or prior difficult hospitalization adds another element to be considered in care planning and delivery. The nurse is again the lead caregiver and, using the nursing process [8, 9] can assess coping mechanisms, patient expectations, and interventions to respond to unique needs. As in all settings, nurses should always identify themselves and explain their role in the patient's care to build safety and trust. Use of a simple whiteboard in a patient's room enhances patient satisfaction scores, improves nurse communication and involvement in decision making on medical wards [44]. Patients can be asked what would help them feel more comfortable or even safer in the inpatient environment. As the relationship is building, simple conversation can delve into past experience, prior coping mechanisms, and potential for re-traumatization during procedures, therapies, or activities. Although it is not possible to allow the patient to control the entire admission, allowing them to discuss their concerns and contribute to the care plan will help give them a sense of engagement and involvement, leading to a better overall sense of control over the events surrounding them [43].

The care plan should include consistent communication to all shifts and caregivers and will reinforce that the patient may be vulnerable and there have been dysfunctional coping mechanisms identified in the patient's behavior. It is important to identify triggers for the patient. Triggers may be related to any of the senses—touch, smell, hearing, sight, and taste. Each patient is an individual, and their strengths for coping in the variety of settings they will face are different. Helping the patient to identify these triggers will make hospital inpatient encounters less stressful for the patient and the staff.

Because many traumas involve violation of the person's bodily integrity, the care given in the hospital may trigger responses that interfere with care. Early recognition of potential triggers, and implementation of safety measures, will minimize potential trauma reactions and bad outcomes that may result. Common triggering experiences in the inpatient setting include being exposed and touched, lack of privacy and frequent incursions by multiple staff, sharing a room with a stranger, being isolated, being restrained by medical equipment (IVs, oxygen lines/masks, monitors, or surgical equipment such as braces and traction devices), limited mobility, sounds and noises, and caregiver gender. The body area being treated may have been a focus of prior maltreatment. Harris and Fallot [35] shared a now classic example of the challenges faced by a breast cancer patient whose grandfather had fondled her breasts in childhood.

Once it is recognized that there is a potential for dysfunctional coping and the situations that may trigger or escalate the person's emotions have been identified, the next step is to work with the patient to identify ways in which they have adapted in the past or the strategies that may be used to help them manage their strong reactions. It may be as simple as a night light or taking a walk or as complex as calling a mental health provider, psychiatric consult liaison service, or social worker. Implementation of the plan of care should include communication of these identified helpful interventions so that all staff are aware of triggers and of the patient's choice of remedies. Consistency of approach will increase the person's sense of security, safety, and control. Evaluation after each encounter will assess the success of the plan and provide reinforcement or necessary change for it. Again, communication across the entire caregiving team is a requisite step.

At the time of discharge, engaging the patient in discharge planning by making appropriate aftercare referrals and providing resources to the patient to ensure success in self-care will also demonstrate to the patient that they have control over future encounters. Communication back to the primary care nurse and team concerning trauma-informed strategies used during the inpatient stay will continue to reinforce the person's feeling of safety and sense of security within the healthcare system. It will also maintain consistency of approach and goal achievement, important aspects of helping patients learn to manage the long-term effects of trauma.

Not surpisingly, burnout and compassion fatigue are common among nurses and must be acknowledged and addressed when delivering TIC. The next chapter addresses these issues and best practices for caring for the healthcare workforce, including nurses [45, 46].

## Conclusion

Trauma-informed nursing care is important for patients in all healthcare settings. Trauma-exposed patients are commonly seen in primary care for a wide range of issues from chronic disease management to routine health promotion. They are seen in ED and UCC for immediate, acute needs or when they lack access to primary care. They are frequently admitted to the hospital for medical and surgical care. Nurses in all care settings must be educated to be trauma-informed holistic caregivers [24], and serve as advocates for patient autonomy and engagement in care. Throughout the health system, the nurse manages patient flow and is typically the first team member to see and assess the patient in all of these settings. Nurses are well-positioned to be leaders in implementing TIC; core principles of nursing practice parallel those of TIC and both must permeate all of our healthcare encounters. Given the prevalence of trauma, it is essential that TIC becomes part of standard nursing undergraduate education and core competencies [15], much work is still needed to identify best practices especially beyond mental health and pediatric settings.

Nursing is naturally aligned with TIC. Hildegard Peplau [47], a prominent nursing theorist, conceptualized the therapeutic relationship as a dominant concept in nursing care, giving importance to the patient's individual story as a foundation for the nurse-patient relationship. She reinforced the establishment of safety and security for the patient through therapeutic relationship by attending to the patient's needs and not simply to their behaviors and actions. This theory, still relevant today, positions nurses in a leadership role to Assess, Diagnose, Plan, Implement, and Evaluate the patient's needs in any setting. The nurse is the ideal team member to lead efforts to promote application of TIC, plan for care, and ensure the most therapeutic encounter occurs for both patients and colleagues.

## References

1. American Association of Colleges of Nursing. Violence as a public health problem [position statement]. Washington, DC; 1999. Accessed 2 June 2018. Available at http://www.aacnnursing.org/News-Information/Position-Statements-White-Papers/Violence-Problem.
2. Schulman M, Menschner C. Laying the Groundwork for Trauma-Informed Care (Brief). Hamilton, NJ: Center for Health Care Strategies; 2018. Accessed 2 June 2018. Available from: https://www.chcs.org/media/Laying-the-Groundwork-for-TIC_012418.pdf.
3. Felitti VJ, Anda RF, Nordenberg D, Williamson DF, Spitz AM, Edwards V, et al. Relationship of childhood abuse and household dysfunction to many of the leading causes of death in adults. The Adverse Childhood Experiences (ACE) Study. Am J Prev Med. 1998;14(4):245–58.
4. Muskett C. Trauma-informed care in inpatient mental health settings: a review of the literature. Int J Ment Health Nurs. 2014;23(1):51–9.
5. Kassam-Adams N, Rzucidlo S, Campbell M, Good G, Bonifacio E, Slouf K, et al. Nurses' views and current practice of trauma-informed pediatric nursing care. J Pediatr Nurs. 2015;30(3):478–84.

6. Reeves E. A synthesis of the literature on trauma-informed care. Issues Ment Health Nurs. 2015;36(9):698–709.
7. Purkey E, Patel R, Phillips SP. Trauma-informed care: better care for everyone. Can Fam Physician. 2018;64(3):170–2.
8. American Nurses Association (ANA). The nursing process. Accessed 15 December 2018. Available from: https://www.nursingworld.org/practicepolicy/workforce/what-is-nursing/the-nursing-process/.
9. Alfaro-LeFevre R. Applying nursing process: a tool for critical thinking. 6th ed. Philadelphia: Lippincott Williams & Wilkins; 2006.
10. Basile K, Hertz M, Back S. Intimate partner violence and sexual violence victimization assessment instruments for use in healthcare settings: Version 1. Atlanta: Centers for Disease Control and Prevention, National Center for Injury Prevention and Control; 2007. Accessed 3 June 2018. Available from: https://www.cdc.gov/violenceprevention/pdf/ipv/ipvandsvscreening.pdf.
11. Stewart KR, Stewart GL, Lampman M, Wakefield B, Rosenthal G, Solimeo SL. Implications of the patient-centered medical home for nursing practice. J Nurs Adm. 2015;45(11):569–74.
12. Shaw RJ, McDuffie JR, Hendrix CC, Edie A, Lindsey-Davis L, Williams JW Jr. VA evidence-based synthesis program reports. Effects of nurse-managed protocols in the outpatient management of adults with chronic conditions. Washington (DC): Department of Veterans Affairs; 2013.
13. Yano EM, Bair MJ, Carrasquillo O, Krein SL, Rubinstein LV. Patient Aligned Care Teams (PACT): VA's journey to implement patient-centered medical homes. J Gen Intern Med. 2014;29(Suppl 2):547.
14. Substance Abuse and Mental Health Services Administration (SAMHSA). SAMHSA's Concept of Trauma and Guidance for a Trauma-Informed Approach. 2014. Accessed 2 June 2018. Available from: https://store.samhsa.gov/shin/content/SMA14-4884/SMA14-4884.pdf.
15. LoGiudice JA, Douglas S. Incorporation of sexual violence in nursing curricula using trauma-informed care: a case study. J Nurs Educ. 2016;55(4):215–9.
16. Strait J, Bolman T. Consideration of personal adverse childhood experiences during implementation of trauma-informed care curriculum in graduate health programs. Perm J. 2017;
17. Girouard S, Bailey N. ACEs implications for nurses, nursing education, and nursing practice. Acad Pediatr. 2017;17(7S):S16–S7.
18. Ulrich YC, Cain KC, Sugg NK, Rivara FP, Rubanowice DM, Thompson RS. Medical care utilization patterns in women with diagnosed domestic violence. Am J Prev Med. 2003;24(1):9–15.
19. Chartier MJ, Walker JR, Naimark B. Separate and cumulative effects of adverse childhood experiences in predicting adult health and health care utilization. Child Abuse Negl. 2010;34(6):454–64.
20. Freeman Williamson L, Kautz DD. Trauma-informed care is the best clinical practice in rehabilitation nursing. Rehabil Nurs. 2018;43(2):73–80.
21. Raja S, Hasnain M, Hoersch M, Gove-Yin S, Rajagopalan C. Trauma informed care in medicine: current knowledge and future research directions. Fam Community Health. 2015;38(3):216–26.
22. Taylor TF. The influence of shame on posttrauma disorders: have we failed to see the obvious? Eur J Psychotraumatol. 2015;6(1):28847.
23. Currier JM, Stefurak T, Carroll TD, Shatto EH. Applying trauma-informed care to community-based mental health services for military veterans. Best Pract Ment Health. 2017;13:1.
24. Cowling WR 3rd. Where is holistic nursing? J Holist Nurs. 2018;36(1):4–5.
25. Halderman F. Ben's story: a case study in holistic nursing and veteran trauma. Holist Nurs Pract. 2013;27(1):34–6.
26. Krejci LP, Carter K, Gaudet T. Whole health: the vision and implementation of personalized, proactive, patient-driven health care for veterans. Med Care. 2014;52(12 Suppl 5):S5–8.

27. Snyderman R, Dinan MA. Improving health by taking it personally. JAMA. 2010;303(4):363.
28. Sinsky C. Pre-visit planning: American Medical Association; 2014, October. Accessed 15 Dec 2018. Available from: https://edhub.amaassn.org/steps-forward/module/2702514.
29. Gerber MR, Wittenberg E, Ganz ML, Williams CM, McCloskey LA. Intimate partner violence exposure and change in women's physical symptoms over time. J Gen Intern Med. 2008;23(1):64–9.
30. Spertus IL, Yehuda R, Wong CM, Halligan S, Seremetis SV. Childhood emotional abuse and neglect as predictors of psychological and physical symptoms in women presenting to a primary care practice. Child Abuse Negl. 2003;27(11):1247–58.
31. Goldstein E, Athale N, Sciolla AF, Catz SL. Patient preferences for discussing childhood trauma in primary care. Perm J. 2017;21:16–55.
32. Wilson JM, Fauci JE, Goodman LA. Bringing trauma-informed practice to domestic violence programs: a qualitative analysis of current approaches. Am J Orthopsychiatry. 2015;85(6):586–99.
33. Simmons LA, Drake CD, Gaudet TW, Snyderman R. Personalized health planning in primary care settings. Fed Pract. 2016;33(1):27–34.
34. Rodriguez HP, Meredith LS, Hamilton AB, Yano EM, Rubenstein LV. Huddle up!: the adoption and use of structured team communication for VA medical home implementation. Health Care Manag Rev. 2015;40(4):286–99.
35. Harris M, Fallot RD. Envisioning a trauma-informed service system: a vital paradigm shift. New Dir Ment Health Serv. 2001;2001(89):3–22.
36. Stephens J, Allen JK, Dennison Himmelfarb CR. "Smart" coaching to promote physical activity, diet change, and cardiovascular health. J Cardiovasc Nurs. 2011;26(4):282–4.
37. Grant R, Greene D. The health care home model: primary health care meeting public health goals. Am J Public Health. 2012;102(6):1096–103.
38. Crothers D. Vicarious traumatization in the work with survivors of childhood trauma. J Psychosoc Nurs Ment Health Serv. 1995;33(4):9–13.
39. Holman EA, Silver RC, Waitzkin H. Traumatic life events in primary care patients: a study in an ethnically diverse sample. Arch Fam Med. 2000;9(9):802–10.
40. Smolowitz J, Speakman E, Wojnar D, Whelan E, Ulrich S, Hayes C, Wood L. Role of the registered nurse in primary health care: meeting health care needs in the 21st century. Nurs Outlook. 2015;63(2):130–6.
41. Matthias MS, Bair MJ, Nyland KA, Huffman MA, Stubbs DL, Damush TM, et al. Self-management support and communication from nurse care managers compared with primary care physicians: a focus group study of patients with chronic musculoskeletal pain. Pain Manag Nurs. 2010;11(1):26–34.
42. Hall A, McKenna B, Dearie V, Maguire T, Charleston R, Furness T. Educating emergency department nurses about trauma informed care for people presenting with mental health crisis: a pilot study. BMC Nurs. 2016;15:21.
43. Berwick DM. What 'patient-centered' should mean: confessions of an extremist. Health Aff (Millwood). 2009;28(4):w555–65.
44. Singh S, Fletcher KE, John Pandl G, Schapira MM, Nattinger AB, Biblo LA, Whittle J. It's the writing on the wall: Whiteboards improve inpatient satisfaction with provider communication. Am J Med Qual. 2011;26(2):127–31. https://doi.org/10.1177/1062860610376088.
45. Hunt PA, Denieffe S, Gooney M. Burnout and its relationship to empathy in nursing: a review of the literature. J Res Nurs. 2017;22(1–2):7–22.
46. Mazzotta CP. Paying attention to compassion fatigue in emergency nurses. AJN The Am J Nursing. 2015;115(12):13.
47. D'Antonio P, Beeber L, Sills G, Naegle M. The future in the past: Hildegard Peplau and interpersonal relations in nursing. Nurs Inq. 2014;21(4):311–7.

# Part IV
# Helping Providers

# Chapter 11
# Trauma-Informed Care: Helping the Healthcare Team Thrive

Jessica Barnhill, Joslyn W. Fisher, Karen Kimel-Scott, and Amy Weil

## Moving from Vicarious Trauma to Compassion Satisfaction for Healthcare Providers

As discussed in Chapter 1 of this volume, traumatic experiences are common, and those experiences reverberate within individuals and throughout communities. Trauma, when understood as a process rather than a discrete event, is both ever present and ever changing. Therefore, trauma-informed care (TIC) seeks to create a set of universal precautions designed to anticipate, acknowledge, and respond to the effects of trauma on people's lives and, in so doing, mitigate the effects and foster healing.

While trauma is common, it manifests itself differently in different populations and settings. Prior chapters have examined the unique challenges and strengths encountered by specific populations. The first section of this chapter explores the ways in which trauma can adversely affect healthcare professionals. The second section describes methods to understand individual and institutional wellness. The

J. Barnhill
Department of Physical Medicine and Rehabilitation, UNC-Chapel Hill, Chapel Hill, NC, USA

J. W. Fisher
Baylor College of Medicine, Houston, TX, USA

K. Kimel-Scott
University of North Carolina at Chapel Hill, Chapel Hill, NC, USA

A. Weil (✉)
University of North Carolina at Chapel Hill School of Medicine,
Beacon Child and Family Program, Chapel Hill, NC, USA
e-mail: amy_weil@med.unc.edu

third section focuses on strategies for building individual, group, and organizational resilience. By recognizing the interconnectedness between our patients' and our own experience with violence, well-being, and resilience, healthcare professionals and organizations have the opportunity to disrupt this cycle of violence, to promote healing and resilience among healthcare workers, and to reconnect healing professionals to the meaning and purpose that drew them to this work. This in turn will improve the health of those we serve [1].

## The Impact of Trauma in the Healthcare Workforce

The healthcare workforce is not immune to the personal experience of trauma. In fact, healthcare workers are more likely than the population at large to have experienced personal trauma [2]. When compared to their cohorts in other industries, they are also more likely to experience workplace violence [3–5]. A third, and perhaps most insidious, experience occurs when healthcare professionals develop vicarious, or secondary, traumatization through exposure to their patients' stories of violence and trauma [5].

## Personal Experience of Violence

Many persons drawn to the helping professions have overcome adversity in their own lives. For example, [6] report that 68% of the healthcare workforce have experienced at least one episode of violence, abuse, or neglect. These personal exposures can become a professional asset, as providers can empathize with patients; however, these exposures can also be a source of vulnerability. While attending to the effects of trauma on patients' lives can be deeply meaningful and inspirational, it can also open deep personal wounds and negatively affect sense of self [5]. Whether or not healthcare workers consciously identify the role that personal trauma plays in their own work, the collective experience of personal trauma exerts itself on the healthcare team. Maunder states:

> A personal history of violence, abuse or neglect is common in healthcare workers. The well-being of healthcare workers is critical to the effectiveness of an over-taxed healthcare system. Although healthcare workers may be resilient as a group, the cumulative impact of stress on abused healthcare workers is substantial. Attitudes of shame and blame have historically led to a silencing of the victims of abuse and have stifled constructive social responses to the problem. An open discussion within the field of healthcare is required which acknowledges the strengths and vulnerabilities that accompany extraordinary personal adversity, and which supports healthcare workers in their efforts to establish and maintain a working environment that is safe, supportive and flexible and facilitates the best possible patient care [6].

In sum, healthcare providers' experiences of violence can both impact patient-provider relationships and patient-healthcare team interactions.

## Workplace Violence

Workplace violence is a sometimes underrecognized form of trauma experienced in the healthcare setting. According to the International Labor Organization (ILO), [7] workplace violence is *"any action, incident, or behavior that departs from reasonable conduct in which a person is assaulted, threatened, harmed, injured in the course of, or as a direct result of, his or her work"*. The Centers for Disease Control and Prevention (CDC) National Institute for Occupational Safety and Health (NIOSH) categorizes workplace violence into four domains [8].

1. Violent acts by criminals who have no other connection with the workplace.
2. Violence directed at employees by customers, clients, patients, students, or any others for whom an organization provides services.
3. Violence against coworkers, supervisors, or managers by a present or former employee.
4. Violence committed in the workplace by someone who does not work there but has a personal relationship with an employee.

The prevalence of workplace violence in the primary care setting is not well categorized and is likely underreported [4]. However, it is well established that healthcare workers experience higher rates of workplace violence than other industries [9, 10]. Nurses, by means of their increased contact with patients, experience some of the highest rates of workplace violence. For example, in the Minnesota Nurses' Study, annual rates of physical violence were 13.2%, and annual rates of verbal abuse were 38.8% [11]. Workplace violence is most commonly perpetrated by patients, current or former employees, someone with a relationship with an employee, and least often someone not connected with the healthcare setting [10]. Attention to the personal dynamics present in the work environment can help mediate destructive and abusive behaviors that undermine the mission of an organization and contribute to loss of wellness for individuals and organizations.

## Secondary or Vicarious Trauma and the Possibility of Posttraumatic Growth

Many terms have been proposed to describe the emotional and psychological effects of working with trauma survivors [12]. What follows are a few examples of how this phenomenon is conceptualized. Secondary exposure to trauma (or vicarious trauma) refers to the indirect experience of trauma as retold by another person. This secondary exposure can lead to secondary traumatic stress as well as secondary posttraumatic growth [13]. As discussed at the beginning of this book, people respond to traumatic events in varying ways, and not all traumatic events lead to the development of posttraumatic stress disorder (PTSD). Similarly, the manner in which healthcare workers receive and respond to vicarious trauma predicts whether they develop secondary traumatic stress or secondary posttraumatic growth. Among healthcare workers, as with the population at large, self-efficacy in the face of traumatic events predicts self-growth [14]. Secondary trauma self-efficacy refers to *the perceived ability to cope with the challenging demands resulting from work with traumatized clients and the perceived ability to deal with the secondary traumatic stress symptoms* [15]. Individual characteristics (both innate and learned) as well as organizational structures can promote health professionals' self-efficacy.

## Compassion Fatigue and the Possibility of Compassion Satisfaction

A similar construct to secondary trauma leading to posttraumatic stress disorder or posttraumatic growth exists between compassion fatigue and compassion satisfaction. Compassion fatigue has varying definitions within the medical literature. In essence, compassion fatigue is the inability to feel compassion and empathy toward patients. It is hypothesized to result from a combination of burnout and secondary traumatic stress [15]. While an understandable reaction of a depleted self in the setting of human suffering, compassion fatigue robs healthcare providers of the satisfaction gained by meaningful connections with patients. In contrast, compassion satisfaction describes the personal and professional rewards derived from providing compassionate care to others. Compassion satisfaction is negatively correlated with burnout, suggesting that it may exert a protective effect [16].

### *Chronic Work Stress and Burnout*

Burnout is a well-recognized syndrome characterized by emotional exhaustion, depersonalization, a feeling of reduced personal accomplishment, loss of work fulfillment, and reduced effectiveness. Manifestations of depersonalization include negativity, cynicism, and inability to express empathy or grief. Clinicians with burnout struggle to perform clinical duties, much less provide empathic trauma-informed care. In addition to poor work performance, according to a recent meta-analysis, they suffer physical and psychological sequelae, similar to others with toxic stress exposures [17]. Many factors may be contributing currently to create a "perfect storm," leading to burnout. One mechanism posits that loss of self-efficacy, fatigue, and depersonalization affect the ability of healthcare providers to derive meaning from their work. As provider well-being declines, quality of care suffers and providers are more prone to make errors. Providers also become more vulnerable to vicarious trauma (aka secondary traumatic stress described above). Personal factors, which can also lead to excellent care provision, such as the inherent perfectionism of those drawn to become providers, may also make clinicians more susceptible. When coupled with increasing demands from our healthcare systems such as administrative pressures associated with use of electronic health records (EHR), the push for greater productivity and efficiencies coupled with rising patient dissatisfaction, and the pressure to balance home demands, one can see how a spiral of burnout occurs. Now that this syndrome is recognized as a problem affecting over half the physicians in the US and similar numbers of other healthcare providers, new attention is being paid to solutions [18]. Providers particularly at risk include female physicians, younger providers (less than age 55), and those with children younger than 21 [19]. So far, no studies have been done to determine the influence of race and ethnicity on reported burnout [20]. On a national level, the National Academy of Medicine has identified a goal of addressing burnout, or the well-being of clinicians, as a "Fourth Aim" (along with the original "Triple Aim": improving health of the population, improving patient experience, and reducing cost) [21].

Hence, healthcare professionals' experiences of personal trauma, workplace violence, and/or vicarious trauma can contribute to compassion fatigue, burnout, and depression which in turn can adversely impact patient care. However, alternatively, individual, group, and organizational strategies such as those described below can foster posttraumatic growth and promote achievement of the "fourth aim" in the pursuit of high-quality, high-value care of our patients and our communities.

These strategies include measuring individual and organizational wellness, building resilient providers and teams, and making the system that they work in supportive [20] (Tables 11.1, 11.4 and Fig. 11.1). Together these efforts can reverse the downward spiral of burnout and compassion fatigue and instead bolster resilience, healing, compassion satisfaction, and ultimately improved patient care.

## Assessing Wellness: Individual and Organizational

In order to provide optimal trauma-informed care, it is important for healthcare professionals to assess their own well-being and to incorporate evidence-based strategies into their routine practice to strengthen their personal resilience. Assessing organizational culture is also key to successful delivery of trauma-informed care as institutional "wellness" supports the well-being of its providers.

To address the state of wellness within individuals and within organizations, it can be helpful to quantify the extent of the problem and the degree to which interventions are improving wellness. To this end, the Research, Data and Metrics Working Group of the National Academy of Medicine's Action Collaborative on Clinician Well-Being and Resilience maintains a list of validated instruments that can be used to measure wellness. Divided into three broad categories, these instruments measure burnout, composite well-being, depression, and suicide risk. The characteristics of each tool, including purpose, format, cost, and validation, are available at the National Academy of Medicine's website. See Fig. 11.1 for examples of validated tools [23].

**Table 11.1** Causes of and solutions for burnout [20]

| Cause | Organization-level solutions | Individual-level solutions |
|---|---|---|
| Excessive workload | Fair productivity targets<br>Duty hour limits<br>Appropriate distribution of job roles | Negotiated expectations<br>Part-time status<br>Informed specialty choices<br>Informed practice choices |
| Work inefficiency and lack of work support | Optimized electronic medical records<br>Non-physician staff support to offload clerical burdens<br>Appropriate interpretation of regulatory requirements | Efficiency and skills training<br>Prioritize tasks and delegate work appropriately |
| Lack of work–home integration | Respect for home responsibilities in setting schedules for work and meetings<br>Include all required work tasks within expected work hours<br>Support flexible work schedules, including part-time employment | Reflection on and active management of life priorities and values<br>Attention to self-care |
| Loss of control and autonomy | Physician engagement in establishing work requirements and structure<br>Physician leadership and shared decision-making | Stress management and resiliency training<br>Positive coping strategies<br>Mindfulness |
| Loss of meaning from work | Promote shared core values<br>Protect physician time with patients<br>Promote physician communities<br>Offer professional development opportunities<br>Leadership training and awareness around physician burnout | Positive psychology<br>Reflection/self-awareness of most fulfilling work roles<br>Mindfulness<br>Engagement in physician small-group activities around shared work experiences |

Burnout
- Maslach Burnout Inventory
- Oldenburg Inventory
- Physician Work-life Study's Single-Item
- Copenhagen Burnout Inventory

Composite well-being
- Stanford Professional Fulfillment Index
- Well-being Index

Depression and Suicide Risk
- Patient Health Questionnaire-9 (PHQ-9)

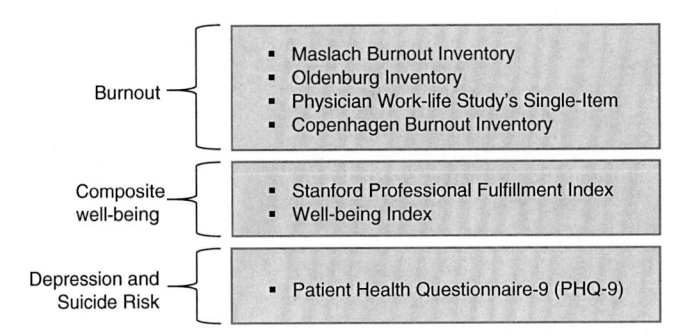

**Fig. 11.1** Validated tools to assess wellness. (Adapted from the Research, Data and Metrics Working Group of the National Academy of Medicine's Action Collaborative on Clinician Well-Being and Resilience. Additional information about each tool, including purpose, format, cost, and validation, are available at https://nam.edu/valid-reliable-survey-instruments-measure-burnout-well-work-related-dimensions. Accessed 7/5/18)

Once a better understanding of specific stressors is established, institutions will be able to craft solutions, creating supports such as scribes, modifying schedules and workload intensity, enhancing job control, increasing the level of participation in decision-making, and fostering a sense of community and teamwork [24, 25]. Interventions that combine several elements such as structural change, fostering communication, cultivating teamwork, and job control have had the most success [26]. Organizations such as the Institute for Healthcare Improvement (IHI) support the development of healthier, safer, and more efficient healthcare environments [27].

## From Trauma-Informed Care to Healing-Centered Engagement: Evidence-Based Solutions to Promote Well-Being

As has been described in prior chapters, there is significant evidence regarding the physical and psychological effects of trauma and stress on the body. These effects are mediated by nervous, endocrine, and immune pathways and can even be inherited epigenetically. The great promise of trauma-informed care (TIC) is threefold in that it (1) provides an understanding of mechanisms that can lead to development of solutions, (2) suggests strategies for undoing the toxic pathways for providers and patients, and (3) enables a way forward to heal and keep providers feeling well so that they can tap into other modalities to continue to be engaged and joyous in their work, in turn contributing to our patients' greater well-being.

The three pillars of trauma-informed care include the teaching of self-management and coping skills, the promotion of healing relationships, and the development of safety [28]. What follows will be a brief review of how these strategies work and a variety of examples of these techniques that can be adapted according to available time. A more extensive resource list, or toolkit, is included for additional study (Table 11.4).

### *What Are the Physiologic Mechanisms Underlying Trauma?*

It is well known that stress and trauma can lead to an overactivation of the hypothalamic-pituitary adrenal (HPA) axis resulting in a "fight or flight" response. While useful as we evolved to activate us to flee from mortal danger, chronic elevation of this system in response to stress has negative health effects over time. One mechanism is thought to be sustained elevation of cortisol, which disrupts other feedback loops in the nervous system. Persistently elevated cortisol at the cellular level can lead to shortened telomeres and early cell death. Remarkably, the perception of being under stress is as important as any objective measure of stress for the health effects it has. This was shown in a study in which caregivers of seriously ill family members, who were more distressed, died earlier independent of the health of the ill family member [29].

As the HPA axis is also involved in cognitive and emotional balance, autonomic dysregulation can lead to myriad difficulties, including with learning, memory, and mood. As was postulated in the adverse childhood experiences (ACEs) study, chronic exposure to stress can also cause people to develop maladaptive coping mechanisms that can lead to poor mental and physical health via increased use of substances such as tobacco, alcohol, drugs, food, and other self-soothing risky behaviors [30].

## What Is Mindfulness and How Are the Mechanisms of Mindfulness Uniquely Suited to Combat the Effects of Trauma?

Mindful practices have historic roots in Buddhist meditation practices from over 2500 years ago and are aimed at spiritual and intellectual development by strengthening concentration. The four prongs of mindfulness according to Jon Kabat Zinn [31] include (Fig. 11.2):

1. Paying attention – focusing one's attention.
2. On purpose – intentionally.
3. In the present moment – not thinking of the past or the future.
4. Non-judgmentally – calmly acknowledging and accepting one's feelings, thoughts, and bodily sensations.

It turns out that these actions activate the parasympathetic nervous system which helps cortisol return to baseline levels, thus offering hope of rebalancing the HPA axis which has been disrupted from acute and chronic stressors. Brain research has shown that mindfulness causes changes throughout the brain in multiple areas (see Table 11.2).

These changes are associated with increased well-being, reduced cognitive reactivity, enhanced immune function, decreased autonomic sensitivity, increased telomerase activity, and increased levels of melatonin and serotonin. Mindful practice has been shown to help with a number of medical conditions including irritable bowel, chronic fatigue, hot flashes, insomnia, and stress-related hyperphagia, and it diminishes craving in substance abuse [33].

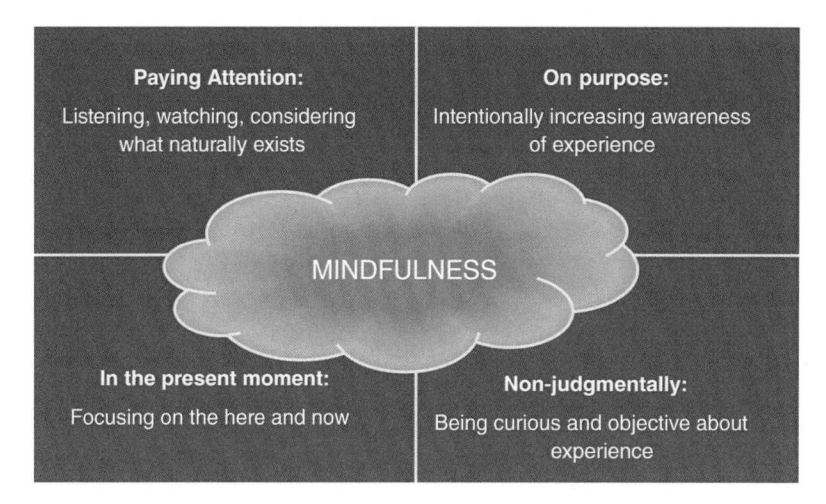

**Fig. 11.2** Four prongs of mindfulness

**Table 11.2** Brain changes associated with mindful practice [32]

| Effect of mindful practice | Regions of brain affected |
|---|---|
| Attention regulation | Cingulate cortex |
| Body awareness | Insula, temporoparietal junction |
| Emotional regulation | Modulation of the amygdala by the lateral prefrontal cortex |
| Cognitive reevaluation | Activation of the dorsal medial prefrontal cortex, hippocampus, amygdala |
| Flexible self-concept | Prefrontal medial cortex, posterior cingulated cortex, insula, temporoparietal junction |

Tang and Hölzel [44]

For providers, mindfulness practice has been shown to reduce psychologic distress and improve well-being and also to reduce burnout and improve psychosocial orientation and empathy. Mindfulness has even been shown to enhance executive function when dealing with moral quandaries. Several meta-analyses have borne out the studies noting increased well-being/decreased stress for health providers who pursue meditative practices [20, 34]. In addition, Epstein noted that mindfulness practice enhanced care provided to patients by enabling physicians to listen attentively to patients' distress, recognize their own errors, refine their technical skills, make evidence-based decisions, and clarify their values so they could act with compassion, technical competence, presence, and insight [35]. An additional study by Beach and colleagues found that patients reported that providers who practiced mindfulness were more patient-centered in their communication skills [36]. Also, a longitudinal training program in mindful communication increased empathy and decreased burnout in primary care physicians [37].

## Individual Strategies to Cultivate Resilience

While no single intervention will work for every provider, a commitment to personal well-being is key. From there can stem many different practices that reconnect people with meaning and purpose in their work as individuals and groups. Well-being and connection with meaning can lead to gratitude and job satisfaction as well as the energy to forge organizational changes [38]. Some examples of individual interventions in the realms of mindfulness, positive psychology, and group support are described in greater detail in this chapter, and we provide a list of other recommended wellness resources below.

## Mindful Practices

A large number of healing practices originate from this understanding of the physiology of mindfulness. A partial list includes:

- Mantra meditation.
- Mindfulness-based stress reduction.
- Mind–body medicine skills.
- Mindful self-compassion.
- Yoga.
- Tai chi.
- Qi gong.

It is also worth noting that any number of practices can be done mindfully including being in nature (so-called forest bathing) [39], playing music, creating art, doing daily chores, and eating. Quite a number of therapies have mindful roots including mindfulness-based cognitive therapy (CBT), acceptance and commitment therapy (ACT), dialectical behavioral therapy (DBT), internal family systems (IFS), mode deactivation therapy, Morita therapy, and others. Detailed exploration of these techniques is beyond the scope of this chapter.

## *So How Can We Harness the Positive Effects of Mindfulness to Help Providers Maintain or Build Their Resilience?*

**Meaning Practices**

Routinely engaging in mindfulness becomes easier over time and cultivates qualities of awe, gratitude, compassion, and equanimity [40]. Mindfulness practices enhance the appreciation of the moment and can lead to an "upward spiral" of positive emotions [41–43].

Similarly, gratitude practices such as remembering three good things that happened on a given day can also foster positive emotions that can improve well-being and build resilience [44]. Research shows that journaling and reflection foster well-being in the general population [45]. A technique called appreciative inquiry, where the focus is on looking at the positive and what worked, rather than what failed, can cultivate more positivity, build resilience, and lead to repeated success. This is similar to Fredrickson's description of the effect of positive emotions [41]. When providers are feeling strong and resilient, they are more able to engage with others in their work and home lives and are more likely to be prepared to care for others safely and effectively (Table 11.3).

**The Power of Group Practice for Resilience**

Having the opportunity to perform meaning practices in the workplace and/or in professional training groups can help providers to cultivate resilience even as they explore and process difficult experiences. Some examples of this practice include Healer's Art (designed for medical students) [46], Passing the Torch [47], and Finding Meaning in Medicine [48] for providers, as well as larger groups such as Schwartz Rounds [49].

## Future Directions: Organizational Strategies

Redesign of the healthcare system is well beyond the scope of this book, its readers, and many of the institutions within which healthcare is delivered. Nonetheless, resilient individuals and groups are best equipped to create healthier work environments within their organizations. Some suggestions to create a more trauma-informed physical environment include walls painted with soft colors, tranquil music or periodic chime as a mindfulness reminder, and welcoming language in all

**Table 11.3** Sample activities to integrate wellness into a busy day

| Time for wellness | Activity |
|---|---|
| **When you have no time** | *****Be present in this moment** |
| **When you have seconds** | *****Take a deep breath. Hold it. Exhale slowly.**<br>*****Smile**<br>*****Feel your feet on the floor.**<br>*(Feel the weight of your body on your feet, feel where your feet rub against your shoes, notice what it feels like to be in your body in this moment)*<br>*****Pause before entering the next exam room. Breathe.**<br>*****Recite a mantra**<br>*(A word that reconnects you to the meaning and purpose of your work, a word that brings you peace of mind or joy, for example, "peace", or "mind", or "joy")*<br>*****Laugh at something funny.**<br>*(Plan ahead and post something funny in a place where you are likely to see it. Depending on your sense of humor, you could post it where other people are likely to see it, too)*<br>*****Greet a coworker. Smile at them.**<br>*****When a coworker greets you and smiles at you, smile back.**<br>*****Stretch to the sky. Touch the floor.** |
| **When you have minutes, take a moment to settle your mind and then…** | *****Try a rooted tree meditation.**<br>*You can search the Internet to find guided meditations on this theme (or see resources below). Find one that you like and practice using it. Once you are familiar with the imagery, you can guide yourself. These meditations often include the following sequence: find your feet, notice what it feels like to be in your body, imagine roots growing from your feet and anchoring you to the floor, then the subfloor, extending down through the building that currently supports you, until you reach the soil. Sink into the earth. Notice what it feels like to be in the ground; when you are ready gently turn your attention back to the room, to the sights and the sounds of this moment.*<br>*****Name three things that bring you joy or for which you are grateful.**<br>*Imagine that these things are each carefully wrapped presents and slowly open them; notice how you feel as you receive each gift.*<br>*****Explore expressive writing.**<br>*Find a pen and paper. Write down what you are feeling in this moment without concern for punctuation or spelling or words for that matter. Try not to edit yourself. Look at what you have created, and then take advantage of the document shredder.*<br>*****Strike a pose.**<br>*Practice a few yoga stretches. For starters, you can google "chair yoga"* |
| **When you have hours and days…** | *****Take a class or a workshop.**<br>There are suggestions in the toolkit.<br>*****Immerse yourself in nature.**<br>*****Spend time with people who bring you joy, in places that make you happy.** |
| **Over weeks and months…** | *****Take advantage of the many wellness resources available to you.**<br>*Stay curious and reward yourself for trying new things. Also pay attention to what works for YOU, and keep doing THAT. There are many paths to wellness.*<br>*****Treat yourself with kindness.**<br>It takes time to build healthy routines, and life is full of interruptions. |

**Table 11.4** A toolkit for fostering resilience in patients and ourselves[a]

| | |
|---|---|
| Books | *Cope, Stephen. *Yoga and the Quest for the True Self*<br>*Epstein, Ronald. *Attending: Medicine, Mindfulness, and Humanity* (2017)<br>Hanh, TN. *The Miracle of Mindfulness: An Introduction to the Practice of Meditation*<br>*Kabat-Zinn, Jon. *Wherever You Go, There You Are: Mindfulness Meditation in Everyday Life*<br>*Remen, Rachel Naomi. *Kitchen Table Wisdom & My Grandfather's Blessings*<br>*Schiffman, Eric. *The Art of Moving into Stillness*<br>*Sood, Amit. *Train Your Brain…Engage Your Heart…Transform Your Life* |
| Websites | *American Psychological Association:<br>http://www.apa.org/helpcenter/road-resilience.aspx<br>*Fostering Resilience in Children:<br>http://www.fosteringresilience.com/7cs_professionals.php<br>*Project Resilience: http://www.projectresilience.com<br>*At my best: http://atmybest.com/<br>*My 31 practices: https://www.my31practices.com/have_a_go/<br>*Office of Patient-centered Care and, Cultural Transformation, Veterans Health Administration:<br>https://www.va.gov/PATIENTCENTEREDCARE/resources/Mobile_Apps_and_Online_Tools.asp<br>*Whole Health Library:<br>http://projects.hsl.wisc.edu/SERVICE/curriculum/index.html<br>*ACP Physician Burnout and Wellness Information and Resources:<br>https://www.acponline.org/about-acp/chapters-regions/united-states/new-mexico-chapter/physician-burnout-and-wellness-information-and-resources<br>*ACGME: http://www.acgme.org/What-We-Do/Initiatives/Physician-Well-Being/Resources<br>*Substance Abuse and Mental Health Services Administration:<br>SAMHSA's Concept of Trauma and Guidance for a Trauma-Informed Approach. HHS Publication No. (SMA) 14-4884. Rockville, MD: Substance Abuse and Mental Health Services Administration, 2014.<br>https://www.samhsa.gov/nctic/trauma-interventions |
| Apps | *Mindfulness Apps: (Number indicates rating by Journal of Medical Internet Research [22]<br>Headspace (Overall Rating 4.0)<br>Smiling Mind (Overall Rating 3.7)<br>iMindfulness (Overall Rating 3.5)<br>Mindfulness Daily (Overall Rating 3.5)<br>Gratitude 365 (gratitude journaling)<br>Guided Mind (has some guided imagery – some in app purchases)<br>*Exercise/Yoga:<br>Seven-minute workout (iphone or android)<br>DDP Yoga Now<br>Office Yoga (or Lite – Free variety) |

(continued)

**Table 11.4** (continued)

| Training | Healer's Art (Naomi Rachel Remen, MD): |
|---|---|
| | http://www.ishiprograms.org/programs/medical-educators-students/ |
| | The Center for Mind Body Medicine: |
| | https://cmbm.org/trainings/mind-body-medicine/ |
| | The Institute for Integrative Health: |
| | https://tiih.org/what-we-do/ |
| | Center for Mindfulness in Medicine, Health Care and Society: |
| | https://www.umassmed.edu/cfm/ |
| | Kripalu: https://kripalu.org/ |
| | Hakomi Institute |
| | See http://www.hakomicalifornia.org/index.shtml. . |
| | Somatic Experiencing® |
| | See http://www.traumahealing.com/somatic-experiencing/ |
| | The Sensorimotor Psychotherapy Institute (SPI) |
| | See http://www.sensorimotorpsychotherapy.org/about.html. |
| **Reflective writing outlets** | *Academic Medicine: Teaching & Learning Moment* |
| | *Annals of Internal Medicine – On Doctoring* |
| | *Bellevue Literary Review* |
| | *Intima: A Journal of Narrative Medicine* |
| | *Journal of Medicine Humanities* |
| | *Literature and Medicine* |
| | *Medical Humanities* |
| | *Survive & Thrive: A Journal for Medical Humanities and Narrative as Medicine* |
| | *The Healing Muse* |
| | *Yale Journal for Humanities in Medicine* |

[a]This toolkit provides examples of available resources and is not meant to be exhaustive

signage. In addition, having values alignment at the organizational level around the alleviation of suffering and cultivation of compassion and humanism are central as exemplified by ongoing training of all clinical and non-clinical personnel in the administration of trauma-informed care, facilitating easy non-stigmatizing access to employee assistance programs, and engaging patients as well as community resources in practice design [50, 51].

## Conclusion

In summary, healthcare staff are more likely than the general population to have experienced both personal and workplace trauma. Workplace violence includes physical and emotional violence inflicted by clients and colleagues. Burnout is common across healthcare roles and manifests itself as exhaustion, depersonalization, and loss of self-efficacy. Burnout also makes employees more vulnerable to secondary traumatic stress and compassion fatigue, rather than satisfaction, and less capable of providing quality care.

As we look to the future, trauma-informed organizations may help build resilience by proactively supporting the health of their employees. Ideally, they will maintain a sense of readiness to recognize the impact of trauma on the lives of their staff and the clients/patients they serve. Healthcare professionals can work collaboratively with organizations to create environments that are physically and emotionally safe, recognize when interventions are needed, adapt to the needs and strengths of their workforce, and provide opportunities for individuals to build their resilience.

We have discussed how resilience can be learned and cultivated. Secondary exposure to trauma can result in secondary traumatic stress or secondary posttraumatic growth, compassion fatigue, or compassion satisfaction. Self-care, including practicing mindfulness, can increase resilience. Resilience practiced individually and in groups, in turn, helps preserve self-efficacy and social support that is crucial to finding meaning and purpose at work. Practicing mindfulness and other self-care strategies that resonate with the individual also equips healthcare providers to teach these skills to colleagues and patients. As a widened circle of resilient healthcare providers grows within a positive, trauma-informed, healing-centered work environment, the health of individuals and populations will significantly benefit [52].

## References

1. Dewa CS, Loong D, Bonato S, Trojanowski L. The relationship between physician burnout and quality of healthcare in terms of safety and acceptability: a systematic review. BMJ Open. 2017;7(6):e015141.
2. Lanctôt N, Guay S. The aftermath of workplace violence among healthcare workers: a systematic literature review of the consequences. Aggress Violent Behav. 2014;19(5):492–501.
3. Hogh A, Hoel H, Carneiro IG. Bullying and employee turnover among healthcare workers: a three-wave prospective study. J Nurs Manag. 2011;19(6):742–51.
4. Phillips JP. Workplace violence against health care workers in the United States. Longo DL, editor. N Engl J Med. 2016;374(17):1661–9.
5. Ellis C, Knight KE. Advancing a Model of Secondary Trauma: Consequences for Victim Service Providers. J Interpers Violence. 2018:088626051877516.
6. Maunder RG, Peladeau N, Savage D, Lancee WJ. The prevalence of childhood adversity among healthcare workers and its relationship to adult life events, distress and impairment. Child Abuse Negl. 2010;34(2):114–23.
7. International Labor Organization. Code of practice on workplace violence in services sectors and measures to combat this phenomenon. Geneva 2003.
8. Centers for Disease Control and Prevention/National Institute for Occupational Safety and Health (NIOSH). Workplace violence prevention strategies and research needs. Report from the Conference, Partnering in Workplace Violence Prevention: Translating Research to Practice. November 17-19, 2004, Baltimore, MD; 2006, September. Contract No.: DHHS (NIOSH) Publication No. 2006–144.
9. Edward K, Ousey K, Warelow P, Lui S. Nursing and aggression in the workplace: a systematic review. Br J Nurs. 2014;23(12):653–9.
10. US Department of Labor, Occupational Safety and Health Administration. Caring for our caregivers caring for our caregivers workplace violence in healthcare. Accessed 23 May 2018. Available from: https://www.osha.gov/Publications/OSHA3826.pdf.

11. Gerberich SG, Church TR, McGovern PM, Hansen HE, Nachreiner NM, Geisser MS, et al. An epidemiological study of the magnitude and consequences of work related violence: the Minnesota Nurses' Study. Occup Environ Med. 2004;61(6):495–503.
12. Newell JM, Nelson-Gardell D, MacNeil G. Clinician responses to client traumas. Trauma Violence Abus. 2016;17(3):306–13.
13. Shoji K, Bock J, Cieslak R, Zukowska K, Luszczynska A, Benight CC. Cultivating secondary traumatic growth among healthcare workers: the role of social support and self-efficacy. J Clin Psychol. 2014;70(9):831–46.
14. Cieslak R, Benight CC, Rogala A, Smoktunowicz E, Kowalska M, Zukowska K, et al. Effects of internet-based self-efficacy intervention on secondary traumatic stress and secondary post-traumatic growth among health and human services professionals exposed to indirect trauma. Front Psychol. 2016;7:1009.
15. Smart D, English A, James J, Wilson M, Daratha KB, Childers B, et al. Compassion fatigue and satisfaction: a cross-sectional survey among US healthcare workers. Nurs Health Sci. 2014;16(1):3–10.
16. Adimando A. Preventing and alleviating compassion fatigue through self-care: an educational workshop for nurses. J Holist Nurs. 2017;089801011772158.
17. Salvagioni DAJ, Melanda FN, Mesas AE, González AD, Gabani FL, de Andrade SM. Physical, psychological and occupational consequences of job burnout: a systematic review of prospective studies. van Wouwe JP, editor. PLoS One. 2017 Oct 4;12(10):e0185781.
18. Dzau VJ, Kirch DG, Nasca TJ. To care is human — collectively confronting the clinician-burnout crisis. N Engl J Med. 2018;378(4):312–4.
19. Dyrbye LN, Shanafelt TD, Sinsky CA, Cipriano PF, Bhatt J, Ommaya A, et al. Burnout among health care professionals: a call to explore and address this underrecognized threat to safe, high-quality care. Washington, DC: National Academy of Medicine; 2017.
20. West CP, Dyrbye LN, Erwin PJ, Shanafelt TD. Interventions to prevent and reduce physician burnout: a systematic review and meta-analysis. Lancet. 2016;388(10057):2272–81.
21. Wright AA, Katz IT. Beyond burnout — redesigning care to restore meaning and sanity for physicians. N Engl J Med. 2018;378(4):309–11.
22. Mani M, Kavanagh DJ, Hides L, Stoyanov SR. Review and evaluation of mindfulness-based iPhone apps. JMIR Mhealth Uhealth. 2015;3(3):e82.
23. National Academy of Medicine. Validated instruments to assess work-related dimensions of wellbeing 2018. Accessed 6 July 2018. Available from: https://nam.edu/valid-reliable-survey-instruments-measure-burnout-well-work-related-dimensions/
24. Sinsky CA, Willard-Grace R, Schutzbank AM, Sinsky TA, Margolius D, Bodenheimer T. In search of joy in practice: a report of 23 high-functioning primary care practices. Ann Fam Med. 2013;11(3):272–8.
25. Epstein RM, Privitera MR. Doing something about physician burnout. Lancet. 2016;388(10057):2216–7.
26. Linzer M, Poplau S, Grossman E, Varkey A, Yale S, Williams E, et al. A cluster randomized trial of interventions to improve work conditions and clinician burnout in primary care: results from the Healthy Work Place (HWP) Study. J Gen Intern Med. 2015;30(8):1105–11.
27. Perlo J, Balik B, Swenson S, Kabcenell A, Landsman J, Feeley D. IHI framework for improving joy in work. IHI White Paper. Cambridge, MA, 2017. Accessed 6 July 2018. Available from: http://www.ihi.org/resources/Pages/IHIWhitePapers/Framework-Improving-Joy-in-Work.aspx
28. National Educational Service (U.S.). Reclaiming children and youth : journal of emotional and behavioral problems. [Internet]. National Educational Service; Accessed 6 July 2018. Available from: http://vb3lk7eb4t.scholar.serialssolutions.com/?sid=google&auinit=H&aulast=Bath&atitle=The+three+pillars+of+trauma-informed+care&title=Reclaiming+children+and+youth&volume=17&issue=3&date=2008&spage=17&issn=1089-5701.
29. Schulz R, Beach SR. Caregiving as a risk factor for mortality. JAMA. 1999;282(23):2215.
30. Adverse Childhood Experiences (ACEs) [Internet]. Accessed 6 July 2018. Available from: https://www.cdc.gov/violenceprevention/acestudy/index.html.

31. Kabat ZJ. Coming to our senses: healing ourselves and the world through mindfulness. New York: Hyperion; 2005.
32. Tang YY, Hölzel BK, Posner MI. The neuroscience of mindfulness meditation. Nat Rev Neurosci. 2015;16(4):213–25.
33. Hempel S, Taylor SL, Marshall NJ, Miake-Lye IM, Beroes JM, Shanman R, et al. Evidence Map of Mindfulness [Internet]. Department of Veterans Affairs (US); 2014. Accessed 6 July 2018. Available from: http://www.ncbi.nlm.nih.gov/pubmed/25577939.
34. Goyal M, Singh S, Sibinga EMS, Gould NF, Rowland-Seymour A, Sharma R, et al. Meditation programs for psychological stress and well-being. JAMA Intern Med. 2014;174(3):357.
35. Epstein RM. Mindful practice. JAMA. 1999;282(9):833–9.
36. Beach MC, Roter D, Korthuis PT, Epstein RM, Sharp V, Ratanawongsa N, et al. A multicenter study of physician mindfulness and health care quality. Ann Fam Med. 2013;11:421.
37. Krasner MS. Association of an educational program in mindful communication with burnout, empathy, and attitudes among primary care physicians. JAMA. 2009;302(12):1284.
38. Shanafelt TD, Noseworthy JH. Executive leadership and physician well-being: nine organizational strategies to promote engagement and reduce burnout. Vol. 92, Mayo Clinic Proceedings; 2017.
39. Li Q. 'Forest bathing' is great for your health. Here's how to do it. Time [Internet]. 2018; Accessed 1 August 2018. Available from: http://time.com/5259602/japanese-forest-bathing/.
40. Crane RS, Brewer J, Feldman C, Kabat-Zinn J, Santorelli S, Williams JMG, et al. What defines mindfulness-based programs? The warp and the weft. Psychol Med. 2017;47(06):990–9.
41. Fredrickson BL, Joiner T. Reflections on positive emotions and upward spirals. Perspect Psychol Sci. 2018;13(2):194–9.
42. Garland EL, Farb NA, Goldin P, Fredrickson BL. Mindfulness broadens awareness and builds eudaimonic meaning: a process model of mindful positive emotion regulation. Psychol Inq. 2015;26(4):293–314.
43. Cohn MA, Fredrickson BL, Brown SL, Mikels JA, Conway AM. Happiness unpacked: positive emotions increase life satisfaction by building resilience. Emotion. 2009;9(3):361–8.
44. Rippstein-Leuenberger K, Mauthner O, Bryan Sexton J, Schwendimann R. A qualitative analysis of the Three Good Things intervention in healthcare workers. BMJ Open. 2017;7(5):e015826.
45. Immordino-Yang MH, Christodoulou JA, Singh V. Rest is not idleness. Perspect Psychol Sci. 2012;7(4):352–64.
46. Remen RN, Rabow MW. The Healer's Art: professionalism, service and mission. Med Educ. 2005;39(11):1167–8.
47. Branch WT, Frankel RM, Hafler JP, Weil AB, Gilligan MC, Litzelman DK, et al. A multi-institutional longitudinal faculty development program in humanism supports the professional development of faculty teachers. Acad Med. 2017;92(12):1680–6.
48. Branch WT, Weil AB, Gilligan MC, Litzelman DK, Hafler JP, Plews-Ogan M, et al. How physicians draw satisfaction and overcome barriers in their practices: "It sustains me.". Patient Educ Couns. 2017;100(12):2320–30.
49. Lown BA, Manning CF. The Schwartz Center Rounds: evaluation of an interdisciplinary approach to enhancing patient-centered communication, teamwork, and provider support. Acad Med. 2010;85(6):1073–81.
50. Kearsley JH, Youngson R. "Tu Souffres, Cela Suffit": the compassionate Hospital. J Palliat Med. 2012;15(4):457–62.
51. Rider EA, Gilligan MC, Osterberg LG, Litzelman DK, Plews-Ogan M, Weil AB, et al. Healthcare at the crossroads: the need to shape an organizational culture of humanistic teaching and practice. J Gen Intern Med. 2018;33(7):1092–9.
52. Ginwright S. The future of healing: shifting from trauma informed care to healing centered engagement Shawn Ginwright Ph.D. [Internet]. Accessed 6 July 2016. Available from: https://medium.com/@ginwright/the-future-of-healing-shifting-from-trauma-informed-care-to-healing-centered-engagement-634f557ce69c.

# Correction to: Trauma-informed Care of Sexual and Gender Minority Patients

Tyler R. McKinnish, Claire Burgess, and Colleen A. Sloan

## Correction to: Chapter 5 in: M. R. Gerber (ed.), Trauma-Informed Healthcare Approaches, https://doi.org/10.1007/978-3-030-04342-1_5

On page 100, in the paragraph "In addition to clinical offerings...," the reference citation [84] was incorrectly mentioned as c.

Incorrect text 'c' is now replaced with the correct reference citation [84].

---

The updated online version of this chapter can be found at
https://doi.org/10.1007/978-3-030-04342-1_5

# Conclusion

> The most beautiful people we have known are those who have known defeat, known suffering, known struggle, known loss, and have found their way out of the depths. These persons have an appreciation, a sensitivity, and an understanding of life that fills them with compassion, gentleness, and a deep loving concern. Beautiful people do not just happen [1].
>
> Elizabeth Kübler-Ross

Trauma is common in human experience, and healthcare personnel and systems must be cognizant of its impact on past, present, and future health. In this book, we have presented an overview of common forms of trauma and provided a theoretical basis for implementing trauma-informed care (TIC). We have reviewed unique considerations in working with populations that experience a high burden of traumatic exposures and have provided strategies for incorporating TIC into aspects of the healthcare system. The final section of this volume reviews the critical need to support and nurture the health of those who care for trauma-exposed patients.

TIC holds great promise for promoting health and healing and is especially critical for populations at high risk for traumatic exposure, as trauma and its impact are not equally distributed in society [2]. As such, an aspirational goal of TIC is to promote health equity and reduce health disparities. At a minimum, application of TIC can build trust and a sense of self-efficacy for those served by health systems. Finally, asking a person "what happened to you?" instead of "what's wrong with you?" also allows us to understand and validate the inherent strengths that the individual possesses and enables us to collaborate in the service of wellness and healing. In healthcare, we have the unique opportunity to witness and assist in this process of growth and recovery.

## References

1. Kubler-Ross E. Death: the final stage of growth. New York: Prentice Hall; 1975.
2. Bowen EA, Murshid NS. Trauma-informed social policy: a conceptual framework for policy analysis and advocacy. Am J Public Health. 2016;106(2):223–9.

# Index

**A**
Abusive violence, 110
Acceptance and commitment therapy (ACT), 206
Accountability, 64
Active case management, 79
Active Duty personnel, 112
Acute stress disorder, 160
Adult primary care
　appointment, 133
　caring for staff, 136, 137
　chronic pain, 127, 128
　clinical environment
　　preplanning, 133
　　staff training, 132
　　trauma histories, 132
　inquiry in, 128
　resilence, 137
　substance use, 128
　TIC
　　guidance for, 131, 132
　　in medical settings, 129
　　patient-clinician relationship, 129
　　PCP encounter and examination, 133–135
　　pelvic and invasive exams/procedures, 135
　　universal trauma screening, 129, 130
　trauma in, 126–127
Advance practice nurses and physician assistants, 125
Adverse childhood experiences (ACEs), 4, 5, 28, 30, 39–40, 46, 73, 112, 126, 130, 148, 158–160
African American men
　culturally focused interventions, 78, 79
　empowering men of color, 78
　epidemiology of violence and trauma, 73
　institutional racism, 75, 76
　interventions, 79, 80
　intrinsic racism, 76, 77
　neighborhood effects, 77
　non-fatal violence estimates, 70
　personally mediated racism, 74, 75
　race and racism, 74
　and trauma, 69–72
　violence estimates, fatal deaths from, 70
Allostasis, 6, 7
Allostatic load, 6, 8
American Academy of Family Physicians (AAFP), 129
American College of Obstetricians and Gynecologists (ACOG), 12, 129, 148
American Medical Association, 90, 129
Amyotrophic lateral sclerosis (ALS), 111
Anxious patient, nursing of, 184, 186–188
Appreciative inquiry, 207
Association of Social Workers, 90
Asylum-seekers, 62, 63
Auditory privacy, 183
Autonomic nervous system (ANS), 161

**B**
B'more fit for babies, 149–152
Behavioral health, 39, 41, 43, 45, 47, 75, 80, 126, 171–177, 184, 185, 187
Behavioral Risk Factor Survey (BRFSS), 108
Behaviorists, Behavioral Health Specialists/Consultants, 173
Birth plan, 148–150

Birth trauma, 146, 147
Bisexual, 14, 86, 88, 92
Breathing techniques, 35, 148
Burnout, 125, 126, 136, 137

## C

California Evidence Based Clearinghouse for Child Welfare (CEBC), 172
Calm, 35–37
Care, 41–44
Catastrophic events, 27
Center for Youth Wellness (CYW) Adverse Childhood Experiences Questionnaire, 171, 175
Centering Pregnancy, 150
Centers for Disease Control (CDC), 11, 14, 69, 108, 112, 129, 146, 158, 159, 199
Centers for Medicare and Medicaid Services, 63
Child abuse, 10, 11
Child-parent psychotherapy, 46
Children, Youth and Families System of Care, 176
Children's Hospital Philadelphia (CHOP), 175
Chronic toxic stressors, 6
Cisgender, 86, 89, 95, 96
Cognitive Behavioral Intervention for Trauma in Schools (CBITS), 174
Cognitive behavioral therapy (CBT), 78, 172
Cognitive therapy (CBT), 78, 79, 172, 175, 206
Collapsible immobility, 161
Communication, 64
Community violence, 12–14, 29, 50, 136, 151, 159, 175
Compassion fatigue (CF), 48, 136, 137, 200
Compassion satisfaction, 48, 137, 200
Complex psychological trauma, 27
Complex PTSD (cPTSD), 46–47
Complex trauma, 27, 160
Contain, trauma-informed care, 38–40
Continuous improvement, cultural humility, 64, 65
Contraceptive coercion, 145
Conversion therapy, 90
Coping, trauma-informed care, 44–47
Cortisol, 5–7, 18, 203, 204
Cultural brokerage, 65
Cultural competence, 60
Cultural humility, 32, 41, 43, 60, 61
communication and language assistance, 64
engagement, continuous improvement, and accountability, 64–66
governance, leadership, and workforce, 63, 64
healthcare delivery, recommendations for, 63
populations of interest, 61
  asylum-seekers, 62
  migrant, immigrant, emigrant, 62
  refugees, 61
principal standard, 63
traumatic experiences and phases of displacement, 62, 63
Culturally focused interventions, 78, 79
Culture change, 32

## D

Defense and Veterans Brain Injury Center, 111
Department of Defense (DoD), 113
Department of Veterans Affairs (VA), 113
Depressed mood, 77
Diagnostic and Statistical Manual of Mental Disorders, 4, 7, 90, 127, 160
Dialectical behavioral therapy (DBT), 206
Displacement phases, 62, 63
Dissociative phenomena, 127
Doula (birth companion) care, 149, 150
Dual care, 108
Duke Health, 100
Dwell time, 111

## E

Economic migrants, 62, 63
Electronic health records (EHRs), 92, 168, 201
Emigrants, 62
Endocrine Treatment of Transsexual Persons, 91
Engagement, 64, 65
Epigenetics, 6, 7, 18, 27–28
Equal Employment Opportunity (EEO) policy, 99
Equity, 30, 37, 43

## F

Fenway Health, 99
Fight or flight responses, 161
Find it/ fix it model, 188
Forest bathing, 206

# Index

Forgotten War, 109
Freeze signal, 161

## G
Gay, 88, 92
Gay and Lesbian Medical Association, 97
Gender dysphoria, 100
Gender expression, 86, 98
Gender fluid, 100
Gender identity, 86, 87, 92–98
Gender-affirming hormone therapy, 96
Gender-neutral language, 96
Genderqueer, 86, 95
Governance, cultural humility, 63, 64
Greatest generation, 109
Guerilla war, 110
Gulf war syndrome, 111
Gun violence, 50

## H
Harmful coping behaviors, 42
Harvard Center for the Developing Child, 28
Head wounds, 109
Healer's Art, 207, 210
Healing, 42, 45, 48, 50
Health outreach/navigator support, 80
Healthcare delivery, recommendations for, 63
Healthcare disparities, 60
Healthcare Equality Index (HEI), 98
Healthcare professionals
    burnout, 200–202, 210
    chronic work stress, 200
    compassion fatigue, 200
    compassion satisfaction, 200
    PTSD, 199
    secondary/vicarious trauma, 199
    TIC
        to healing centered engagement, 203
        mindful practices, 204–206
        organizational strategies, 207, 210
        physiologic mechanisms, 203, 204
        positive psychology, 207
        resilence, 206, 207
    trauma impact on, 198
    violence personal experience, 198
    wellness assessment, 201–203
    workplace violence, 199
Healthcare providers, 38, 45, 46, 80
Healthcare systems, 50
Healthy Environments and Response to Trauma in Schools (HEARTS) program, 174
Heteronormativity, 86
Hispanic Black Gay Coalition, 99
Historical trauma, 17, 18, 27, 33, 136, 145, 161
Historical Trauma/transgenerational trauma, 161
Holistic nursing, 184, 186, 191
Holocaust survivors, 161
Home Front workers, 109
Homeless Veterans, 115
    barriers to TIC, 115
    incidence, 114
    PTSD, 115
    rurals, 115
    women, 115
Homosexuality, 90
Hospital Violence Intervention Programs (HVIPs), 79
Human trafficking, 14–16, 27, 145
Humiliation, Afraid, Rape, Kick (HARK) measure, 129
Hurt, Insult, Threaten, Scream (HITS) measure, 129
Hypothalamic-pituitary adrenal (HPA) axis, 5, 203

## I
I-HELP framework, 49
Immune system, 5
Incarcerated, 15, 145
Inequity, 75, 76
Institutional racism, 75, 76
Integrated Behavioral Health Providers, 173
Internal family systems (IFS), 206
Interpersonal trauma, 9–10, 126
Interpersonal violence, 10, 27, 38, 42, 43, 69, 72, 77, 89, 112–113, 128
Interpreting skills, 151
Intersectionality, 86
Intersex, 86
Intimate partner violence (IPV), 11, 12, 38, 39, 49, 112, 129, 145, 148
Intimate Partner Violence and Sexual Violence Victimization Assessment Instruments, 129
Intrinsic racism, 76, 77

## K

Kaiser Permanente Adverse Childhood Experiences Study, 4, 159
Korean war, 109, 110

## L

Language assistance, 64
Leadership, cultural humility, 63, 64
LGBT Aging Project, 99
Loma Linda Whole Child Assessment (WCA), 171

## M

Maine Thrive, 176
Maltreatment, 7–11, 14, 28, 145, 151
Marine Corps, 114
Massachusetts Child Trauma Project (MCTP), 175
Maternity care
   B'more fit for babies, 151, 152
   PTSD, 147, 148
   Survivor Mom's Companion, 151
   TIC
      ACEs screening, 148
      Centering Pregnancy, 150
      goals of, 146
      principles, 148–150
      SDM, 148, 150
      women-centered maternity care, 148
   trauma and women's reproductive health, 146
Mayors' Challenge to End Veteran Homelessness, 114
Mental health care, 78
Mental health providers, 75
Metabolic syndrome, 7, 8
Meyer's Minority Stress Model, 88
Migrant worker, 62
Military culture, 107, 109, 113
Military sexual trauma (MST)
   coordinator, 114
   definition, 113
   incidence, 113
   interpersonal trauma history, 113
   medical care, 114
   men *vs.* women, 113, 114
   prevalence, 113
Mindfulness meditation, 46
Mode deactivation therapy, 206
Modelling reliable, 40
Modified Childhood Trauma Questionnaire–Short Form, 129
Montefiore Children's Hospital, 176
Montefiore HealthySteps, 176
Morita therapy, 206

## N

National Academy of Medicine, 201
National Academy of Medicine's Action Collaborative on Clinician Well-Being and Resilience, 201
National Center for Cultural Competence, 66
National Child Traumatic Stress Network (NCTSN), 172, 173, 175
National Crime Victimization Survey (NCVS), 13
National Culturally and Linguistically Appropriate Services (CLAS), 63, 64
National Guard and Reserve Veterans, 114
National Guard/Reserves, 112
National Health Study, 114
National Home for Disabled Volunteer Soldiers, 107
National Institute for Occupational Safety and Health (NIOSH), 199
National MST program, 114
National Neighborhood Crime Study (NNCS), 13
National Registry of Evidence-Based Programs and Practices (NREPP), 172
National Survey of Children's Exposure to Violence (NatSCEV), 11
National Transgender Discrimination Survey (NTDS), 87
The Network/La Red, 99
New Generation of Us Veterans (NewGen), 114
Nursing care
   assessment, 182
   diagnosis, 182
   implementation, 182, 183
   personal experiences, 182
   planning, 182
   safe environment
      communication, 183
      family or friends, 184
      privacy, 183
   TIC
      during the visit, 185–187
      emergency department/ urgent care nursing, 188–189
      holistic nursing, 184
      inpatient care, 189–190

# Index

patient-centered care, 184, 186
   preparing for the visit, 185
   between visits, 187–188
   Whole Health approach, 186
trauma histories, 181

## O

Office of Juvenile Justice and Delinquency Prevention (OJJDP), 10
Operation Iraqi Freedom, 111
Operation New Dawn, 111
Operation Enduring Freedom, 111
Organizational culture transformation, 43
Organization-wide or system-wide programs, 79
Outpatient obstetrics and gynecology (OB-GYN) practice, 145

## P

Pansexual, 92–93
Parasympathetic nervous system, 204
Patient Centered Medical Home, 185
Patient navigators, 49
Patient-Aligned Care Team (PACT), 185
PC-PTSD-5 questions and scoring, 131
Pediatric care
   adverse childhood experiences, 159, 160
   care-focused initiatives
      BCHC-CYW, 175
      CHOP, 175
      MCTP, 175
      PACTS, 175
   PTSD, 160–161
   Sanctuary Model, 161, 176
   SFDPH TIS initiative, 176, 177
   sociocultural stressors, 159
   systems-focused initiatives
      Maine thrive, 176
      Montefiore HealthySteps, 176
   toxic stress, 158
   trauma-informed system
      capacity building methods, 173–174
      champions recruitment, 170
      collaboration and empowerment, 168
      compassion and dependability, 167
      cultural and racial humility, 168, 169
      healing, 162
      leader role, 165–166
      levels, 163
      organizational assessments, 169, 170
      organizational growth plan, 170
      organizational practices, 163
      pediatric providers role, 170
      principles and competencies, 166
      raising awareness, 164–165
      resilience and recovery, 169
      safety and stability, 167, 168
      Sanctuary Model, 161
      screening, 171
      symptoms, 163
      treatment, 163, 172–173
      understanding trauma, 167
      voice and choice, 164
Pentagon, 111
Persian Gulf war (Gulf war I), 111
Personally mediated racism, 74, 75
Philadelphia Alliance for Child Trauma Services (PACTS), 175
Polaris Project, 15
Police action, 109
Posttraumatic stress disorder (PTSD), 4, 7–8, 18, 25, 39, 44–48, 71–73, 75, 77, 79, 88–90, 108, 110–113, 115–116, 126–127, 130, 146–147, 151, 160, 199–200
   adolescents, 160
   African American men, 71
   children
      historical trauma/transgenerational trauma, 161
      neurobiology and, 160, 161
      vicarious traumatization, 161
   maternity care, 147–148
   SGM, 89
   trauma specific screening *vs.*, 130
Power imbalance, 26
Primary care providers (PCP)
   burnout, 126
   caring for staff, 136, 137
   dissociation symptoms, 127
   encounter and examination, 133–135
   patient trauma histories, 128
   pelvic and invasive exams/procedures, 135
   shortages, 125
   staff training, 133
   training for, 128
Protective factors, 30
Pseudoseizure, 127
Psychological First Aid (PFA), 173
PTSD Coach, 45, 113

## Q

Queer, 87, 97

## R

Race/racism, 18, 27, 33, 42–43, 48, 74, 151, 161, 175
Race-related stresses, 76, 77
Reactance theory, 76
Reaction skills, 151
Redwood Health System, 36–39, 43, 44, 50
Refugees, 61
Relative value unit (RVU), 165
Renewal House of the Unitarian Universalist Urban Ministry, 99
Resilience, 28, 30, 42, 48, 50

## S

Safety, Emotion management, Loss and Future (SELF), 176
San Francisco Department of Public Health (SF DPH), 165, 166
San Francisco Department of Public Health (SFDPH) TIS initiative, 176, 177
San Francisco Department of Public Health Trauma Informed Principles and Competencies, 31, 32
Sanctuary Model, 32, 161, 176
Schwartz Rounds, 207
Secondary traumatic stress (STS), 48
Self-harm, 42
Self-injury, Veterans, 111
Sexual abuse
    childhood, 148
    in expectant women, 146
Sexual and gender minorities (SGM)
    adolescent gender care clinic, 100
    clinical environment, 94
    clinical personnel, 94, 95
    documentation, 96, 97
    electronic health record, 97
    Fenway Health, 99
    Gender Minority Stress Model, 88
    healthcare systems, 96
    HIV and, 88
    interpersonal trauma and, 85
    outreach and visibility, 97–98
    PTSD, 88, 89
    screening for trauma, 93, 94
    stressors, 89
    substance abuse, 88
    suicide, 88
    trauma informed care
        clinical environment, 92
        identity disclosure, 92, 93
        medical competencies in, 91, 92
        privacy, 93

    stressor, 90–91
    Veteran's Health Administration, 98, 99
    violence, 89
Sexual assault, 11–14, 87, 89, 112, 114, 117, 128–129, 136, 145, 184–185, 188
Sexual orientation, 86, 87, 92, 96, 98, 99
SF Department of Public Health (SF DPH) TIS Initiative, 166
Shared decision-making (SDM), 148, 150
Skills for Psychological Recovery (SPR), 173
Social determinants of health, 75, 76
Socioeconomic status (SES), 7, 75
Soldiers' homes/military homes, 108
Soothing skills, 151
Structural violence, 26, 27
Substance Abuse and Mental Health Services Administration (SAMHSA), 27, 42, 64, 131
Substance use, 5, 13, 15, 18, 28, 40, 42, 44–47, 50, 63, 88–89, 127
Substance use disorder (SUD), 110
Suicides, 111
Survey of Exposure to Community Violence (SECV), 10, 13
Survivor childbirth, 147, 148, 150, 151
Survivor Mom's Companion, 151

## T

Task-centered disclosure, 130
Telomeres, 7, 18, 203
TOD@S program, 99
Tool for a Trauma Informed Work Life, 169
Top Performer/Leader in LGBTQ Healthcare Equality, 98
Top-down decision-making processes, 164
Transgender, 87, 88, 95–97, 99, 100
Transgender Health Conference, 99
Transgender non-conforming (TGNC), 90, 91
Trauma, 26
    ACEs study, 4, 5
    African American men and, 71–73
    allostatic load, 6, 7
    child abuse and maltreatment, 10, 11
    community violence, 12–14
    definition of, 4, 27
    early, 28–30
    environment and epigenetics, 6, 7
    historical trauma, 17, 18
    human trafficking, 14–16
    IPV, 11, 12
    prevention, 50, 51
    process/biology of, 5, 6

# Index

PTSD and metabolic syndrome, 7, 8
sexual assault, 12
socioeconomic status and cortisol, 7
traumatic exposures, prevalence of, 8, 9
Trauma-focused cognitive behavioral therapy (TF-CBT), 46, 175
Trauma-informed Advisory Board, 41
Trauma-informed Agency Assessment, 169
Trauma-informed care (TIC), 3, 30, 70, 109
    calm, safety and compassion, 33
    4 C's, 34
        calm, 35–37
        care, 41–43
        contain, 38–40
        coping, 44–47
    healthcare organization, 33
    maladaptive behaviors, 32
    mission and principles, 31, 32
    practical application of, 33
    vicarious traumatization, 33, 47–49
Trauma-Informed Program Self-Assessment Scale (TIPS), 169
Traumatic amputations, 109
Traumatic brain injury (TBI), 111
Traumatic events, 3–8, 17, 26, 27, 40, 61, 62, 71, 73, 110, 130, 147, 151, 160, 170, 171, 199, 200
Traumatic experiences, 27, 42, 47–49, 62–63
A truce, 109
Trustworthy behavior, 40, 45
Type 2 trauma/t trauma, 160

## U

UCLA-PTSD-Reaction Index (RI), 171
UCSF Benioff Children's Hospitals, 175
Undocumented immigrants, 63
United Nations, 62
United States Preventative Services Task Force (USPSTF), 12, 129
United States Transgender Survey (USTS), 87, 88, 90
Universal Education (UE), 38, 49
Universal trauma precautions, 18, 129, 183
Urban ACE score, 29
Urgent Care Clinics, 133, 188
Urgent care nursing, 188–189
US Interagency Council to End Homelessness (USICH), 114

## V

VA Medical Centers, 114
Veteran Care Coordinator, 99
Veteran Enrollees' Health and Use of Health Care, 108
Veteran's Health Administration (VA), 98, 99
Veterans
    healthcare usage of, 108
    homeless veterans
        barriers to TIC, 115
        incidence, 114
        PTSD, 115
        rurals, 115
        women, 115
    interpersonal violence exposure, 112, 113
    Korean war, 109, 110
    mental health and primary care, 115, 116
    military sexual trauma
        definition, 113
        incidence, 113
        interpersonal trauma history, 113
        medical care, 114
        men *vs.* women, 113
        prevalence, 113, 114
    Operation Enduring Freedom, 111
    Operation Iraqi Freedom, 111
    Operation New Dawn, 111
    Persian Gulf war, 111
    trauma-informed care, 116, 117
    traumatic brain injury, 111
    Vietnam war, 110
    women Veterans, 112
    WWII, 109
Veterans Choice Act, 108
Vicarious resilience, 48
Vicarious traumatization, 33, 37, 47–49, 136, 137, 160, 161, 185, 187
Vietnam war, 4, 110, 115
Violence, African American men, 73
Violence Recovery Program, 99

## W

Web-based Injury Statistics Query and Reporting System (WISQARS), 69
Whole Health approach, 184, 186
Women
    expectant mother (*see* Maternity care)
    interpersonal trauma, 145
    PTSD, 146
    reproductive health, 146
    Veterans, 112
Women-centered maternity care, 148
Workforce, cultural humility, 63, 64

World Professional Association for
    Transgender Health (WPATH)
    Standards of Care, 91
World Trade Center, 111
World War II (WWII), 109

**Y**
Yoga, 46, 206
Youth Risk Behavior Surveillance System
    (YRBSS), 14
Youth Violence Prevention Centers (YVPCs), 14